The Final FRCR
Complete Revision Notes

The Final FRCR
Complete Revision Notes

VINCENT HELYAR AND AIDAN SHAW

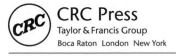

CRC Press
Taylor & Francis Group
Boca Raton London New York

CRC Press is an imprint of the
Taylor & Francis Group, an **informa** business

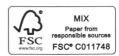

Contents

Foreword

The transition from the FRCR Part 1 to FRCR Part 2 is always a challenge. The first part of the examination demands encyclopaedic knowledge of several subjects. Although understanding is important, there is no getting away from the fact that in order to pass this examination a candidate needs to extensively read and absorb many details. Part 2 is very different—although wide reading and extensive knowledge would help, this examination is mainly a test of a candidate's ability to use his or her knowledge to make appropriate clinical diagnoses and management decisions.

Many candidates find it difficult to switch from 'MCQ mode' to the pragmatic and sensible approach required for the second part of the FRCR examination. Although there is no substitute for clinical practice for making this necessary transition, this excellent book by Dr. Aidan Shaw and Dr. Vincent Helyar will help FRCR Part 2 candidates to focus on real clinical issues in a sensible way and to think like practising radiologists in real clinical situations. It adopts a succinct, accessible style peppered with the kind of pertinent points which trainees usually only pick up as they move through a sub-specialty. Plain radiographs and cross-sectional imaging examinations of excellent quality are annotated clearly and are accompanied by the main differential diagnoses presented in a format that is easy to read and memorise.

I anticipate that the book will be used as an adjunct to major textbooks for the purposes of revision, and as a self-testing aid as the examination approaches. It is enjoyable to read and easy to use, and its authors can take pride in a challenging task extremely well accomplished.

Andreas Adam, CBE
Professor of Interventional Radiology
Guy's and St. Thomas' NHS Foundation Trust
London, UK

Acknowledgements

I dedicate this book to my family, my wife Sinéad and my daughters Clara and Elizabeth for their love and support. I am very grateful to my parents for giving me my love of words and to my mother for the inspiration to write.

Vincent Helyar

I would like to dedicate this book to my amazing wife Juliette and my son Edward for their continuing love, support and understanding throughout the writing of this book and my career. I would also like to thank my legendary parents, Bryn and Ozden. Without their continual love and support, I would not be where I am today.

Aidan Shaw

Introduction

This book is the product of several years of hard labour, the aim being to produce a definitive revision manual for the unfortunate souls preparing for the final Fellowship of the Royal College of Radiologists (FRCR). The aim of the book is to support you in preparation both for the written '2a' exams as well as the oral and written '2b' component. In each topic covered in this book, we hope that you will find enough information to understand the clinical context of a condition and its key imaging characteristics. Some information that you may find particularly useful is highlighted throughout in boxes.

To help you pass the 2a modules, we suggest you:

1. Over-prepare—do not underestimate how much work these exams require!
2. Start early and read widely (expect about 3 months of preparation per module if working in the evenings and occasional weekends).
3. Do as many multiple choice questions (MCQs) as you can and read up on everything you do not know.

For the 2b modules, we suggest you:

1. Over-prepare.
2. Report lots of plain films.
3. Read some case study texts early on (e.g. 4–6 months pre-exam).
4. Focus on viva practice, especially in the last 2–3 months.
5. Avoid burnout—know when to have time out!
6. Do at least 70 dedicated rapid-reporting plain film packs.
7. Use a checklist for rapid reporting.
8. Rehearse spiels for classic cases—whether or not you use them, it will build your confidence in presenting a case.
9. Practice with your peers.

The FRCR examination is a great challenge to prepare for, not least because of the sheer volume of information. You will be expected to have both a breadth and depth of knowledge, and in the dreaded final viva, you will be expected to assimilate all of this under pressured conditions in order to proffer a handful of sensible differential diagnoses—good luck! Rest assured that your hard work will pay off and you will emerge with a very robust qualification.

Authors

Dr Vincent Helyar, FRCR EBIR is a Consultant Interventional Radiologist at Hampshire Hospitals NHS Foundation Trust. After a successful career in information technology, Vincent graduated from Guy's, King's and St Thomas' School of Medicine in 2009 with Distinction. He completed his Foundation years in the South West of England and then began specialty training in Clinical Radiology at Guy's and St Thomas' NHS Foundation Trust. He completed specialty training in 2017 following a 2-year Fellowship in Interventional Radiology.

Vincent trained as an Interventional Radiologist at Guy's and St Thomas' NHS Foundation Trust. His practice includes a broad range of both vascular and non-vascular intervention. He has a keen interest in teaching and has authored several book chapters, numerous articles and has presented widely at national and international conferences. He is a member of the Royal College of Radiologists, the British Society of Interventional Radiology, the European Society of Radiology and the Cardiovascular and Interventional Radiological Society of Europe.

Dr Aidan Shaw, MRCS FRCR is a Consultant Interventional Radiologist at Maidstone and Tunbridge Wells NHS Trust. He completed his specialty training at Guy's and St Thomas' NHS Foundation Trust including a two-years Interventional Radiology fellowship. He has a particular interest in uterine artery embolisation, ovarian vein embolisation and prostate artery embolisation.

He has authored books as well as book chapters, has been published extensively in a number of international peer-reviewed journals and has won awards and fellowships in the field of surgery and radiology. He is a member of the Royal College of Radiologists, the Royal College of Surgeons, the British Society of Interventional Radiology and the Cardiovascular and Interventional Radiological Society of Europe.

CHAPTER 1

Cardiothoracic and Vascular

CARDIOVASCULAR

ABERRANT LEFT PULMONARY ARTERY

Occurs due to the failure of formation of the sixth aortic arch. Blood to the left lung arises from an aberrant left pulmonary artery that arises from the right pulmonary artery. The vessel passes between the trachea and oesophagus and causes narrowing of the trachea in a caudal direction. Associated with other anomalies (e.g. patent ductus arteriosus).

PLAIN FILM
- Bronchial obstruction causes lung emphysema (right lung, middle lobe, lower lobes, left upper lobe)

BARIUM SWALLOW
- Anterior indentation on the oesophagus, just above the level of the carina

AORTIC ANEURYSM

Considered either true (aneurysm bound by all three walls of the vessel) or false (i.e. pseudoaneurysm, part of the wall of the aneurysm is formed by surrounding soft tissue). Aneurysms are described as being saccular or fusiform.

- Saccular aneurysms are eccentric in shape, the aneurysm only forming from part of the circumference of the vessel wall. Associated with mycotic aneurysms (Figure 1.1).
- Fusiform aneurysms involve the full vessel circumference and feature cylindrical dilatation. More commonly seen with atherosclerotic aneurysms (Figure 1.2).

CT
- Thoracic aortic aneurysms are mostly atherosclerotic and calcified in 75%. Other causes include cystic medial necrosis (a disorder of the large arteries with

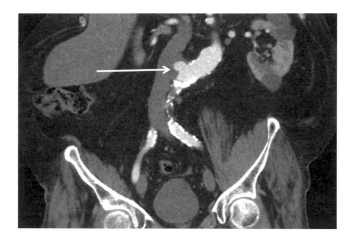

Figure 1.1 Saccular aneurysm. CT angiogram demonstrating a saccular aneurysm arising from the abdominal aorta.

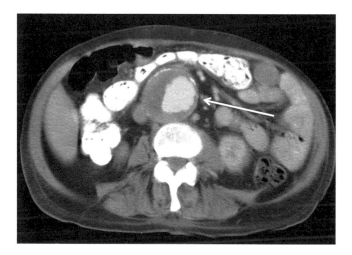

Figure 1.2 Fusiform aneurysm. CT angiogram demonstrating a fusiform abdominal aortic aneurysm.

formation of cyst-like lesions in the media, associated with e.g. Marfan and Ehlers–Danlos syndromes) and syphilis (expect extensive calcification).
- Abdominal aortic aneurysms (AAAs)—mostly atherosclerotic.
- Popliteal aneurysms, associated with an AAA in 30%–50%.

INTERVENTION
- Advised when diameter >5.5 cm (the risk of rupture is greatly increased over this).
- Endovascular stents are generally oversized by 10%. The presence of perigraft air is a common finding in the immediate post-operative period; however, if present >1 week after surgery, suspect infection.
- Endoleak is defined as the continued perfusion of the aneurysm despite placement of a stent graft (Table 1.1).

Table 1.1 The classification of endovascular stent graft endoleaks

Type of endoleak	Site
Type 1	Leak from the stent/graft attachment due to an inadequate seal
1a	Proximal
1b	Distal
Type 2 (most common, 80%)	Filling of the sac from retrograde flow through aortic branches (e.g. lumbar arteries, inferior mesenteric)
Type 3	Structural failure of the stent graft/leak from mid-graft component junction
Type 4	Porosity of the graft (corrects with reversal of anticoagulation)
Type 5	Endotension (i.e. aneurysm sac enlargement without demonstrable leak)

AORTIC COARCTATION

Narrowing of the aortic isthmus, mostly occurs in males (80%). Associated with multiple congenital anomalies, most commonly a bicuspid aortic valve (seen in 80%). Other associations include Turner syndrome (15%–20%), posterior fossa malformations–hemangiomas–arterial anomalies–cardiac defects–eye (PHACE) syndrome and intracerebral berry aneurysms and bleeds. Causes heart failure in infancy and hypertension later.

PLAIN FILM (FIGURE 1.3)

- Cardiomegaly with left ventricular hypertrophy.
- Look for the 'reverse 3 sign,' formed by pre-stenotic aortic dilatation, the coarctation and post-stenotic dilatation.
- **Inferior rib notching** (large collateral intercostal vessels), most commonly affecting the fourth to eighth posterior ribs after 5 years of age.

AORTIC DISSECTION

Blood under arterial pressure enters a tear in the intima and tracks along in the media. A total of 60% of dissections involve the ascending aorta (Stanford type A and DeBakey

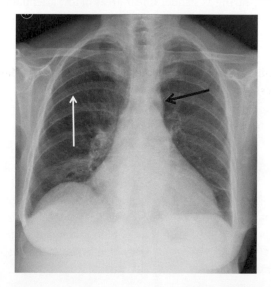

Figure 1.3 Coarctation of the aorta. Chest x-ray demonstrating cardiomegaly, a reverse 3 sign (red arrow) and inferior rib notching (white arrow).

Table 1.2 Stanford and DeBakey classifications of thoracic aortic dissection

Stanford	DeBakey
Type A	Type I
Affects the ascending aorta and/or arch and possibly into the descending aorta	Involves ascending and descending aorta
	Type II
	Involves the ascending aorta only
Type B	Type III
Affects the descending aorta and/or arch beyond the left subclavian artery	IIIA—descending aorta only without extension below the diaphragm
	IIIB—descending aorta with extension below the diaphragm

type I and II) and will require surgical management. They mostly originate from the right anterolateral wall of the ascending aorta, just distal to the aortic valve. They are associated with connective tissue disorders (Marfan and Ehlers–Danlos syndromes), bicuspid aortic valves, coarctation, relapsing polychondritis, Behçet disease, Turner syndrome, trauma and pregnancy (Table 1.2).

PLAIN FILM
- Widened mediastinum (over 8 cm)
- Double aortic contour
- Displacement of aortic knuckle calcification by 10 mm
- May manifest as lower lobe atelectasis

CT (FIGURE 1.4)
- Dissection flap separating true and false lumens (can be hard to tell which is which).
- The false lumen tends to be larger, enhances more slowly and may be thrombosed. The 'beak' sign (wedges around the true lumen) and 'cobweb' sign (remnant ribbons of media appearing as slender linear areas of low attenuation) are also clues.

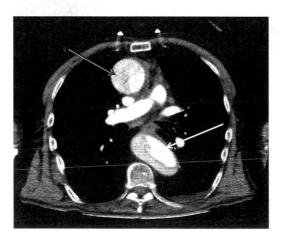

Figure 1.4 Aortic dissection. CT angiogram demonstrating a dissection of the ascending and descending thoracic aorta—Stanford type A and DeBakey type I. Red arrow—false lumen of the ascending aorta. White arrow—true lumen of the descending thoracic aorta.

AORTIC TRANSECTION

Occurs following major blunt trauma, 90% in the proximal descending aorta at the level of the isthmus (mobile aortic arch moves against the fixed descending aorta at the level of the ligamentum arteriosum). The diaphragmatic hiatus and aortic root are other risk areas.

PLAIN FILM (FIGURES 1.5 AND 1.6)

- Widened mediastinum (over 8 cm above the level of the carina and more than 25% of the width of the chest) or indistinct arch contour.
- Left apical pleural cap is classic, due to pleural haematoma.
- Look for rightward deviation of the trachea and depression of the left main bronchus.

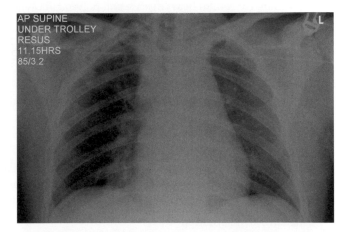

Figure 1.5 Transection of the aorta. Chest x-ray demonstrating widening of the mediastinum, a left apical pleural cap with slight deviation of the trachea to the right. There is also a fracture of the right second rib in keeping with high-energy trauma.

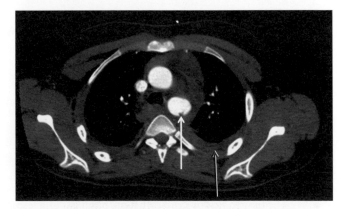

Figure 1.6 Transection of the aorta. CT demonstrating a transection of the aorta (white arrow) with mediastinal haematoma and pleural haematoma (red arrow), which creates the apical pleural cap on the chest x-ray.

AORTIC REGURGITATION

The causes are congenital (e.g. bicuspid aortic valve) or acquired. Acquired regurgitation is more common and may be divided into processes affecting the valve (e.g. rheumatic fever and endocarditis) or just the ascending aorta (e.g. syphilis, Reiter syndrome, Takayasu arteritis, etc.).

PLAIN FILM
- Non-specific cardiomegaly with left ventricular enlargement
- Apex blunted and inferolateral displacement of the left heart border

AZYGOS CONTINUATION OF THE INFERIOR VENA CAVA

Absent hepatic segment of the inferior vena cava (IVC). Commonly associated with IVC duplication, congenital heart disease and polysplenia syndromes.

Box 1.1 ANOMALIES ASSOCIATED WITH POLYSPLENIA SYNDROME

Pulmonary
- Bi-lobed continuation of the lungs
- Bilateral hyparterial bronchi

Cardiac
- Bilateral superior vena cava (SVC)
- Dextrocardia/cardiac malposition
- Anomalous pulmonary venous return
- Atrial septal defect/ventricular septal defect (ASD/VSD)

Abdominal
Small bowel malrotation
Absent gallbladder
Stomach malposition

BEHÇET DISEASE

Behçet disease is a multi-systemic immune-mediated vasculitis affecting both arteries and veins, more common (by four- to five-fold) in young women. The classic presentation is with a triad of oral ulceration, genital ulceration and ocular inflammation.

CT (FIGURES 1.7 AND 1.8)
- Cardiovascular system involved in up to 30%. Look for aortic pseudoaneurysms and occlusion/stenosis of distal vessels.
- Pulmonary artery aneurysms and haemorrhage.

MRI
- Central nervous system (CNS) involved in up to 20%.
- The best indicator is a brainstem/basal ganglia lesion (bright on T2) in the right clinical context.

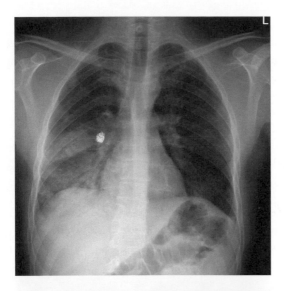

Figure 1.7 Behçet disease. Chest x-ray demonstrating coil embolisation of a pulmonary artery aneurysm and dense airspace opacification in keeping with haemorrhage.

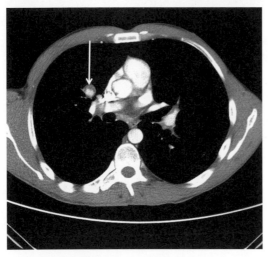

Figure 1.8 Behçet disease. CT pulmonary angiogram (CTPA) demonstrating a right pulmonary artery aneurysm (with arrow).

BUERGER DISEASE

Also known as thromboangiitis obliterans. It is a non-atherosclerotic vascular disease affecting medium- and small-sized vessels of the upper and lower limbs. It affects the distal vessels first and then progresses proximally.

INTERVENTION

- Characteristic appearance on angiography of arterial occlusions with multiple corkscrew shaped collaterals.
- Skip lesions are also a recognised feature—occlusions with normal intervening arteries.

CARDIAC TRANSPLANTATION

Complications post-cardiac transplantation include infection and post-transplant lymphoproliferative disorder (PTLD).

INFECTION

This is the most common complication following cardiac transplant. Infections in the first month post-transplant are more likely bacterial. After that, opportunistic viral and fungal infections are more common.

Plain film
- Single or multiple pulmonary nodules may represent *Nocardia* or *Aspergillus* infection.
- *Aspergillus* is more common 2 months post-transplant. *Nocardia* tends to occur later (e.g. 5 months).

PTLD

Non-specific complication mostly occurring within 1 year of transplant. Affects about 10% of solid organ recipients. It is due to B- or T-cell proliferation, usually following Epstein–Barr virus (EBV) infection. Responds rapidly to a reduction in immunosuppression or alternatively rituximab.

Plain film
- Single or multiple well-defined, slow-growing lung nodules
- Consolidation less common
- Hilar or mediastinal lymph node enlargement

CARDIAC ANGIOSARCOMA

More frequently affects middle-aged males. Typically involves the pericardium (80%) and the right atrium, which explains the presentation with right heart failure or tamponade.

CT
- Diffusely infiltrating mass extending along the pericardium and extending into the cardiac chambers/pericardiac structures
- Or, a low-attenuation mass in the right atrium showing heterogeneous enhancement and central necrosis

CARDIAC LIPOMA

This is the second most common benign cardiac tumour of adulthood, usually discovered incidentally. They can grow to a large size without causing symptoms.

CT
- Homogeneous low-attenuation mass in the pericardium or a cardiac chamber

CARDIAC METASTASES

Most commonly from lung, breast or melanoma.

CARDIAC MYXOMA

This is the most common primary cardiac tumour of adulthood. It is typically found in the left atrium (75%–80%). Associated with the Carney complex (a rare multiple endocrine syndrome featuring multiple cardiac myxomas and skin pigmentation).

ECHOCARDIOGRAPHY

- Mobile echogenic mass with a well-defined stalk—may obstruct the mitral valve

PLAIN FILM/CT

- Cardiomegaly with left atrial enlargement (splaying of the carina)
- Signs of mitral valve obstruction (pulmonary hypertension and pulmonary oedema from increased left atrial pressure)
- Soft tissue mass within the left atrium (Figure 1.9)

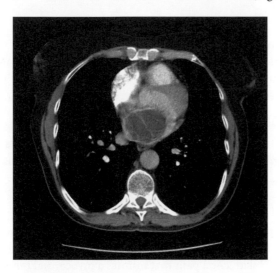

Figure 1.9 Atrial myxoma. CT image demonstrating a soft tissue mass within the left atrium; this was proven to be an atrial myxoma.

CARDIAC RHABDOMYOMA

Most common childhood cardiac tumour, mostly diagnosed incidentally (usually asymptomatic) at <1 year of age. They tend to be multiple. Associated with tuberous sclerosis (50% of patients with cardiac rhabdomyomas later diagnosed with tuberous sclerosis).

ECHOCARDIOGRAPHY

- Hyperechoic mass, most commonly arising from the interventricular septum (can be found anywhere)
- May obstruct a valve

MRI

- Useful for characterising an abnormality/aiding surgical planning

CARDIOMYOPATHY

ARRHYTHMOGENIC RIGHT VENTRICULAR DYSPLASIA

Rare cause of fatal arrhythmia and sudden death, typically in young males. Familial association. Variants described include a fatty (myocardium replaced by fatty tissue) and a fibrofatty form (myocardium replaced by fibrofatty tissue).

MRI

- High T1 infiltration of the right ventricular wall
- Dilatation of the right ventricle with thinning of the ventricle, aneurysmal bulging

DILATED CARDIOMYOPATHY

This is a diagnosis of exclusion and relates to dilatation of the ventricles of unknown aetiology. It implies systolic dysfunction.

HYPERTROPHIC CARDIOMYOPATHY

Asymmetric left ventricular hypertrophy (>12–15 mm, commonly located at the base of the interventricular septum) leads to narrowing of the outflow tract. Affects flow dynamics and gives rise to systolic anterior motion of the mitral valve.

MRI
- Useful for assessing the distribution of disease and wall thickness.
- Note—fibrotic tissue within the interventricular septum leads to patchy, delayed enhancement post-contrast.

RESTRICTIVE CARDIOMYOPATHY

Any disease that restricts diastolic filling—restrictive cardiomyopathy is a diastolic problem, so atria are large and ventricles small. Causes include sarcoidosis, amyloidosis and haemochromatosis.

TAKOTSUBO CARDIOMYOPATHY

Transient cardiac syndrome predominantly involving postmenopausal women (90%). There is left ventricular apical akinesis and dysfunction, with normal coronary arteries. The typical presentation is with chest pain that mimics a myocardial infarction (troponin enzymes are mildly elevated) following a physically/emotionally stressful event.

Plain film
- Pulmonary oedema

MRI
- Left ventricular dyskinesia and ballooning
- High T2 signal (oedema) in the ventricular wall
- No significant delayed contrast enhancement of the ventricular wall (distinguishing from myocardial infarction)

CAROTID ARTERY STENOSIS

Box 1.2 CAROTID ARTERY STENTING

There are specific indications for carotid artery stenting (rather than endarterectomy; e.g. restenosis following surgery, radiation stenosis and previous neck surgery on the ipsilateral side). Stent is placed within 2 weeks of a stroke.

This is a major cause of stroke, typically caused by atherosclerosis at the carotid bulb and the proximal segment of the internal carotid artery. Note that the internal carotid artery is also the second most common site for fibromuscular dysplasia stenosis after the kidneys.

DOPPLER ULTRASOUND (US)

- More than 70% stenosis increases systolic and diastolic flow velocity.
- Systolic flow >230 cm/second and diastolic flow >110 cm/second are significant.

MYOCARDIAL ISCHAEMIA

HIBERNATING MYOCARDIUM

This is viable myocardial tissue that has adapted over time to reduced perfusion. The tissue may be a target for revascularisation.

Nuclear medicine

- Abnormal perfusion and abnormal wall motion

MYOCARDIAL INFARCTION

Nuclear medicine

- Matched rest and stress perfusion defect, does not normalise.
- Note: Myocardial ischaemia shows a perfusion abnormality that reverses on rest.

MRI

- Infarcted tissue is indicated by delayed hyper-enhancement.
- In the first few days after infarction, there is high T2 signal in the affected myocardium.

STUNNED MYOCARDIUM

Temporary, acute severe ischaemia causes an abnormality of wall motion.

Nuclear medicine

- Normal perfusion, abnormal wall motion.
- Repeated stunning may cause myocardial hibernation.

PERICARDIAL CYST

Mostly an incidental finding, typically found at the right anterior cardiophrenic angle.

PLAIN FILM (FIGURE 1.10)

- Well-demarcated, rounded mass at right cardiophrenic angle.

CT (FIGURE 1.11)

- Low-attenuation (Hounsfield unit [HU25]) rounded mass adjacent to the pericardium

MRI

- Low T1 signal, high on T2

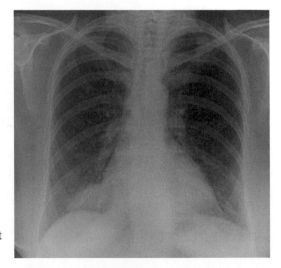

Figure 1.10 Pericardial cyst. Chest x-ray demonstrating a well-demarcated mass at the right cardiophrenic angle.

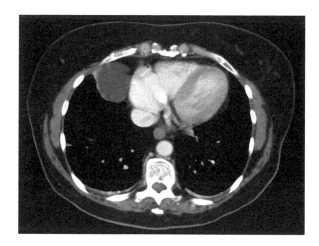

Figure 1.11 Pericardial cyst. Computed tomography image demonstrating a low-attenuation mass adjacent to the pericardium.

PERICARDITIS

Most pericarditis is idiopathic and may be due to an undiagnosed viral infection. Restrictive pericarditis is associated with myocardial thickening.

ACUTE PERICARDITIS

Look for evidence of a pericardial effusion. Symptoms (cardiac tamponade) relate to both the volume of the effusion and speed of accumulation.

Plain film
- Normal until fluid volume >250 mL.
- Bilateral hila overlay sign, globular enlargement of the heart (gives a 'water bottle' appearance).
- On a lateral chest x-ray, the signs are the epicardial fat pad sign (epicardial fat separated from pericardial fat by a lucent line) and filling in of the retrosternal space.

CONSTRICTIVE PERICARDITIS

Thickened pericardium restricts diastolic ventricular filling, and the end result is cardiac failure. The aetiology includes sarcoidosis, tuberculosis (TB), chronic renal failure, rheumatic fever, trauma and radiation.

Plain film
- Pericardial calcification (50%) and pleural effusions
- Pericardial effusion
- No pulmonary oedema

CT
- Pericardial thickening >4 mm suggests pericarditis (normal 2 mm, excludes pericarditis).
- Pericardial effusion.
- Findings may be isolated to one side of the heart.
- Pericardial enhancement with contrast.

MRI
- Useful for distinguishing pericardial thickening from pericardial effusion.

POLYARTERITIS NODOSA

This is a vasculitis of the small- and medium-sized arteries and is more common in males. Fever, malaise and weight loss are almost always present, due to ischaemic complications. Most (80%) have renal involvement. The gastrointestinal (GI) tract is affected in about 60%.

CT/INTERVENTION (FIGURES 1.12 AND 1.13)

- 1–5-mm microaneurysms, typically peripheral and intra-renal.
- Aneurysms tend to occur where vessels bifurcate.

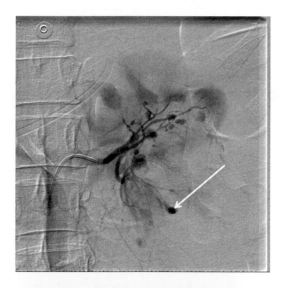

Figure 1.12 Polyarteritis nodosa. Left renal artery angiogram demonstrating multiple small renal artery aneurysms (white arrow).

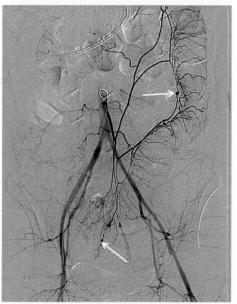

Figure 1.13 Polyarteritis nodosa. Inferior mesenteric artery angiogram demonstrating multiple small aneurysms (white arrows).

- Stenoses also occur.
- Vasculitis causes distal ischaemia (renal infarcts, gut ischaemia, etc.).
- May present with haemorrhage.

POPLITEAL ARTERY ENTRAPMENT SYNDROME

Symptomatic deviation and compression of the popliteal artery secondary to an abnormal relationship with the medial head of gastrocnemius/popliteus (rare). Affects young sportsmen and is bilateral in up to two-thirds. May present as intermittent claudication or acute thrombosis. The management is surgical.

MRI

- Most useful for demonstrating artery–muscle relationship and vessel lumen.

INTERVENTION

- Medial deviation or compression of the artery on plantar or dorsi flexion of the ankle.

POST-EMBOLISATION SYNDROME

This arises as a complication of transarterial chemoembolisation or arterial embolisation (e.g. liver lesion treatment or uterine artery embolisation). Incidence increases with increasing lesion size. It usually occurs within the first 3 days and eases over the next 3 days, and is usually self limiting. The symptoms are mild fever, nausea/vomiting and pain.

CT

- Commonly demonstrates gas within the embolised lesion—does not imply infection.

RENAL ARTERY STENOSIS

Accounts for <5% of hypertension in adults. In the elderly, it is mostly due to atherosclerosis (90%); in the young, consider fibromuscular dysplasia. Presents with severe refractory hypertension, renal impairment and raised intracranial pressure. Biochemistry shows raised plasma renin (captopril test).

DOPPLER US

- Raised peak systolic velocity, mild 100–200 cm/second and severe >200 cm/second.
- Damped systolic waveform ('parvus–tardus').
- Affected side may show an elevated resistive index if measured proximal to the stenosis.

INTERVENTION

- Focal or segmental stenosis, atherosclerotic lesions tend to be at the ostium or proximal 2 cm.
- Angioplasty effective in 80% for proximal lesions, 30% for ostial lesions.

RHEUMATIC HEART DISEASE

Heart disease arising from rheumatic fever (a complication of a streptococcal pharyngitis). May affect the myocardium, pericardium or valves (mitral valve affected most often).

PLAIN FILM

- Enlarged left atrial appendage/left atrium is classic (splaying of the carina with left atrial enlargement).
- Mitral stenosis—look for evidence of pulmonary oedema, left atrial enlargement, alveolar haemorrhage and pulmonary ossification (due to pulmonary haemosiderosis).
- Mitral regurgitation—look for left ventricular enlargement.
- Also look for pericardial calcification, valvular calcification and global cardiomegaly.

SARCOIDOSIS

Suspected in patients with sarcoidosis and arrhythmias, affects about 5% of sarcoidosis patients. Associated with poorer outcomes and up to a quarter of deaths from sarcoidosis.

MRI

- In acute sarcoidosis, there may be delayed enhancement (also with ischaemia) or T2 hyperintense nodules at the base of the septum and left ventricle.
- Look for high T2 signal in the epicardium with or without wall thickening secondary to oedema; subendocardium is spared.
- Pericardial effusion.

SUBCLAVIAN STEAL SYNDROME

Severe stenosis of the proximal subclavian artery causes retrograde flow in the ipsilateral vertebral artery (to bypass the stenosis by collaterals). In partial steal, there is antegrade flow in the vertebral artery in systole, with retrograde flow in diastole. Associated with cerebral ischaemic symptoms (e.g. vertigo, dizziness and syncope). Mostly due to atherosclerosis, but also linked to vasculitis. Mostly occurs on the left.

US

- Retrograde ipsilateral vertebral artery flow with evidence of a subclavian stenosis (parvus–tardus and monophasic waveform in the distal subclavian artery)

CT/MR ANGIOGRAPHY

- Subclavian stenosis/occlusion
- Delayed enhancement/retrograde flow in ipsilateral vertebral artery

INTERVENTION

- Angioplasty and stenting preferred to surgical bypass in symptomatic patients

TAKAYASU ARTERITIS

This is a large-vessel arteritis tending to affect young women. There is granulomatous inflammation of the vessel wall, with vessels ultimately becoming stenotic, occluded or aneurysmal.

CT

- Vessel wall thickening and enhancement.
- Aorta (thoracic particularly) and its branches are mostly affected.
- Pulmonary arteries affected in 50%, peripheral pulmonary arteries may be 'pruned', trunk dilated.
- Vessels calcify in chronic disease (otherwise they are more likely to become aneurysmal).

MRI

- Look for high signal on the short tau inversion recovery (STIR) in the vessel wall, indicating oedema.

RESPIRATORY

ADULT RESPIRATORY DISTRESS SYNDROME (ARDS)

Box 1.3 THE BASIC PRINCIPLES OF HRCT OF THE THORAX

Why?
HRCT of the chest is the *only* way to demonstrate the secondary pulmonary lobule (i.e. the basic anatomical structure responsible for gas exchange composed of acini, bronchioles, lymphatics and vessels).

When?
Any diffuse lung disease including interstitial lung disease, pulmonary eosinophilias and obstructive lung disease and to investigate patients with symptoms and a normal chest x-ray.

How?
The key aspects of HRCT are thin collimation (1–2-mm slices) and high spatial resolution reconstruction. Slices may be taken at staggered intervals ('interspaced'; e.g. six to eight images total) or as a volumetric dataset (e.g. every 10 mm)—the merits of each are debatable. Patients are usually scanned supine; prone positioning is useful to differentiate disease from 'dependent' changes (i.e. atelectasis in older patients and smokers). Images are usually gathered in full inspiration. Expiratory scans are used to demonstrate air-trapping or to differentiate between vascular and airway disease as a cause of air-trapping.

Read more:
Kazerooni, E. 2001. High-resolution CT of the lungs. *American Journal of Roentgenology* 177:501–519.

Box 1.4 WHAT IS GROUND-GLASS ATTENUATION?

An amorphous increase in lung attenuation that does not obscure vessels. Vessels are obscured by consolidation.

Also known as 'acute respiratory distress syndrome', this is an acute condition characterised by bilateral pulmonary infiltrates and severe hypoxaemia in the absence of cardiogenic pulmonary oedema. The underlying problem is diffuse alveolar damage.

PLAIN FILM

- Normal for the first 24 hours, then septal lines and peribronchial cuffing, but no effusions.
- Unlike pulmonary oedema, infiltrates are initially peripheral rather than central, and air bronchograms are more commonly seen.
- May be complicated by pneumonia.

HIGH-RESOLUTION CT (HRCT)

- After months, the consolidative pattern gives way to reticulation in the non-dependent lung and, finally, honeycombing.

α1 ANTITRYPSIN DEFICIENCY

α1 antitrypsin is an inhibitor of a protease for elastin. The deficiency is also associated with cirrhosis, necrotising panniculitis and Wegener granulomatosis. It causes a pan-lobar emphysema in the lungs in young patients (aged 40–50 years).

PLAIN FILM (FIGURE 1.14)

- Normal in mild disease
- Later on, lucent, hyperinflated lungs in a young patient

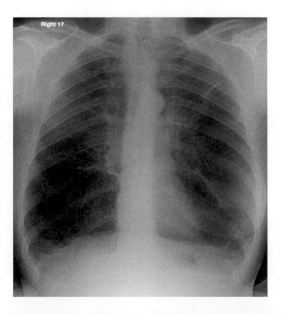

Figure 1.14 α1 antitrypsin deficiency. Chest x-ray demonstrating hyperexpanded lungs and predominant lower zone emphysema.

HRCT (FIGURE 1.15)

- Pan-lobular emphysema (i.e. enlarged and destroyed secondary pulmonary lobule) tending to affect the lower lobes bilaterally
- Associated with bronchiectasis

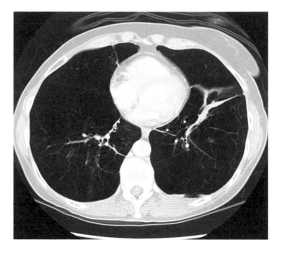

Figure 1.15 α1 antitrypsin deficiency. Computed tomography image demonstrating marked pan-lobular emphysema.

AMIODARONE LUNG DISEASE

Box 1.5 DIFFERENTIALS FOR A HYPERDENSE LIVER
Amiodarone
Gold
Thorotrast (old contrast agent)
Haemochromatosis
Haemsiderosis (spleen affected, too)
Glycogen storage disease

An interstitial lung disease affecting patients after amiodarone treatment. It occurs 1–12 months following at least 6 months of treatment.

HRCT

- Peripheral, hyperdense consolidation and patchy ground-glass opacification (i.e. alveolar infiltrates)
- Peripheral/basal fibrosis
- Hyperdense liver and heart—this is classic

ARTERIOVENOUS MALFORMATION (AVM)

Affects up to 15% of people with hereditary haemorrhagic telangiectasia (Osler–Weber–Rendu syndrome). Patients may present with orthodeoxia (postural hypoxaemia accompanied by breathlessness) or stroke due to paradoxical emboli.

PLAIN FILM/CT
- Well-defined, lobulated nodules with a feeding artery and draining vein
- May contain phleboliths
- Most are unilateral and two-thirds are in the lower lobes.

ASBESTOS-RELATED LUNG DISEASE

Box 1.6 CAUSES OF LOWER ZONE FIBROSIS
Asbestosis **C**onnective tissue diseases (rheumatoid, scleroderma and systemic lupus erythematosus) **I**diopathic pulmonary fibrosis (usual interstitial pneumonia [UIP]) **D**rugs (methotrexate, bisulfan and bleomycin) Look for soft tissue calcification, dilated oesophagus, distal clavicular osteolysis, pleural plaques, diaphragmatic calcification and sympathectomy clips to help diagnose the cause.

This refers to a spectrum of lung disease resulting from asbestos exposure. It may be a benign pleural disease, usually occurring >20 years after exposure. More common in males (occupational).

PLAIN FILM
- Pleural effusion first.
- Then, often (80%) pleural plaques affecting both parietal pleura (posterolateral/lateral/costophrenic angles/mediastinal).
- Diaphragmatic plaques are pathognomonic, the apices are spared.
- Plaques are not always calcified.

CT (FIGURE 1.16)
- Look for areas of round atelectasis ('pseudotumour' appearance) next to a pleural plaque. The bronchovascular bundle typically converges into the lesion ('comet tail' sign).

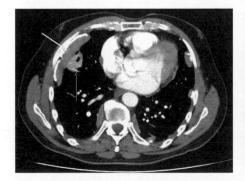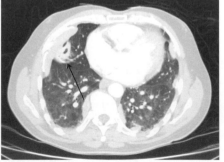

Figure 1.16 Rounded atelectasis. CT images demonstrating calcified pleural plaques with rounded atelectasis (pseudotumour; red arrow) overlying a calcified pleural plaque (white arrow). The bronchovascular bundles form the comet tail sign (red arrow).

ASBESTOSIS

This is an interstitial lung disease due to asbestos exposure. There is progressive dyspnoea and a strong association with malignancy (adenocarcinoma more likely).

Plain film
- Lower zone fibrosis (due to inhalation gradient)
- Pleural plaques
- Effusions

HRCT
- Initially small, sub-pleural, round or branching opacities a few millimetres from the pleura—this is peri-bronchiolar fibrosis.
- Sub-pleural curvilinear opacities, parallel to the chest wall—may represent atelectasis or be associated with honeycombing later on.
- Late disease is characterised by parenchymal bands and reticulation with distortion of the lung parenchyma and traction bronchiectasis.
- As the disease progresses, there is basal honeycombing, appearing similar to UIP.
- No lymph node enlargement.

ASPERGILLOSIS

Aspergillosis refers to a spectrum of abnormalities caused by infection with the *Aspergillus* fungus. The severity of the disease depends partly on the patient's immune status (Note: AIDS alone does not count).

ASPERGILLOMA

Affects patients with normal immunity but abnormal lungs. Fungal infection occurs within a pre-existing cyst, cavity, bulla or area of bronchiectasis. Commonly referred to as mycetoma.

Plain film (Figure 1.17)
- Typically upper lobe abnormality, mass within a cavity frequently accompanied by pleural thickening.
- 'Monad'/air crescent sign—the fungus ball is frequently surrounded by a crescent of air.

CT
- Fungus ball (may calcify) lying dependently within a cavity or thin-walled cyst.

Intervention
- Bronchial arteries supplying the abnormal lung become hypertrophied and are liable to bleed.
- Bronchial artery embolisation may be performed for haemoptysis.

ALLERGIC BRONCHOPULMONARY ASPERGILLOSIS (ABPA)

Usually occurs in the context of chronic asthma or cystic fibrosis. *Aspergillus* organisms are inhaled by an atopic host and cause a hypersensitivity reaction. It is the most common pulmonary cause of an eosinophilia. Treatment is with steroids.

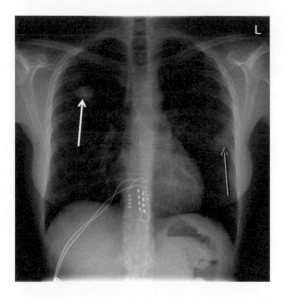

Figure 1.17 Cystic fibrosis with aspergilloma. Chest x-ray demonstrating a right upper zone cavity with a soft tissue focus outlined by a crescent of air (Monad sign; white arrow) in keeping with an aspergilloma. A further aspergilloma is identified within the left mid-zone (red arrow).

Plain film (Figure 1.18)

- Migratory patchy foci of consolidation.
- 'Tram track' appearance (i.e. gross bronchiectasis), central/upper zones is classic.
- Tubular opacities are classic—these are dilated airways plugged with mucous, known as the 'finger in glove' appearance.
- Atelectasis from airway obstruction.

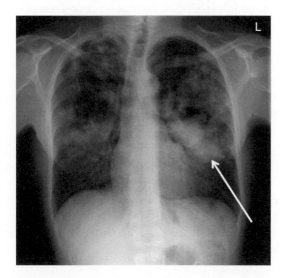

Figure 1.18 Allergic bronchopulmonary aspergillosis. Chest x-ray demonstrating gross central bronchiectasis with tubular opacities. These represent mucous-filled bronchi known as the 'finger in glove' appearance.

HRCT (Figure 1.19)

- Hyperdense mucoid impaction of central and upper lobe airways giving rise to bronchiectasis.
- Bronchiectasis is varicose or saccular.
- Centrilobular nodules and masses are features, not pleural effusions.

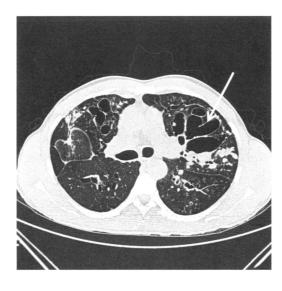

Figure 1.19 Allergic bronchopulmonary aspergillosis. CT image demonstrating gross central varicose bronchiectasis (white arrow) with mucous-filled bronchi.

- Chronic disease leads to upper zone fibrosis.
- Air-trapping—gives a mosaic pattern of attenuation.

SEMI-INVASIVE PULMONARY ASPERGILLOSIS

Also known as 'chronic necrotising pulmonary aspergillosis'. It may affect those with mild immunosuppression; overall prognosis is good. Treatment is with anti-fungals.

CT
- Typically upper zone nodules that then cavitate—a necrotic area then separates the nodule from the surrounding lung (the 'air crescent' sign).

ANGIOINVASIVE ASPERGILLOSIS

The most common fungal infection to affect the severely immunosuppressed (commonly post-transplant, leukaemia and post-chemotherapy). Invades blood vessels and causes pulmonary infarction. Rapid progression and high mortality.

CT
- Nodules with a rim of ground-glass opacification (haemorrhage)—known as the 'halo' sign

AIRWAY-INVASIVE ASPERGILLOSIS

Aspergillosis that affects the airways. It may manifest as acute tracheobronchitis, bronchiolitis or bronchopneumonia. There is ulceration of the airways.

CT
- Nodular opacities, centrilobular nodules or consolidation

ASPIRATION

Location depends on the position of the patient at the time of aspiration. The left lung may be spared.

PLAIN FILM
- Most commonly the lower lobes are affected if erect; posterior upper lobe and superior lower lobe are affected if supine.

CT
- Consolidation, material in the airway
- May be complicated by necrosis or abscess formation

BRONCHIECTASIS

Box 1.7 CAUSES OF BRONCHIECTASIS
Idiopathic • Most common cause overall *Congenital* • Cystic fibrosis—most commonly congenital *Bronchial atresia* • Primary ciliary dyskinesia *Acquired* • Post-infectious (including ABPA)—most commonly acquired • Aspiration (including foreign body obstruction) • Inflammation—rheumatoid, sarcoid

Defined as abnormal, irreversible airway dilatation often associated with thickening of the bronchial wall. Subtypes are cylindrical, varicose and cystic.

CYLINDRICAL
Relatively uniform, mild airway dilatation with parallel bronchial walls. Most common and least severe. Causes include cystic fibrosis (pan-lobar), hypogammaglobulinaemia (lower lobe) and Japanese pan-bronchiolitis (pan-lobar).

Plain film
- Tram-track appearance (en face dilated airways) or ring shadows (axial appearance of dilated airways)
- Bronchial wall thickening

HRCT
- 'Signet ring' sign describes the axial view of a dilated airway of larger diameter than the accompanying artery.
- Airways do not taper as they approach the lung periphery (airways can be seen in the peripheral third of lung).

VARICOSE
Bronchial lumen assumes a beaded ('string of pearls') configuration with sequential dilatation and constriction. Causes include ABPA.

Plain film

- Beaded airway dilatation with or without mucous impaction ('finger in glove').
- ABPA tends to affect the upper lobes.

CYSTIC

A string or cluster of cyst-like bronchi, the most severe kind of bronchiectasis. Causes include post-infectious (e.g. pertussis and unilobar), post-obstruction and Mounier–Kuhn syndrome.

Plain film/HRCT (Figure 1.20)

- Cysts in clusters or strings
- Air-fluid levels commonly seen within the cysts

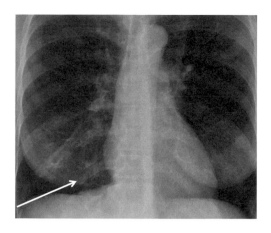

Figure 1.20 Cystic bronchiectasis. Chest x-ray demonstrating ring shadows in keeping with cystic bronchiectasis.

BRONCHIOLITIS OBLITERANS

Box 1.8 MOSAIC PERFUSION OF THE LUNG

Subtle pattern of variable lung attenuation with a slight decrease in the calibre and number of pulmonary vessels within the areas of low attenuation.

Expiratory HRCT differentiates between the two causes (i.e. small airways disease vs. pulmonary vascular abnormalities).

Bronchiolar and peribronchiolar inflammation of the bronchioles leads to submucosal and peribronchiolar fibrosis. This causes an obstruction of the bronchial lumen, also known as obliterative bronchiolitis. Associated with transplantation (e.g. bone marrow/graft vs. host—up to 10%; lung transplant), viral infection (known as Swyer–James or MacLeod syndrome in children), toxin inhalation, rheumatoid arthritis, inflammatory bowel disease and drug reactions (bleomycin, gold, cyclophosphamide, methotrexate and amiodarone).

HRCT

- Air-trapping on expiratory scans (i.e. mosaic perfusion pattern)—this is classic and due to obstruction of the small airways.
- Bronchiectasis (i.e. dilated and thick-walled).
- Centrilobular ground-glass opacification.

BRONCHOGENIC CYST

This is the most common foregut malformation in the thorax. It constitutes up to 20% of mediastinal masses. It is an abnormality of the ventral diverticulum of the primitive foregut and is associated with other congenital anomalies, spina bifida, extra-lobar sequestration and congenital lobar emphysema.

> **Box 1.9 CAUSES OF A MIDDLE MEDIASTINAL MASS**
>
> Look for:
>
> - Widened paratracheal stripe
> - Mass in the aortopulmonary window
> - Displacement of the azygo-oesophageal line
>
> Common differentials include:
>
> 1. Foregut duplication cyst (bronchogenic or oesophageal)—most common
> 2. Lymph node
> 3. Lung cancer
> 4. Aortic aneurysm

PLAIN FILM

- Posterior or middle mediastinal mass, typically subcarinal and more common on the right
- Can be intrapulmonary—most commonly located in the medial lower lobes

CT

- Well-circumscribed spherical mass, usually with an internal density of 0–25 HU (may be higher)
- May contain an air–fluid level if communicating with an airway
- Rim-enhancement may be seen, calcification is not typical

BRONCHOPLEURAL FISTULA

This is an abnormal communication between the pleural space and the bronchial tree caused by lobectomy, pneumonectomy, lung necrosis, TB, etc.

PLAIN FILM

- The pleural cavity is expected to fill with fluid post-pneumonectomy—a fistula is suspected if this does not occur, if there is an abrupt decrease in the air–fluid level or there is a new gas in a previously fluid-filled pleural cavity.
- Contralateral shift of the mediastinum.

NUCLEAR MEDICINE

- Xenon ventilation study will show activity in the pleural space.

CARCINOID TUMOUR (FIGURE 1.21)

Carcinoid tumours are neuroendocrine tumours with low malignant potential; overall prognosis is good. They are associated with multiple endocrine neoplasia type-1. They are well-vascularised, endobronchial lesions, so commonly present with haemoptysis. Cough and recurrent pneumonia are also common.

- Diffuse idiopathic pulmonary neuroendocrine cell hyperplasia—may be a precursor to a bronchial carcinoid. Characterised by small lung nodules, air-trapping, ground-glass opacification and bronchiectasis.

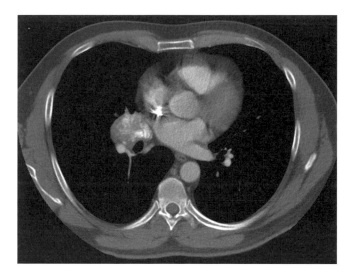

Figure 1.21 Carcinoid tumour. CT image demonstrating an avidly enhancing central mass with foci of calcification.

PLAIN FILM

● Atelectasis commonly, a nodule (typically perihilar) may be seen.

CT

● Avidly arterial enhancing endobronchial lesion.
● Rounded appearance and mostly found centrally (20% are peripheral).
● A third calcify, no fat content and rarely cavitate.
● Check lymph nodes for evidence of metastasis—Note: Lymph nodes may be enlarged from concurrent infection.

NUCLEAR MEDICINE

● Cold on fludeoxyglucose positron emission tomography (PET).
● Gallium 68 PET is used to stage carcinoid.

Box 1.10 A DIFFERENTIAL FOR ENHANCING LYMPH NODES

Benign
● Castleman disease
● Sarcoid

Neoplastic
● Renal cell carcinoma
● Thyroid
● Small-cell carcinoma

CASTLEMAN DISEASE

Benign B-cell lymphoproliferation, more common in patients with HIV or AIDS.

CT

- Multiple, enhancing lymph nodes—usually axillary or supraclavicular
- Mediastinal or hilar nodes—rare
- Centrilobular lung nodules and ground-glass opacification that mimics lymphocytic interstitial pneumonia (LIP)—rare

CHURG–STRAUSS SYNDROME

Also known as eosinophilic granulomatosis with polyangiitis, this is a variant of polyarteritis nodosa affecting small to medium vessels. It is a necrotising vasculitis. Almost all patients have asthma, and eosinophilia and p-ANCA is positive in 75%. Cardiac involvement (including infarction) is common.

Diagnostic criteria (four required): asthma, eosinophilia, neuropathy, migratory or transient pulmonary opacities, paranasal sinus abnormalities and/or extravascular eosinophils at biopsy.

PLAIN FILM

- Transient peripheral consolidation and small pleural effusions

HRCT

- Non-segmental, transient peripheral consolidation/ground glass
- Interlobular thickening
- Centrilobular nodules (less commonly)

CYSTIC FIBROSIS

This is an autosomal recessive defect in the gene regulating chloride transport, resulting in thick secretions. The lungs and pancreas are affected most severely.

PLAIN FILM (FIGURE 1.22)

- Bronchiectasis (cylindrical at first).
- Bronchial wall thickening.
- Hyperinflation (due to air-trapping).
- Any part of the lungs may be affected, but particularly central zones, upper lobes and apical lower lobes.
- Look for mucous impaction with atelectasis.
- Spontaneous pneumothorax.
- Pulmonary artery enlargement.

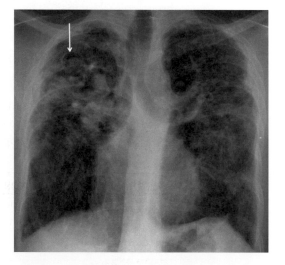

Figure 1.22 Cystic fibrosis. Chest x-ray demonstrating hyperexpanded lungs with upper zone fibrosis, bronchial wall thickening and bronchiectasis affecting the central and upper zones. There is a cavity with a soft tissue focus outlined by a crescent of air (Monad sign; white arrow) in keeping with an aspergilloma.

HRCT
- Most sensitive for detecting early change

DIAPHRAGMATIC RUPTURE

Usually occurs due to blunt abdominal trauma, with the left side three-times more likely to rupture (the liver shields the right side).

PLAIN FILM
- Abnormal contour to the diaphragm, abdominal contents in the chest and deviation of an enteral tube

CT
- Discontinuity of the left hemidiaphragm.
- 'Collar' sign describes a focal constriction of the herniating viscera at the site of rupture.
- The 'dependent viscera' sign is where abdominal viscera lie dependently against the posterior ribs due to loss of diaphragmatic support.

EXTRINSIC ALLERGIC ALVEOLITIS

See 'Hypersensitivity pneumonitis' section.

EMPHYSEMA

Defined as abnormal, permanent enlargement of the airspaces distal to the terminal bronchiole, accompanied by destruction of their walls without obvious fibrosis.

CENTRILOBULAR
This is the most common subtype, mostly caused by smoking.

Plain film
- Normal unless advanced
- Hyperinflated lucent lungs and flattened diaphragms
- More common in the upper zones
- Check for bullae

HRCT
- Multiple small, round foci of abnormally low attenuation without visible walls that are scattered throughout normal-appearing lung parenchyma

PAN-LOBULAR
Associated with various causes, including α1-antitrypsin deficiency and drug reaction (e.g. Ritalin and intravenous drug users).

Plain film
- Insensitive—look for diffuse simplification of the lung architecture.

HRCT
- Diffusely low-attenuation lungs without clear demarcation of normal lung
- Loss of vascular markings

PARASEPTAL

Lucent, cystic spaces arranged beneath the pleural surfaces, including the interlobar fissures. Associated mostly with smoking.

Plain film
- Rarely detectable
- May be complicated by pneumothorax

HRCT
- Cystic spaces arranged beneath the pleural surfaces including the interlobar fissures.
- The borders of the secondary pulmonary lobule are intact.

EOSINOPHILIC LUNG DISEASE

Idiopathic subtypes are described below: namely, simple pulmonary eosinophilia, acute, chronic and hypereosinophilic syndrome.

SIMPLE PULMONARY EOSINOPHILIA (LÖFFLER SYNDROME)

Initially described as due to parasitic infection, may be associated with other pathology (e.g. ABPA) or drug reaction. It is benign and self-limiting. There is mild blood eosinophilia.

Plain film
- 'Reverse bat's wing' appearance is classic (i.e. bilateral peripheral airspace opacification).

HRCT
- Peripheral ground-glass opacification/consolidation
- Nodules with surrounding ground-glass opacity ('halo' sign)

ACUTE EOSINOPHILIC PNEUMONIA

Mean age of onset about 30 years, may be smoking related. Rapid onset of symptoms, fever and hypoxaemia. Marked eosinophilia on bronchoalveolar lavage (BAL)/pleural samples, but normal blood levels. Rapid response to steroids.

Plain film
- Bilateral densities with effusions, with or without consolidation

HRCT
- Bilateral, patchy, ground-glass opacities
- Interlobular septal thickening and pleural effusions

CHRONIC EOSINOPHILIC PNEUMONIA

Insidious onset of night sweats, pyrexia, cough and weight loss. More common in middle age and 50% have asthma. Mild blood eosinophilia and high eosinophilia on BAL. Responds to steroids.

Plain film
- Bilateral, non-segmental, upper peripheral lobe airspace opacification (so-called 'photographic negative of pulmonary oedema' or 'reverse bat's wing' appearance)

Box 1.11 CAUSES OF THE BAT'S WING APPEARANCE

Simple pulmonary eosinophilia
Chronic eosinophilic pneumonia
Cryptogenic organising pneumonia
Pulmonary vasculitis
Pulmonary infarction
Pulmonary contusion

HRCT
- Dense peripheral consolidation
- With or without ground glass, nodules and reticulation
- Rarely effusions

IDIOPATHIC HYPEREOSINOPHILIC SYNDROME

Rare condition with marked eosinophilia and end-organ eosinophilic infiltration and damage. Heart (endocardial fibrosis, cardiomyopathy, etc.) and nervous system most affected.

Plain film
- Non-specific findings—multiple opacities, usually related to pulmonary oedema

HRCT
- Nodules with a ground-glass halo
- Pleural effusions due to cardiac failure

FAT EMBOLUS

Lung embolus of fat-containing material (may also travel to the brain or skin), the vast majority are in patients 1–2 days following severe trauma or long bone fracture. Resolves in 1–4 weeks, often asymptomatic.

PLAIN FILM/CT
- Bilateral, widespread, ill-defined peripheral infiltrates similar to ARDS in a patient with a recent history of major trauma

FIBROSING MEDIASTINITIS

Non-malignant proliferation of fibrous tissue affecting the mediastinum. Wide range of causes including infectious (histoplasmosis and TB), inflammatory (retroperitoneal fibrosis and orbital pseudotumour) and iatrogenic (radiotherapy and drug reaction). Tends to affect the young. Described as focal (80%—usually secondary to TB or histoplasmosis) or diffuse (20%—mostly inflammatory). It is the most common benign cause of SVC obstruction.

FOCAL
CT
- 2–5-cm calcified (80% calcified) mass compressing pulmonary vasculature leading to right heart strain

- Peribronchial cuffing, septal thickening and wedge-shaped areas of pulmonary infarction

DIFFUSE FORM
CT

- Soft tissue encasement of mediastinal structures with infiltration of fat planes

FLEISCHNER SOCIETY GUIDELINES FOR PULMONARY NODULES

The purpose of the guidelines is to help with the management of small lung nodules detected incidentally. The likelihood of malignancy depends on nodule size and patient factors.

- A low-risk patient has minimal/no smoking history and no other known risk factors (e.g. significant family history, asbestos exposure, etc.).
- The likelihood of malignancy is thought to be 0.2% for nodules of <3 mm, 0.9% for nodules of 4–7 mm and 18% for nodules of 8–20 mm (Table 1.3).

Table 1.3 Fleischner Society guidelines 2013

Size (mm)	Low risk	High risk
≤4	No follow-up	12 months
>4–6	12 months	6 months, then 18–24 months
>6–8	6–12 months, then 18–24 months	3–6 months, 9–12 and 24 months
>8	3, 9 and 24 months + positron emission tomography ± biopsy	Same as low risk

Solid nodules: McMahon, H. et al. 2005. Guidelines for management of small pulmonary nodules detected on CT scans: A statement from the Fleischner Society. *Radiology* 237:395–400.

Sub-solid nodules: Naidich, D. et al. 2012. Recommendations for the management of subsolid pulmonary nodules detected at CT: A statement from the Fleischner Society. *Radiology* 266:304–317.

Box 1.12 A DIFFERENTIAL FOR SOLITARY PULMONARY NODULES

Granuloma
Organising pneumonia
Bronchogenic cyst
Infection/inflammation
Tumour
Carcinoid
Hamartoma

GOODPASTURE SYNDROME

Autoimmune disease characterised by glomerulonephritis and pulmonary haemorrhage—note that pulmonary features occur before renal manifestations. The pathology is antiglomerular basement membrane antibodies; these attack the alveolar basement membrane in the lung. Associated with a positive p-ANCA (anti-neutrophil cytoplasmic antibody) or c-ANCA in about 30%.

PLAIN FILM
- Bilateral consolidation with sparing of the costophrenic angles and lung periphery.
- Progression to an interstitial/fibrotic pattern in chronic disease.

HRCT
- Patchy ground-glass opacification with peripheral and costophrenic angle sparing.
- Airspace disease clears within a couple of weeks.
- Pulmonary fibrosis may develop in the long term.

HAMARTOMA

This is a common, benign lung neoplasm peaking in the sixth decade. A minority (10%) are endobronchial.

PLAIN FILM
- Smooth, marginated nodule, frequently calcified.
- Two-thirds in the lung periphery.
- Look for atelectasis/consolidation, suggesting an endobronchial lesion.

CT
- Fat attenuation of the nodule (50%)
- Or a combination of fat and calcification
- Diffuse popcorn calcification (classic)

NUCLEAR MEDICINE
- Note: Up to 20% are hot on PET

HEREDITARY HAEMORRHAGIC TELANGIECTASIA

Also known as Osler–Weber–Rendu syndrome. It is an autosomal dominant disorder characterised by multiple AVMs with a classic triad of telangiectasia, epistaxis and a positive family history. A total of 20% of patients have multiple pulmonary AVMs, causing cyanosis, dyspnoea, stroke and brain abscess. Other sites of AVMs include the brain, spinal cord, GI tract and liver.

PLAIN FILM/CT
- Rounded/lobulated nodule with feeding vessels

HISTOPLASMOSIS

Fungal infection from North America and inhaled from bird and bat faeces. In immunocompetent individuals, infection almost always resolves without treatment.

PLAIN FILM/CT
- Calcified pulmonary nodules 2–5 mm in size (miliary appearance).

- Enlarged lymph nodes with peripheral 'egg shell' calcification is classic.
- Look for a broncholith—this is a calcified lymph node that has eroded into the airway.

Box 1.13 CAUSES OF CALCIFIED LYMPH NODES IN THE THORAX
The six 'osis's' Silicosis Sarcoidosis Histoplasmosis Amyloidosis Coal worker's pneumoconiosis Blastomycosis Treated lymphoma

HIV/AIDS—PULMONARY MANIFESTATIONS (TABLE 1.4)

Table 1.4 CD4 count narrows the differential for potential causes of pulmonary infection in the context of HIV and AIDS

>200 cells/μL	<200 cells/μL = AIDS, high risk for opportunistic infection and malignancy	<50 cells/μL
Histiocytosis	Pneumocystis pneumonia	*Mycobacterium avium*
Lymphoma (non-Hodgkin mostly)	Tuberculosis	
Cytomegalovirus	Kaposi's sarcoma	
Recurrent bacterial pneumonia (AIDS-defining illness)		

CRYPTOCOCCUS
Plain film/CT
- Small pulmonary nodules (solitary or multiple) that may cavitate. Segmental and lobar consolidation.
- Check for hilar and subcarinal lymph node enlargement.
- Pleural effusions are common.

KAPOSI'S SARCOMA
This is the most common AIDS-related neoplasm and is more common in men.

Plain film/CT (Figure 1.23)
- Numerous ill-defined perihilar/peribronchovascular nodules, surrounded by ground glass.
- Less commonly, there is interlobular septal thickening.
- Look for enhancing hilar lymph node enlargement.
- Pleural effusions atypical.

Nuclear medicine
- Note: Lymphoma is gallium avid, Kaposi lesions are not.

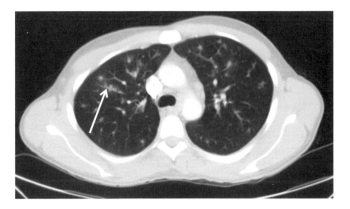

Figure 1.23 Kaposi sarcoma. Computed tomography image demonstrating the typical ill-defined peribronchovascular 'flame-shaped' ground-glass opacities (white arrow).

LYMPHOMA

Mostly non-Hodgkin and usually associated with more disseminated extra-nodal disease involving the CNS, GI tract and bone marrow.

Plain film/CT

- The most common finding is multiple pleural or intrapulmonary masses.

PNEUMOCYSTIS PNEUMONIA (PCP) (FIGURE 1.24)

Fungal infection, the most common opportunistic infection.

Plain film

- May be normal.
- Look for diffuse, bilateral airspace opacification.
- Check for a pneumothorax—this would be nearly pathognomic for PCP in the right setting.

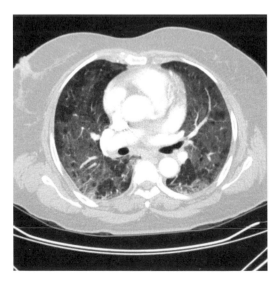

Figure 1.24 Pneumocystis pneumonia. Computed tomography image demonstrating diffuse, bilateral ground-glass opacification.

CT

- Diffuse, ground-glass pattern of airspace opacification (most typical) with or without reticulation.
- Upper lobe cysts are common and prone to pneumothorax.
- No lymph node enlargement or pleural effusion.

PNEUMONIA

Bacterial pneumonia is most common (*Streptococcus* or *Haemophilus*), though TB infection is the most common worldwide.

Plain film

- Focal or lobar consolidation

HODGKIN VERSUS NON-HODGKIN LYMPHOMA

Box 1.14 COTSWOLDS MODIFICATION OF THE ANN ARBOR STAGING SYSTEM

Staging lymphoma

I: Single node group affected
II: Multiple node groups, same side of diaphragm
III: Multiple node groups, both sides of the diaphragm
IV: Multiple extra-nodal sites of disease, **or** nodes and extranodal disease
X: Denotes mass >10 cm
E: Denotes extra-nodal extension or single extra-nodal site of disease

Hodgkin and non-Hodgkin lymphomas are staged using the same system.

HODGKIN LYMPHOMA

Most present with enlarged supraclavicular/cervical lymph nodes, often with no symptoms. Diagnosis confirmed by presence of Reed–Sternberg cells. More common in the chest than non-Hodgkin.

Plain film (Figure 1.25)

- Masses, consolidation and nodules
- Pleural effusions are common

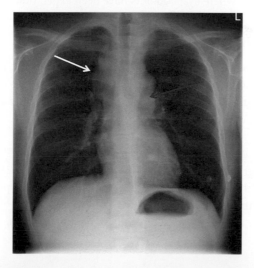

Figure 1.25 Lymphoma. Chest x-ray demonstrating mediastinal lymphadenopathy with widening of the paratracheal stripe (white arrow) and loss of the aortopulmonary window (red arrow).

CT

- Parenchymal disease accompanied by intrathoracic adenopathy
- Expect enlarged mediastinal lymph nodes (paratracheal and anterior mediastinum), hila nodes atypical

NON-HODGKIN LYMPHOMA

Tends to present with slowly growing lymph nodes and B symptoms (i.e. fever, night sweats, weight loss). Far more common than Hodgkin lymphoma. About three-quarters in the thorax are diffuse large B-cell lymphoma (DLBCL).

Plain film

- Classic appearance is hilar or mediastinal lymph node enlargement with a pleural effusion.

CT

- Pattern of lymph node enlargement varies with lymphoma subtype (e.g. in DLBCL, prevascular/pretracheal nodes are most commonly affected).
- May present with miliary nodules.

HYDATID INFECTION

The lungs are the second most common site (about 15%) after the liver to be affected. Up to 15%–25% show no symptoms. Diagnosis made with Casoni skin test or serological antigens. Expect blood eosinophilia.

PLAIN FILM

- Multiple well-defined, rounded masses (up to 20 cm).
- More common in the lower lobes, may have an air–fluid level (due to communication with the bronchial tree).

CT

- Cyst with low-density contents, rarely calcification.
- 'Water lily' sign describes the floating cyst membrane within cyst fluid.
- 'Empty cyst' sign occurs where cyst contents have been expectorated.

HYPERSENSITIVITY PNEUMONITIS

Also known as extrinsic allergic alveolitis, it is a granulomatous response to an inhaled antigen. The antigens involved include animal proteins (e.g. bird fancier's lung), microbes (e.g. farmer's lung, hot tub lung, etc.), chemicals, etc. Presentation may be acute (e.g. 6–8 hours after exposure) or chronic after years of exposure.

PLAIN FILM

- A normal chest radiograph is the most common finding.
- Look for multiple poorly defined small opacities, patchy/diffuse airspace shadowing.
- Pleural effusions are unusual.
- In chronic cases, there may be fibrosis, typically in the upper zones.

HRCT

- Patchy ground-glass change and small ill-defined centrilobular nodules.
- Look for air-trapping giving a mosaic pattern of attenuation (i.e. trapped air in secondary lobules).

IDIOPATHIC INTERSTITIAL PNEUMONIA

Box 1.15 MAKE SENSE OF IDIOPATHIC INTERSTITIAL PNEUMONIA
Mueller-Mang, C. et al. 2007. What every radiologist should know about idiopathic interstitial pneumonias. *Radiographics* 27:595–615.
Hansell, D. et al. 2008. Fleischner society: Glossary of terms for thoracic imaging. *Radiology* 246:697–722.

This is a group of seven diffuse lung diseases. They are rare, and each has its own pattern on HRCT that correlates with histological findings. Patients typically present with non-specific cough or dyspnoea.

In approximate order of frequency:

USUAL INTERSTITIAL PNEUMONIA (UIP)

The UIP pattern is seen with idiopathic pulmonary fibrosis (IPF; the clinical syndrome). It typically affects those >50 years of age, often with a smoking history. The UIP pattern is also seen with rheumatoid lung, systemic sclerosis (can have UIP or non-specific interstitial pneumonia [NSIP] pattern), asbestosis and other connective tissue diseases. Response to steroids and prognosis is poor in IPF.

Plain film

- Normal at first, then decreased lung volumes with sub-pleural, basal reticulation.

HRCT

- The classic trio is: (1) apicobasal gradient of (2) sub-pleural reticular opacities, and (3) macrocystic honeycombing and traction bronchiectasis.
- Ground-glass attenuation less extensive than the reticular opacities.
- Check for an irregular pleural surface.
- Typically, abnormal lung is seen next to normal lung.
- The pattern is typical, biopsy may not be required for diagnosis.
- 10% of IPF patients develop lung cancer.

NON-SPECIFIC INTERSTITIAL PNEUMONIA (NSIP)

Primarily idiopathic, but the pattern may also be associated with connective tissue disorders (e.g. systemic lupus erythematosus [SLE] and systemic sclerosis), other autoimmune diseases (rheumatoid arthritis) and may be drug induced (e.g. gold). Affects younger patients than IPF and responds well to steroid treatment.

Plain film

- Normal at first, then diffuse airspace opacities.

HRCT

- Bilateral, symmetrical, sub-pleural ground-glass change with reticular opacities.
- Traction bronchiectasis and consolidation later in the disease.
- Ground-glass opacification dominates—not reticulation as with UIP.
- There may be honeycombing late in the disease (microcystic).

CRYPTOGENIC ORGANISING PNEUMONIA (COP)

Previously known as bronchiolitis obliterans organising pneumonia. It is characterised by the onset of cough, dyspnoea and low-grade pyrexia over several weeks. Wide age range affected, more common between 40 and 70 years of age.

Plain film

- Bilateral, peripheral patchy consolidation.
- Fleeting/migratory consolidation is classic.

HRCT

- Typically multifocal, transient, patchy, dense consolidation with a predominantly sub-pleural, mid-lower zone distribution (80%).
- Small centrilobular nodules and peribronchial thickening.
- The 'atoll' sign is characteristic (not pathognomic), lesion with central ground glass and rim of consolidation.
- Adenopathy (25%) and effusions (30%) are less common.
- Dense consolidation helps to distinguish COP from desquamative interstitial pneumonia (DIP)—ground-glass opacification dominates in DIP

RESPIRATORY BRONCHIOLITIS-ASSOCIATED INTERSTITIAL LUNG DISEASE (RB-ILD)

This is the interstitial lung disease of smokers, more common in men aged 30–40 years. Treatment is with steroids and smoking cessation.

HRCT

- Centriolobular nodules with ground glass, bronchial wall thickening and air-trapping.
- Expect background centrilobular emphysema (due to smoking history).

DESQUAMATIVE INTERSTITIAL PNEUMONIA (DIP)

Strongly associated with smoking (90% are smokers), considered the end of the RB-ILD spectrum. More common in men, the prognosis is good with steroids and smoking cessation.

Plain film

- Non-specific, hazy opacities

HRCT

- Diffuse ground-glass opacification not respecting fissures—this is classic.
- Deep parenchymal cysts.
- More commonly a peripheral pattern.

ACUTE INTERSTITIAL PNEUMONIA (AIP)

Unlike the other idiopathic interstitial pneumonias (IIPs), symptom onset is acute and rapidly progressive to requiring ventilation in 3 weeks. Steroids are effective early on, but mortality remains 50%.

Plain film

- Diffuse patchy airspace disease (similar to ARDS), but sparing the costophrenic angles.

HRCT

- Ground-glass opacities and dependent consolidation (from oedema and haemorrhage).
- For survivors of the acute disease, there may be non-dependent honeycombing and traction bronchiectasis (consolidation is thought to be protective against this).

LYMPHOCYTIC INTERSTITIAL PNEUMONITIS (LIP)

Very rare when idiopathic. The pattern is more commonly seen in patients with Sjögren syndrome or who are immunocompromised (e.g. HIV) and have chronic, active hepatitis. More common in women.

Plain film

- Non-specific, reticular or reticulo-nodular opacities

HRCT

- The classic duo is: (1) diffuse ground-glass opacification; and (2) thin-walled perivascular cysts.
- Centrilobular nodules, septal thickening and pleural effusions are less common.

KARTAGENER SYNDROME

This is a type of primary ciliary dyskinesia with autosomal recessive inheritance. It comprises a triad of dextrocardia, bronchiectasis and sinusitis. The problem is due to ciliary dysfunction; in the lungs, this leads to bronchitis, recurrent pneumonia, etc. It usually presents in childhood and is associated with infertility, corneal abnormalities, transposition of the great vessels, pyloric stenosis, post-cricoid web and epispadias.

PLAIN FILM

- Classic findings are bronchiectasis and dextrocardia.
- Check also for bronchial wall thickening, collapse and consolidation.

LUNG CANCER

Lung cancer is the most common cause of cancer death worldwide. Mostly diagnosed when the disease is advanced, a minority (about 10%) are picked up incidentally. Lung cancer is divided broadly into two groups: non-small-cell lung cancer (NSCLC; 85%) and small-cell lung cancer (SCLC) (Table 1.5).

Table 1.5 Basic staging of non-small-cell lung cancer

Management	T	Characteristics
Lobectomy	1	Up to 3 cm in size, no bronchial invasion
	2	3–7 cm, >2 cm from carina, lobar atelectasis
Pneumonectomy	3	>7 cm, <2 cm from carina, whole lung collapse, nodules in same lobe, invasion of chest wall, diaphragm, pericardium, etc.
Non-operative	4	Tumour in the carina, invasion of heart/great vessels and nodules in ipsilateral lobes

Note: Ipsilateral nodes are considered N1–2, or N3 if contralateral or supraclavicular. Nodules in the contralateral lung are classified M1a, or M1b if distant metastases.

NSCLC

This is further sub-divided into squamous cell carcinoma (SCC) (35%), adenocarcinoma (30%) and large-cell carcinoma (15%).

Plain film

- Lung mass.
- Lung/lobar collapse denoting an obstructing endobronchial mass.
- Pleural effusion.
- SCC tends to cavitate, adenocarcinoma may appear as consolidation resistant to antibiotics.
- Check for mediastinal or hilar lymph node enlargement and bone destruction.

CT

- Ill-defined, peripheral, spiculated and irregular nodules are high risk.
- Air bronchogram and focal lucency in a nodule also suggest malignancy.
- Cavitation is non-specific, but a cavity wall >15 mm thick is worrying.
- Nodules enhancing >15 HU are 98% sensitive, 73% specific for malignancy.
- Common sites for metastases include adrenal glands, liver, brain, bones and soft tissues.

Nuclear medicine

- PET is superior for staging (92% accuracy, 25% for CT) and assessing bone disease (92% vs. 87%).
- False positives may arise due to inflammatory processes.

SCLC

This used to be known as oat-cell carcinoma. It is very aggressive and rapidly fatal without treatment (chemotherapy/radiotherapy). It is a disease of smokers and typically presents once systemic.

Plain film

- Large central mass involving at least one hilum
- Lung/lobar collapse, pleural effusion

CT

- Large central/hilar mass with associated lymph node enlargement.
- Encasement of the heart and great vessels—note that a quarter of all superior vena cava obstruction is due to SCLC.

Nuclear medicine

- Bone scan is useful for detecting bone metastases.
- PET is used for staging.

LUNG TRANSPLANT PULMONARY COMPLICATIONS

Box 1.16 COMPLICATIONS OF LUNG TRANSPLANTATION

Acute complications
- Reperfusion syndrome
- Acute transplant rejection
- Anastomotic dehiscence

Any time
- Infection

Chronic
- Bronchiolitis obliterans
- PTLD

REPERFUSION SYNDROME

This is the most common immediate complication and occurs within 48 hours of transplant.

Plain film

- Perihilar airspace opacification
- Bibasal pleural effusions

ACUTE TRANSPLANT REJECTION

Occurs at approximately 10 days post-transplant.

Plain film

- Normal in 50%
- Otherwise heterogeneous peri-hilar opacification, septal thickening and right pleural effusion
- Absence of upper lobe blood diversion

BRONCHIOLITIS OBLITERANS

This is a leading cause of death after approximately 2 years; onset is chronic from about 3 months post-transplant. Cytomegalovirus (CMV) is a predisposing factor.

Plain film/CT

- Normal chest x-ray initially, then decreased vascular markings and increasing bronchiectasis
- Hyperinflated lungs with bronchial thickening and dilatation
- Air trapping, mosaic perfusion and bronchiectasis

POST-TRANSPLANT LYMPHOPROLIFERATIVE DISEASE (PTLD)

Non-specific complication within 2 years of a bone marrow or solid organ transplant. It is due to B- or T-cell proliferation, usually following EBV infection. Responds rapidly to a reduction in immunosuppression or, alternatively, rituximab.

Plain film

- Single or multiple well-defined, slow-growing nodules
- Consolidation less commonly
- Often hilar or mediastinal lymph node enlargement

INFECTION

Most commonly bacterial, also CMV (nodules, consolidation and ground-glass opacification at 3–4 months post-transplant) and aspergillosis.

LYMPHANGIOLEIOMYOMATOSIS (LAM)

This is a rare interstitial lung disease that is more common in non-smoking women of child-bearing age. Symptoms worsen in pregnancy or with smoking. May present with spontaneous pneumothorax. Associated with tuberous sclerosis (up to 40% of tuberous scleroses).

PLAIN FILM

- Normal initially, then hyper-expansion and small cysts.
- Check for a pneumothorax.

HRCT

- Uniform, thin-walled cysts with normal intervening lung.
- Chylous pleural effusions.
- Pneumothorax.
- Nodules are unusual.
- HRCT commonly abnormal in affected children with tuberous sclerosis.

LYMPHANGITIS CARCINOMATOSIS

> **Box 1.17 CAUSES OF DIFFUSE RETICULATION**
>
> **Sar**coidosis
> **C**onnective tissue disease, cardiac and cancer
> **C**ystic lung disease (lymphangioleiomyomatosis and Langerhans cell histiocytosis [LCH])
> **O**ccupational
> **I**diopathic pulmonary fibrosis
> **D**rug induced

Lymphangitis carcinomatosis is the permeation of the lymphatics by neoplastic cells. This may occur due to tumour emboli or by direct extension from the hila or bronchogenic carcinoma.

PLAIN FILM

- Classically, there is coarse/nodular reticulation.

CT

- Nodular interlobular septal thickening and thickening of the bronchovascular lymphoid tissue.
- Unilateral lymphangitis is most commonly associated with a lung primary, bilateral usually suggests extra-thoracic malignancy (breast most commonly).

MACLEOD SYNDROME

Box 1.18 CAUSES OF A UNILATERAL HYPERLUCENT HEMITHORAX

Work from chest wall inwards to remember them:
Rotation
Chest wall
- Poland syndrome
- Mastectomy
Pleura
- Pneumothorax
Lung
- Endobronchial obstruction (tumour, foreign body)
- MacLeod syndrome
- Bullae
- Congenital lobar emphysema
- Pneumonectomy
- Contralateral pleural effusion
Vascular
- Large pulmonary embolus

Also known as Swyer–James syndrome. It is often an incidental finding in an adult and follows previous childhood infectious bronchiolitis.

PLAIN FILM (FIGURE 1.26)

- Hyperlucent lung with a paucity of vascular markings.
- Normal or small-volume lung and hilum on the affected side.

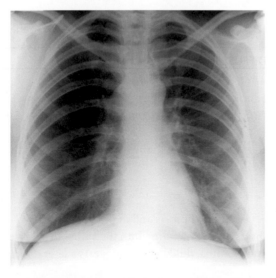

Figure 1.26 MacLeod syndrome. Chest x-ray demonstrating hyperlucency of the right hemithorax with paucity of the vascular markings.

HRCT
- Hyperlucent lung with a paucity of vessels.
- Bronchiectasis and bronchial wall thickening are common.

NUCLEAR MEDICINE
- Expect a matched ventilation/perfusion defect (non-specific).

MESOTHELIOMA

Mesothelioma accounts for about 1% of thoracic neoplasms, but it is the most common pleural malignancy. Mostly it is nodular (70%), with the rest being diffuse, and it originates in the parietal pleura. There is a strong association with previous asbestos exposure, with a latency period of up to 40 years.

PLAIN FILM
- Unilateral pleural effusion, pleural thickening and volume loss
- Calcified pleural plaques

CT
- Nodular pleural thickening with encasement and mediastinal involvement.
- Check for extension below the diaphragm, which denotes T4 disease (rare).

MOUNIER–KUHN SYNDROME

This is congenital tracheobronchomegaly. It leads to reduced clearance of secretions and recurrent infection.

CT
- Tracheal diameter >3 cm, the outline has a corrugated appearance.
- Look for bronchial or tracheal diverticulosis and distal bronchiectasis.

NEUROFIBROMATOSIS

The chest may be involved in neurofibromatosis type 1 (Von Recklinghausen disease), either from neurofibromata, meningocele or parenchymal lung disease.

PLAIN FILM (FIGURE 1.27)
- Large posterior mediastinal mass (meningocele or neurofibroma).
- Ribbon ribs/posterior scalloping of the vertebral bodies (due to adjacent neurofibroma).
- Look for lung nodules—these may actually be cutaneous neurofibromata.
- Fibrosis at the lung bases.

HRCT/CT
- Progressive, symmetrical basal fibrosis and upper lobe bullae.
- Look for paravertebral masses extending into the spinal canal—soft tissue/some fat density suggests neurofibroma, fluid density suggests a lateral meningocele.

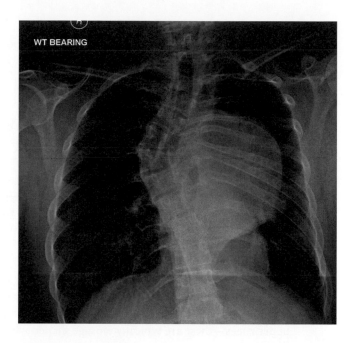

WT BEARING

Figure 1.27 Neurofibromatosis. Chest x-ray demonstrating a large posterior mediastinal mass with splaying and thinning of the ribs.

PECTUS EXCAVATUM

Congenital deformity of the sternum/anterior chest wall associated with Marfan syndrome, neurofibromatosis type 1 (NF1) and Ehlers–Danlos syndrome. Surgical options include insertion of a rod to displace the sternum anteriorly—the Nuss procedure.

PLAIN FILM

- Blurring of the right heart border and displacement of the heart to the left.
- Mimics middle lobe consolidation.
- Posterior ribs appear more horizontal than expected and the anterior ribs more vertical.

PNEUMOCONIOSIS

This is a collection of lung diseases resulting from a local reaction to inhaled particulates. It is broadly classified as fibrotic (coal worker's pneumoconiosis [CWP], silicosis, asbestosis, berylliosis and talcosis) and non-fibrotic (tin oxide: stannosis; iron oxide: siderosis). Requires a long period of exposure.

FIBROTIC
CWP
Due to exposure to coal dust. Increased risk of chronic obstructive pulmonary disease (COPD) and progressive massive fibrosis (PMF). Caplan syndrome is CWP with features of rheumatoid arthritis.

Plain film
- Small, well-defined nodules of 1–5 mm with an upper lobe predominance
- Calcification on chest x-ray in up to 20%

CT
- Diffuse nodules
- Hilar or mediastinal lymph node enlargement with or without central node calcification (eggshell calcification also sometimes present)

Silicosis
Due to exposure to silica (e.g. sandblasting or mining). Acute exposure to large volumes of silica causes acute silicosis ('silicoproteinosis')—classic silicosis is a chronic form. Becomes complicated (i.e. PMF) more commonly than CWP.

Plain film (Figure 1.28)
- Small (<10 mm) calcified nodules, more commonly in the upper zones.
- Check for bilateral mediastinal or hilar lymph node enlargement.
- PMF occurs where the nodules grow and coalesce, forming large opacities in the upper zones—these are typically sausage shaped with fewer adjacent nodules and eventually migrate towards the hilum.
- Upper lobe fibrosis.

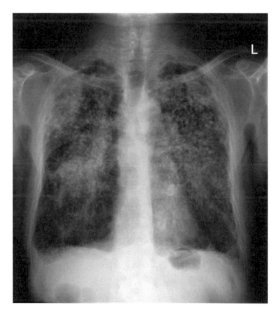

Figure 1.28 Silicosis. Chest x-ray demonstrating multiple small calcified nodules. In the right mid-zone, nodules coalesce, in keeping with progressive massive fibrosis. There is upper lobe fibrosis with volume loss and ascent of the hila bilaterally.

CT
- Hyperdense/calcified nodules.
- Eggshell lymph node calcification is practically pathognomonic of silicosis.
- Acute silicoproteinosis has a similar appearance to pulmonary alveolar proteinosis.

NON-FIBROTIC

Siderosis

Most commonly seen in those exposed to metal fumes (e.g. welders). Changes in the lung are reversible.

Plain film
- Small perihilar nodules

HRCT
- Small centrilobular nodules and branching linear structures (iron oxide particles in the lymphatics)
- Extensive ground-glass opacification less common

Stannosis

Due to deposition of tin oxides in the lung. They are very dense on imaging, but induce little reaction from the lung.

Plain film
- Widespread, high-density miliary nodules

PNEUMONIA

Box 1.19 A DIFFERENTIAL FOR CHRONIC AIRSPACE OPACIFICATION

Focal
- Lipoid pneumonia
- Adenocarcinoma (i.e. bronchoalveolar cell carcinoma)
- Lymphoma

Diffuse
- Adenocarcinoma (i.e. bronchoalveolar cell carcinoma)
- Pulmonary alveolar proteinosis
- Alveolar sarcoid
- Lipoid pneumonia

In most adults, follow-up at 6 weeks is appropriate to check for resolution of consolidation.

Opacity typically appears rapidly (within 12 hours) on radiography and resolves slowly (>2 months in some cases) after successful treatment. Immunosuppression and the coexistence of diabetes, neutropenia, etc., delay infiltrate formation. Cavitation suggests infection with *Staphylococcus*.

PNEUMOCOCCAL PNEUMONIA

Due to *Streptococcus*, it accounts for >50% of bacterial pneumonia.

Plain film
- Consolidation with or without air bronchograms, it may be multi-lobar or bilateral.
- Pleural effusions are common.

- In children, consolidation may be mass-like, 'round pneumonia'—more common in the lower zones.

CT
- Consolidation appears more extensive than on plain radiography.
- Lymph node enlargement is common.
- Look for small nodules or 'tree in bud' opacities (small airway inflammation).
- Pleural effusions are common; pleural enhancement suggests empyema.

VARICELLA-ZOSTER PNEUMONIA

The appearance depends on the stage of the disease.

Plain film/CT
- Multiple small nodules, some of which coalesce to form areas of consolidation when acute
- Miliary (i.e. small calcified) nodules in the chronic phase

LIPOID PNEUMONIA

Due to inadvertent inhalation of mineral oil.

Plain film
- Chronic lower lobe consolidation, may be focal/mass-like or multi-focal

CT
- Fat density attenuation/consolidation

PNEUMOMEDIASTINUM

Box 1.20 THE CRITICAL REVIEW AREAS FOR CHEST X-RAYS—THE THREE PS
Pneumothorax Pneumomediastinum Pneumoperitoneum

Mostly due to alveolar rupture from increased intra-alveolar pressure (e.g. asthma, aspiration of foreign body, mechanical ventilation or trauma). Other causes include disease affecting the alveolar wall directly (e.g. pneumonia, ARDS or COPD), tracheal perforation and oesophageal rupture.

PLAIN FILM
- Look for air giving the heart/mediastinum a more crisp outline than normal.
- Gas in the soft tissues of the neck.
- Large volumes dissect inferiorly into the retroperitoneum/peritoneum.

PNEUMOTHORAX

Appearances on a supine radiograph can be challenging and may underestimate the extent of pneumothorax. Air collects in one or more of the pleural recesses—most common locations are subpulmonic and anteromedial.

PLAIN FILM (SUPINE CHEST X-RAY)

- Hyperlucent right upper quadrant
- 'Deep sulcus' sign, an excessively sharp contour to the hemidiaphragm

POLAND SYNDROME

Congenital, unilateral absence of part or whole of the pectoralis major. Associated with deformity of the fingers, ribs and pectus excavatum.

PLAIN FILM

- Apparent hyperlucent lung (underlying lung is actually normal) due to the absence of overlying soft tissue

PULMONARY ALVEOLAR MICROLITHIASIS

Asymptomatic in 70% of patients (despite florid appearances on imaging!). Typically presents at age 30–50 years, more common in Turkey.

PLAIN FILM

- Diffuse, dense miliary calcification, which may obscure borders with the mediastinum, diaphragm, etc.
- Sub-pleural cyst formation may give the pleura a lucent appearance on chest x-ray.

CT

- Numerous bilateral calcifications, may be most conspicuous in the mid-lower zones and along the microvascular bundles.

PULMONARY ALVEOLAR PROTEINOSIS

Typically affecting middle-aged men, they present with a dry cough and clubbing. There is a strong association with smoking. It is mostly primary (90%). The rest arises due to acute silicosis, haematological malignancy or in the context of infection with immunosuppression (e.g. *Cryptococcus*, *Nocardia* or *Aspergillus*). Characterised by the filling of airspaces with proteinaceous fluid—the interstitium is not affected.

PLAIN FILM

- Symmetrical peri-hilar ground-glass opacification, mimics pulmonary oedema
- No pleural effusion or cardiomegaly

HRCT

- A crazy-paving appearance is classic (less common in secondary disease)—a combination of ground-glass opacification and smooth interlobular septal thickening.
- Ground-glass opacification predominates (the 'black bronchus' sign is useful for demonstrating ground-glass opacification).

PULMONARY EMBOLISM

Patients are typically risk stratified first with the modified Wells score, with those at high risk proceeding to CT pulmonary angiography and low-risk patients having a D-dimer test. CTPA sensitivity is 83% (increased slightly by doing a CT venogram at the same time) and specificity is 96%.

US

- Used to assess the deep veins of the legs, as most pulmonary embolisms (PEs) originate here.
- Expanded, non-compressible vessel.
- Reduced venous flow on calf compression.

CT

- Occlusive/non-occlusive filling defect that forms an acute angle with the vessel wall.
- Look for peripheral wedge-shaped foci of consolidation (pulmonary infarct) and, more rarely, mosaic attenuation of the lung (pulmonary oligaemia).
- Chronic PE—forms an obtuse angle with the vessel wall, crescentic arrangement within the vessel. There may be webs, calcification or collateralisation. Mosaic attenuation (Figure 1.29) is seen more commonly than with acute PE.
- Check for evidence of acute right heart strain (e.g. enlarged right ventricle, reflux of contrast to the hepatic veins, bowing of the intraventricular septum towards the left ventricle and pulmonary hypertension).

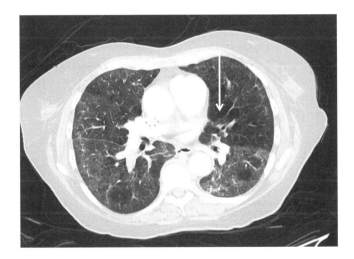

Figure 1.29 Chronic thromboembolism. High-resolution computed tomography image demonstrating mosaic attenuation. The hypoattenuating regions are abnormal and reflect oligaemia. The vessels within the hypoattenuating regions are small (white arrow).

NUCLEAR MEDICINE

- Sensitivity is similar to a CTPA test, but less specific.
- V/Q is now usually performed either in pregnancy (depending on local guidelines) or when renal failure precludes the use of intravenous contrast.

INTERVENTION

- Catheter-directed thrombolysis/mechanical thrombectomy may be considered for certain patients with life-threatening PE.

PULMONARY HYPERTENSION

Divided into primary and secondary causes. Secondary pulmonary hypertension is due to either increased pulmonary blood flow (e.g. left to right shunt), decreased cross-sectional area of the pulmonary vasculature (e.g. pulmonary embolism) or increased resistance to pulmonary venous drainage (commonly due to left-sided heart disease).

PLAIN FILM

● Look for an enlarged right descending pulmonary artery (>25 mm).
● Peripheral oligaemia.

CT

● Main pulmonary artery wider than the ascending aorta (or >28–30 mm)
● Mosaic attenuation of the lungs due to variations in perfusion

PULMONARY LANGERHANS CELL HISTIOCYTOSIS

Rare disease that is most common in smokers aged 30–40 years, thought to be due to antigen exposure (hence it predominates in the upper zones of the lungs).

HRCT

● Early on, nodules are most common in the mid-upper zones.
● As the disease progresses, the nodules undergo cystic degeneration.
● Eventually, the cysts may coalesce to form a honeycomb pattern (Figure 1.30).
● The presence of 3–10-mm nodules and cysts in the upper zones in a smoker is strongly suggestive of histiocytosis.

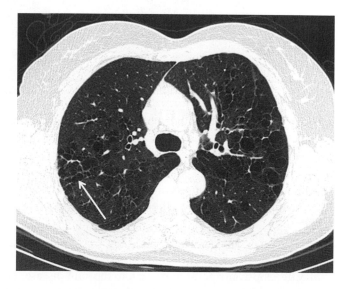

Figure 1.30 Langerhans cell histiocytosis. HRCT image demonstrating bilateral lung cysts with coalescence into a honeycomb pattern (white arrow).

PULMONARY OEDEMA

The accumulation of extravascular fluid in the lung. It is either due to increased fluid pressure (leading first to increased interstitial fluid, then to alveolar flooding) or to increased membrane permeability.

PLAIN FILM

- Initially, there is vascular redistribution—'upper lobe diversion'.
- Then, interstitial fluid and Kerley lines (Kerley A lines are 2–6 cm long, extend from the hila; Kerley B lines are <2 cm long, peripheral extending to the pleural surface).
- Bilateral pleural effusions.
- Finally, airspace opacities indicating alveolar flooding.
- Cardiomegaly.

PULMONARY SEQUESTRATION

This is a non-functioning lung segment with no communication to the bronchial tree and a systemic arterial supply. It is more common in males. There are intralobar and extralobar types (Table 1.6).

Table 1.6 Imaging characteristics of intra- and extra-lobar sequestration

Type	Intra-lobar	Extra-lobar
Percentage	75% of cases	25% of cases
Presentation	Presents in adulthood with pain, infection and haemoptysis	Presents in infancy with feeding difficulties, respiratory distress, cyanosis and heart failure
Venous drainage	Central drainage ('intra' = 'centra[l]' drainage)	Systemic drainage via inferior vena cava, azygos or hemiazygos
Arterial supply	Systemic feeding vessels from the descending thoracic aorta	Systemic feeding from aorta or from the splenic, gastric or intercostal arteries
Pleural relationship	Enclosed in visceral pleura	Own pleura

RHEUMATOID ARTHRITIS

Box 1.21 DIFFERENTIALS FOR UNILATERAL PLEURAL EFFUSION—'VITAL'
Virus/non-tuberculous mycobacteria **I**mmunological (e.g. lupus or rheumatoid arthritis) **T**umour (e.g. lung or mesothelioma) or tuberculosis **a**nd **L**ymphoma

May develop at any point in relation to the joint disease. Typically affects patients who are positive for rheumatoid factor. The chest is more likely to be affected in male patients with rheumatoid.

PLAIN FILM

- Most have a unilateral pleural effusion.
- Bilateral pleural thickening is also common.
- Lower zone volume loss/fibrosis.

HRCT

- The most common interstitial patterns are UIP and NSIP.
- Nodules (<7 cm) may cavitate and be multiple; however, this is rare.
- A third have bronchial abnormalities—bronchiectasis and bronchiolitis obliterans.
- Check for evidence of pulmonary arterial hypertension and heart failure.

SARCOIDOSIS

Box 1.22 SILTZBACH STAGING OF SARCOIDOSIS

1. Normal chest radiograph
2. Bilateral hilar lymph node enlargement
3. Bilateral hilar lymph node enlargement, parenchymal infiltration
4. Parenchymal infiltration
5. Parenchymal volume loss as a result of pulmonary fibrosis—20% get to stage 4 with irreversible fibrosis

Read more:
Criado, E. et al. 2010. Pulmonary sarcoidosis: Typical and atypical manifestations at high-resolution CT with pathologic correlation. *Radiographics* 30:1567–1586.

Sarcoidosis is a multi-system granulomatous disease that is more common in women and those of African descent. Typically presents at <40 years of age. Up to 50% are asymptomatic; otherwise, symptoms are non-specific—cough, chest pain, weight loss, etc. The lungs are affected in 90% and pulmonary complications account for most morbidity and mortality.

PLAIN FILM

- Bilateral hilar lymph node enlargement plus right paratracheal lymph node enlargement ('Garland triad')—this is classic.
- Also check for airspace infiltration, nodules and fibrosis (upper zones).

HRCT (FIGURE 1.31)

- Upper/mid zone tiny nodules 2–4 mm or larger and coalescing in a perilymphatic distribution (i.e. along sub-pleural surfaces, fissures and peribronchovascular bundles).
- Nodular, interlobular septal thickening.
- Fibrosis with traction bronchiectasis.
- Note: The above are the abnormalities most commonly associated with pulmonary sarcoidosis. There are a myriad of alternative abnormalities—sarcoid is a great mimicker!

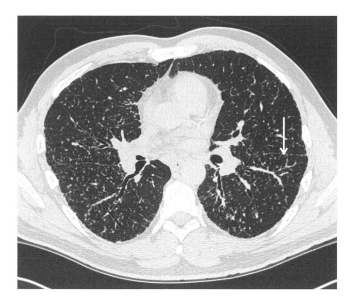

Figure 1.31 Typical sarcoidosis. High-resolution computed tomography image of sarcoidosis, demonstrating small nodules in a perilymphatic distribution (i.e. along the fissure; fissural beading) (white arrow) and along bronchovascular bundles (red arrow).

SEVERE ACUTE RESPIRATORY SYNDROME

Atypical pneumonia caused by a coronavirus. The imaging features are non-specific and indicative of diffuse alveolar damage. About 20% require intensive therapy unit (ITU) treatment; overall mortality about 10%.

PLAIN FILM

● May be normal initially, progressing to airspace opacification.

CT

● Ground-glass opacification/consolidation initially affecting the lower zones (commonly bilateral), then becoming widespread in severe cases.

SCLERODERMA

Also known as systemic sclerosis, this is a connective tissue disease affecting multiple organs. The thorax is commonly affected (most commonly the lungs or oesophagus). May be part of CREST syndrome (calcinosis, Raynaud's, oesophageal dysmotility, scleroderma and telangiectasia).

PLAIN FILM

● The classic appearance is a dilated oesophagus with basal fibrosis.

HRCT

● Basal interstitial lung disease is common (65%, though only a third have symptoms), most commonly NSIP pattern (also UIP).
● Check for evidence of pulmonary hypertension.

SOLITARY PULMONARY NODULE

Box 1.23 CAUSES OF A SOLITARY LUNG NODULE
Granuloma **O**rganising pneumonia **B**ronchogenic cyst **I**nflammation/infection **T**umour **C**arcinoid **H**amartoma

In the absence of malignancy elsewhere, small nodules are risk stratified using the Fleischner Society guidelines. Masses >4 cm are usually malignant. PET is 96% sensitive for lung nodules >1 cm. Nodules <2 cm are benign in about 80% of cases. Features suggesting benignity include:

- Lack of interval growth over 2 years
- Calcification (diffuse, central, popcorn or laminar)
- <15 HU enhancement

SYSTEMIC LUPUS ERYTHEMATOSUS

This is a collagen vascular disease commonly affecting the lungs, characterised by the deposition of autoantibodies and immune complexes in tissues (usually idiopathic, may be drug induced). It is 10-times more common in women. Treatment is with steroids and immunosuppression.

PLAIN FILM
- Pleural thickening (up to 50%, often painful) and pleural effusions.
- Check for a pericardial effusion.

HRCT
- Interstitial lung disease is common in patients with respiratory symptoms, the pattern is most commonly UIP.
- Check for a pulmonary embolism.
- Acute lupus pneumonitis—look for ground-glass opacification/bilateral consolidation. This is a diagnosis of exclusion (pneumonia and haemorrhage are differentials that may also complicate SLE).

TUBERCULOSIS

Box 1.24 THE 'TREE IN BUD' PATTERN
This is a non-specific pattern of tiny centrilobular nodules of soft tissue density attached to branches arising from a single stalk seen on HRCT. The branches and stalk represent dilated, thick-walled lobular bronchioles (normally too small to be seen) filled with mucous, pus, fluid or tumour cells.

Causes include infection (bacterial, fungal or viral), congenital (cystic fibrosis [CF] or mucociliary disorders), aspiration, connective tissue disease, malignancy, etc.

Read more:
Gosset, N. et al. 2009. Tree-in-bud pattern. *AJR* 193:472–477.

Due to inhaled *Mycobacteria tuberculosis.* This is very common worldwide. Initial infection in the naïve host is known as primary TB; secondary/reactivation TB occurs due to immunocompromised status or reinfection. Miliary disease may occur with primary or secondary TB.

PLAIN FILM

- Classic acute appearance is middle/lower lobe consolidation with ipsilateral lymph node enlargement and effusion.
- Apical consolidation is typical of post-primary TB (i.e. healed primary TB).
- Miliary nodules (Figure 1.32).

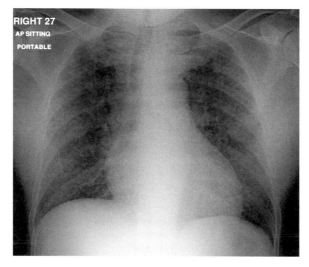

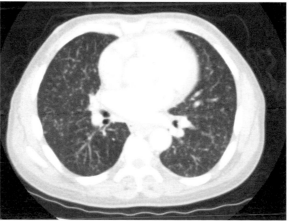

Figure 1.32 Miliary tuberculosis. Chest x-ray and CT image demonstrating multiple miliary nodules due to pulmonary tuberculosis.

CT

- Classically, lobar consolidation with ipsilateral hilar lymph node enlargement.
- Lymph nodes have central low density and peripheral enhancement with intravenous contrast (i.e. lymph node necrosis, fairly specific for TB).
- Look for 'tree in bud', suggesting endobronchial dissemination (i.e. bronchiolitis)—this is relatively specific for active TB.

TERATOMA

Box 1.25 DIFFERENTIALS FOR AN ANTERIOR MEDIASTINAL MASS
All the T's   1. Teratoma   2. Thymoma   3. Thyroid   4. 'Terrible' lymphoma   Look for increased lucency/low attenuation (fat) and calcification for teratoma.   Lobulation and other lymph nodes for lymphoma.   Pleural metatases for thymoma.   Superior mediastinal extension for thyroid.

This is a benign germ cell tumour usually presenting in children or young adults. Derived from two or more germ cell layers. Rarely malignant (prognosis then very poor). Mediastinal teratomas are mostly (95%) found in the anterior mediastinum.

PLAIN FILM (FIGURE 1.33)

- Well-defined mass in the anterior mediastinum
- Widened mediastinum, rounded margins with or without calcification
- With or without pleural effusion

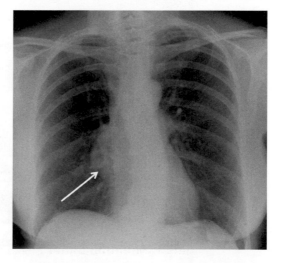

Figure 1.33 Teratoma. Chest x-ray demonstrating a mediastinal mass (white arrow). The hilum can be visualised (hilum overlay sign). The mass is inseparable from the heart border, which indicates that it must lie within the anterior mediastinum.

CT (FIGURE 1.34)

- Most are cystic (fluid density), often with a fatty component (a fat-fluid level is pathognomic).
- There is commonly calcification (sometimes in the form of a tooth).
- Thickened, enhancing soft tissue components suggest malignancy.

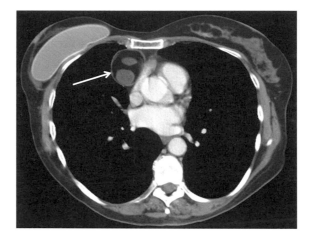

Figure 1.34 Teratoma. Computed tomography image of the same patient as in Figure 1.33, demonstrating that the mass (white arrow) contains soft tissue and fat in keeping with a teratoma.

THYMOMA AND THYMIC CARCINOMA

Thymoma is the most common neoplasm of the anterior mediastinum. It affects those aged 50–60 years most commonly. Associated with myasthenia gravis (35% of patients with thymomas have myasthenia gravis), red cell aplasia (50% develop thymoma) and hypogammaglobulinaemia.

CT (FIGURE 1.35)

- Imaging is not reliable for distinguishing thymoma from thymic carcinoma.

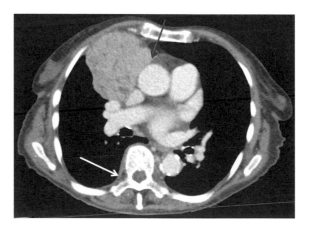

Figure 1.35 Thymic carcinoma. CT image demonstrating a soft tissue anterior mediastinal mass invading the mediastinum/pericardium (red arrow). There is focal pleural thickening in keeping with pleural metastases (white arrow).

- Rounded enlargement of the thymus is seen in both, commonly with calcification (up to a quarter of cases).
- Lymph node enlargement and local invasion suggest malignancy.
- Drop metastases to the pleura—but more common with thymoma.

PET/CT
- Useful for surveillance and staging

THYMOLIPOMA

Rare, benign, slow-growing neoplasm composed of mature thymic tissue and adipose tissue.

CT
- Fat and soft tissue appear as linear strands and whorls of soft tissue embedded in fat or rounded islands of soft tissue surrounded by fat.
- Most have equal amounts of fat and soft tissue.
- Calcification is rare (unlike teratoma).

THYMUS HYPERPLASIA

Mostly acquired due to recent stress (e.g. chemotherapy). Initially, there is thymic atrophy, then the thymus 'rebounds' once the stressor has gone. Other causes include Addison disease, Grave disease and acromegaly.

CT
- Diffuse symmetrical enlargement of the thymus

MRI
- Loss of signal on out-of-phase images due to the chemical shift artefact (not seen in thymic malignancy)

TRACHEOBRONCHIAL INJURY

Traumatic injury with high mortality. Rupture is most commonly near the carina, which is fixed.

PLAIN FILM
- Persistent pneumothorax in spite of drainage.
- Check for a fracture of the first rib.
- 'Fallen lung' sign—lung sags towards the floor of the hemithorax away from the hilum with rupture of the main bronchus.

WEGENER GRANULOMATOSIS

Also known as granulomatosis with polyangiitis (the preferred term due to Friedrich Wegener's links to the Nazi Party), it is a necrotising granulomatous vasculitis of the upper and lower respiratory tracts and renal glomeruli, affecting the small arteries and veins. Common clinical features are rhinitis, sinusitis, focal glomerulonephritis and otitis media. There is cardiac involvement (coronary vasculitis, pancarditis and valvular lesions) in up to 30%. Associated with c-ANCA antibodies.

PLAIN FILM

- Multiple cavitating lung nodules with a lower zone predilection

CT

- Multiple cavitating nodules (larger nodules cavitate more) with lower lobe predominance.
- Nodules are <10 cm and may be surrounded by a halo of ground-glass opacification (haemorrhage).
- Pleural effusions are seen in up to 25%.
- Basal fibrosis and tracheal and bronchial wall thickening are also seen.
- Lymph nodes are not enlarged.

CHAPTER 2

Musculoskeletal

GENERAL MUSCULOSKELETAL (MSK)

ACROMEGALY

Due to an excess of growth hormone (GH) in a mature skeleton ('gigantism' results from GH excess in an immature skeleton). Most commonly due to a benign pituitary adenoma. Associated with an increased heel pad thickness >25 mm.

SPINE X-RAY
- Posterior vertebral scalloping
- Increased anterior–posterior (AP) and transverse diameters of the vertebral bodies
- Narrowed interpedicular distance
- Spur formation
- Calcified discs

HAND X-RAY
- Spade appearance of terminal tufts of phalanges

MRI
- Enlarged, enhancing pituitary gland (note microadenomas enhance less than surrounding gland)
- Macroadenoma if >10 mm

Box 2.1 CAUSES OF INCREASED HEEL PAD THICKNESS (>21 MM)
<ul><li>**M**yxoedema</li><li>**A**cromegaly</li><li>**D**ilantin (phenytoin) therapy</li><li>**C**allus</li><li>**O**besity</li><li>**P**eripheral oedema</li></ul>

ADHESIVE CAPSULITIS

Also known as 'frozen shoulder'—more common in females and between 40 and 70 years of age. Clinically characterised by a restriction of both active and passive elevation/external rotation. Associated with previous trauma and diabetes. It arises due to thickening of the coracohumeral ligament and joint capsule.

MRI (WITH OR WITHOUT ARTHROGRAPHY)

- Thickened coracohumeral ligament
- Synovial/joint capsule thickening
- Obliteration of the fat triangle inferior to the coracoid

ALKAPTONURIA

A rare autosomal recessive enzyme defect (homogentisic acid oxidase) resulting in homogentisic acid deposition, particularly in the joints. This leads to joint degeneration and inflammation, known as 'ochronosis'. Ochronosis tends to affect large joints. It may also affect the eye and can cause urinary calculi, renal failure and cardiac failure.

SPINE X-RAY

- Marked calcification and loss of height of multiple intervertebral discs predominantly in the lumbar spine (then thoracic, then cervical)
- No syndesmophytes (unlike ankylosing spondylitis [AS])
- Intervertebral disc calcification

KNEE X-RAY

- Premature osteoarthritis
- Chondrocalcinoisis

AMYLOID ARTHROPATHY

Results from deposition of amyloid protein in the joints. Mostly it occurs secondary to end-stage renal failure and amyloid protein not being filtered by standard dialysis membranes (a primary type also exists). Classically stains with Congo red. Common clinical features are shoulder pain and carpal tunnel syndrome. Three patterns are described: amyloid arthropathy, diffuse marrow deposition and focal destructive lesion ('amyloidoma'—rare).

PLAIN FILM

- Multiple small lucencies in the medulla or bone cortex—may cause cortical destruction.
- Usually found in periarticular bone, often bilateral.
- Look for subtle cortical irregularity or foveal enlargement.

ULTRASOUND (US)

- Thickening of supraspinatus (>7 mm) or the biceps tendon (>4 mm) or cuff tears
- Joint/bursa effusion

MRI

- Bone lesions are low signal on T1 (variable T2 signal) and enhance following gadolinium.
- Thickened synovium of low signal on T2.
- Intrarticular nodules, which are low signal on T1 and T2, communicate with the subchondral bone lesions.

ANKYLOSING SPONDYLITIS

Box 2.2 COMMON CAUSES OF SACROILIITIS
Tends to affect the lower joint (i.e. the synovial portion)
Symmetrical
Anklyosing spondylitis   **I**nflammatory bowel disease   **R**heumatoid arthritis
Asymmetrical
Osteoarthritis   **P**soriasis/reactive arthritis   **S**eptic arthritis

This is the most common seronegative (i.e. rheumatoid factor-negative) spondyloarthropathy leading to progressive joint fusion. It is more common in males and has a predilection for the sacroiliac joints and spine. It is commonly associated with the *HLA-B27* gene.

SACROILIAC JOINT X-RAY

- First joint affected, typically bilateral and symmetrical
- Periarticular osteoporosis and joint widening initially
- Sclerosis as the disease progresses
- Complete joint fusion in late disease (Figure 2.1)

SPINE X-RAY

- Sclerosis at the edge of the discovertebral joints ('shiny corner') and erosion ('Romanus lesions') are early signs.
- Squared vertebral bodies (more obvious in the lumbar spine).
- Progressive growth of syndesmophytes (ossification of the outer fibres of the annulus fibrosus)—these eventually bridge the disc and cause ankylosis. As more bone forms, the spine develops a smooth, undulating contour 'bamboo spine'.
- Prominent thoracic kyphosis and limited lumbar lordosis.
- Erosion of the endplate.
- Facet joint ankyloses.
- Look for three-column fractures—the ankylosed spine is very susceptible to fracture.
- Signs: 'dagger' sign (ossification of the supraspinous and interspinous ligaments on frontal radiographs) and 'trolley track' (denotes three vertically orientated dense lines corresponding to ossified supraspinous and interspinous ligaments; Figure 2.2).

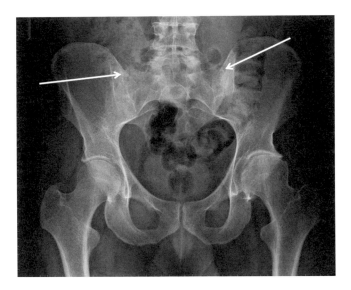

Figure 2.1 Ankylosing spondylitis. Pelvic x-ray demonstrating fusion of the sacroiliac (white arrows) joint.

MRI

- Useful to aid early diagnosis and monitor disease activity.
- Periarticular high signal at the sacroiliac joints on STIR (i.e. oedema), marrow/ sacroiliac (SI) joint enhancement with gadolinium.
- The hyperaemia and oedema at the anterior corners of the vertebral body cause high T2 signal—Romanus lesions (Figure 2.3).

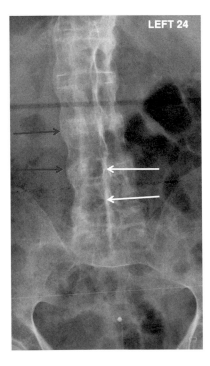

Figure 2.2 Ankylosing spondylitis. Frontal lumbar spine radiograph demonstrating the dagger sign (flowing ossification of the supraspinous and interspinous ligaments in a single dense line [white arrows]) and the trolley track sign (ossification of the apophyseal joints [red arrows] as well as the supraspinous and interspinous ligaments).

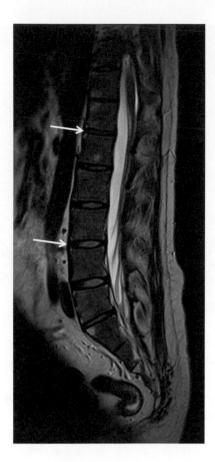

Figure 2.3 Ankylosing spondylitis. Sagittal T2-weighted magnetic resonance image demonstrating high T2 signal/oedema at the anterior corners of the vertebral body—Romanus lesions (white arrows).

● Look for fractures (low signal on T1, high signal on T2/STIR); these commonly occur horizontally through the intervertebral disc and may cause disc herniation and cord compression.

Box 2.3 SYNDESMOPHYTES VERSUS OSTEOPHYTES
1. Syndesmophytes have a vertical orientation
2. Osteophytes arise a few millimetres from the discovertebral junction
3. Osteophytes are triangular in shape
4. New bone formation in diffuse idiopathic skeletal hyperplasia arises from the anterior longitudinal ligament and is prolific

AVASCULAR NECROSIS (AVN)

Box 2.4 EPONYMOUS NAMES FOR AVASCULAR NECROSIS
Hip (Perthe disease)
Medial tibial condyle (Blount disease)
Metatarsal head (Freiberg infarction)
Lunate (Kienbock malacia)
Navicular (Köhler disease; Figure 2.4)
Capitellum (Panner disease)
Scaphoid (Preiser disease)
Vertebral body (Kummel disease)

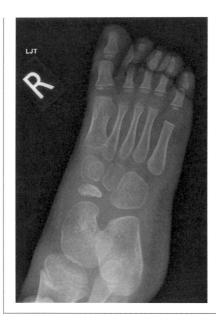

Figure 2.4 Köhler disease. Foot x-ray demonstrating sclerosis and flattening of the navicular in keeping with avascular necrosis (Köhler disease).

Interruption of blood supply causes the cell death of the bone constituents, mostly due to an arterial problem (it can also be due to venous insufficiency). It can affect any bone, but the hip is most commonly affected. It affects the epiphysis (if it affects the diaphysis or metaphysis, it is known as bone infarction). Causes include trauma, haematological conditions (systemic lupus erythematosus [SLE], Gaucher disease or sickle cell anaemia), Cushing syndrome, steroid use, alcoholism, pancreatitis, pregnancy, Caisson disease, etc. Patients taking steroids and transplant recipients are especially at risk.

PLAIN FILM (FIGURE 2.5)
- Focal radiolucencies
- Sclerosis
- Bone collapse
- Loss of joint space

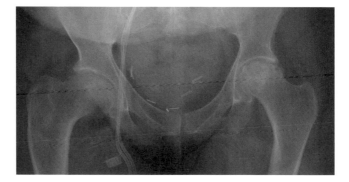

Figure 2.5 Avascular necrosis. Pelvic x-ray demonstrating bony sclerosis with irregularity and flattening of the left femoral head. Note the pelvic clips, anastomosis and femoral line in keeping with renal failure/transplant with steroids, therefore being the likely cause of the avascular necrosis.

MRI

- Most sensitive for diagnosis.
- Low signal on T1 and intermediate signal on T2 (reflects adipocyte death).
- Surrounding high signal on T2/STIR indicates oedema (suggesting an acute event).
- Oedema localises to the subchondral surface with increased severity, with an irregular rim of low T1 signal.
- 'Double line' sign (paired rims of low and high signal on T2 demonstrating the interface of viable/dying bone marrow).

BONE SCAN

- 80%–85% sensitive.
- Early disease is demonstrated by a focus of reduced tracer uptake.
- In late disease, there is a focus of reduced uptake surrounded by a ring of increased uptake ('doughnut sign') due to capillary revascularisation and bone synthesis.

BASILAR INVAGINATION

Occurs where the tip of the dens protrudes above the basion–opisthion line (the opening of the foramen magnum, also known as the McRae line). Commonly associated with rheumatoid arthritis (RA; 10% affected) and platybasia (flattening of the skull base, cranial basal angle >136°), as well as rickets, osteomalacia, osteogenesis imperfecta, Paget disease, fibrous dysplasia, Klippel–Feil syndrome and hyperparathyroidism.

CT

- Sagittal reformat shows tip of the dens <5 mm below the basion–opisthion line.

BAKER CYST

This is the most common cause of a mass in the popliteal fossa. It represents fluid from an over-filled bursa lying between the semimembranosus and the medial head of the gastrocnemius. Most commonly associated with osteoarthritis.

PLAIN FILM

- Soft tissue mass in the posteromedial compartment
- Small foci of calcification

US

- Anechoic collection communicating with the knee joint
- Posterior acoustic enhancement
- Loose bodies within the cyst
- No vascularity (unlike a popliteal artery aneurysm)

BONE INFARCT

Refers to infarction occurring in the diaphysis or metaphysis. Causes include steroid use, sickle cell disease, transplant recipient, trauma, Gaucher disease, etc. Infarction occurring in the epiphysis is known as AVN.

PLAIN FILM

- Typically metadiaphyseal
- Medullary calcification—a serpentine rim of dense sclerosis surrounding a central area calcified to varying degrees
- Sparing of the corticomedullary junction
- Mild remodelling of the bone

MRI

- Low signal on T1, high T2
- Margins enhance with contrast

BONE SCAN

Bone scans are highly sensitive and of variable specificity (like many nuclear medicine scans). The most common radiotracer is technetium-99m, which has a half-life of 6 hours. Images are often acquired 3 hours after injection (delayed phase) when tracer localises to the bone. However, imaging may be performed immediately (vascular phase) or after a few minutes (blood pool/tissue phase).

ABNORMAL BONE SCAN, NORMAL X-RAY

- Osteomyelitis
- Lymphoma
- Primary hyperparathyroidism
- Paget disease
- Metastases

NORMAL BONE SCAN, ABNORMAL X-RAY

- Metabolically inactive bone lesions (e.g. bone cysts, bone islands and exostosis)
- Recent fracture (<48 hours)
- Multiple myeloma
- Osteoporosis
- Metastases with no osteoblast activity

FOCI OF REDUCED TRACER UPTAKE (PHOTOPOENIA)

- Radiotherapy field
- Internal or external artefact (e.g. joint prosthesis)
- Avascular lesions
- Multiple myeloma
- Haemangioma
- Malignant fibrous histiocytoma (MFH)
- Advanced carcinoma

FOCI OF INCREASED TRACER UPTAKE

- Metastases
- Benign: joint disease, fracture (>48 hours)/post-operative, Paget disease, metabolic bone disease, fibrous dysplasia, brown tumour, aneurysmal bone cyst (ABC), osteoid osteoma, chondroblastoma, dental infection
- Physiological: artefact, soft tissue uptake

SUPERSCAN

- There is skeletal tracer uptake, but little or no tracer uptake in the soft tissues or urinary tract (i.e. absent kidneys).
- The most common cause is diffuse bone metastases (e.g. prostate, breast or lung).
- Metabolic bone disease also common (e.g. renal osteodystrophy; look for lack of radiotracer in the bladder—a classic appearance)
- Other causes: osteomalacia, hyperthyroidism, Paget disease, myeloproliferative disorders, myelofibrosis, lymphoma, mastocytosis, leukaemia

CALCIUM PYROPHOSPHATE DEPOSITION (CPPD)

This is widespread in the older population and is the most common crystalline arthropathy. It is caused by deposition of crystals in synovial fluid and cartilage and is associated with four clinical patterns: pyrophosphate arthopathy, pseudogout (the acute manifestation), rheumatoid-like and asymptomatic crystal deposition. Crystals show weak positive birefringence on polarised light microscopy.

PSEUDOGOUT

An acute synovitis arising from crystal release from the articular cartilage. The presentation mimics gout; the knee is most commonly affected. It may be precipitated by surgery, trauma, medical illnesses or joint injection.

PYROPHOSPHATE ARTHROPATHY
Plain film

- Mimics osteoarthritis—joint space narrowing, bone sclerosis, prominent subchondral cysts ('geodes').
- Tendency to affect non-weight-bearing joints (e.g. elbow, radiocarpal joint and patella–femoral compartment of the knee).
- Bilateral and symmetrical.
- Variable osteophyte formation and chondrocalcinosis.
- Joint destruction with subchrondral collapse, fragmentation and loose bodies (similar to a Charcot joint).

CARPAL TUNNEL SYNDROME

Most cases are idiopathic; also associated with diabetes, hypothyroidism, pregnancy, etc.

US

- Cross-sectional area of the median nerve >15 mm^2

MRI

- The most specific sign is an abrupt change in the diameter of the median nerve.
- Increased signal intensity of the median nerve on T2.
- Median nerve enhances with gadolinium.
- Compression and flattening of the median nerve.
- Volar bowing of the flexor retinaculum.
- Pseudoneuroma of the median nerve.

CHARCOT ARTHROPATHY (NEUROPATHIC JOINT)

Box 2.5 THE D'S OF A NEUROPATHIC (CHARCOT) JOINT
Destruction of the articular cartilage
Degeneration (joint space loss)
Debris (loose bodies)
Dislocation
Distension of the joint (i.e. effusion)
Density of bone normal for the patient

This is a destructive joint process arising from nerve damage, most commonly secondary to diabetes. The involvement of particular joints may indicate the underlying aetiology.

- Ankle/foot—diabetes
- Shoulder—syringomyelia
- Spine—spinal cord injury
- Knee—diabetes/syphilis

PLAIN FILM

- The D's (see Box 2.5).
- The presence of loose bodies and subchondral cysts favours a neuropathic joint over septic arthritis.

MRI

- Subchondral enhancement following gadolinium
- Non-specific bone marrow oedema

CHONDROMALACIA PATELLA

This typically occurs in adolescents and young adults. It is a common cause of anterior knee pain associated with trauma, chronic stress and patella instability. There is softening and oedema of the articular cartilage (grade I); this may progress to fissure/fragmentation <1.3 cm diameter (grade II), fissure/fragmentation >1.3 cm (grade III) and full-thickness cartilage loss (grade IV). May heal or progress to osteoarthritis.

PLAIN FILM

- Insensitive, shows non-specific loss of joint space.

MRI

- Axial T2-weighted/intermediate-weighted imaging with fat suppression.
- Thinning of the cartilage in the patella–femoral joint.
- Joint fluid extends to the bone with full-thickness cartilage defects.
- Look for bone oedema and subchondral cystic change.

CYSTICERCOSIS

Due to *Taenia solium*, a tapeworm found in pork. It can affect any organ, most commonly the brain, eye and muscle.

PLAIN FILM

- Characteristic multiple rice-like calcifications aligned in the direction of the muscle fibres

DERMATOMYOSITIS

This is an idiopathic inflammatory myopathy with deposition of complement or inflammatory infiltrate in the skeletal muscle and subcutaneous tissue. It affects children and adults. It is associated with malignant neoplasms in up to 25%, particularly genitourinary, gynaecological, oesophageal, lung and melanoma. There is also an increased risk of venous thromboembolism and myocardial infarction.

PLAIN FILM (FIGURE 2.6)

- Non-specific subcutaneous calcification.
- Sheet-like calcifications along fascial or muscle planes of the proximal large muscles are less common; however, these are pathognomonic.

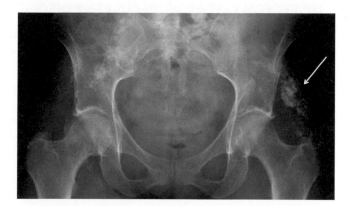

Figure 2.6 Dermatomyositis. Pelvic x-ray demonstrating sheet-like calcification along muscular/fascial planes, particularly above the left hip (white arrow).

HIGH-RESOLUTION CT (HRCT)

- 67% have interstitial lung disease.
- Most commonly there is subpleural consolidation (bronchiolitis obliterans organising pneumonia [BOOP]).
- BOOP may progress to subpleural honeycombing and usual interstitial pneumonia.
- Bronchiolitis ('tree in bud'), ill-defined airspace opacification suggests chronic aspiration pneumonia.

MRI

- Muscle oedema early, followed by calcification and atrophy.
- High T2 signal intensity seen in the muscles suggests oedema, enhancement seen on T1 post-contrast.
- Fatty infiltration late in the disease (high signal on T1 and T2).

DIFFUSE IDIOPATHIC SKELETAL HYPERPLASIA

This is an ankylosing disorder of the spine. Symptoms are mild, consisting of restricted motion and tendinitis from enthesopathy.

X-RAY SPINE/CT

- Undulating soft tissue calcification and hyperostosis along the anterolateral aspect of the spine ('dripping candle wax').
- For diagnosis: affects four or more adjacent vertebrae; intervertebral disc height is preserved; the sacroiliac joints and apophyseal joints (spine) are spared.

OTHER X-RAYS

- 'Whiskering' of the iliac crest (fluffy calcification representing enthesopathy); may also affect the calcaneum (spurs) and olecranon.
- Ossification of the iliolumbar, sacroiliac and sacrotuberous ligaments and patella tendon.
- Soft tissue calcification adjacent to the lateral epicondyle (tennis elbow).

DISCECTOMY (SCAR VS. RECURRENT DISC)

In patients with continued back pain post-discectomy/laminectomy, the cause may be either post-operative epidural fibrosis (i.e. scar tissue) or recurrent disc herniation.

MRI

- Pre- and post-contrast T1 imaging
- Scar: epidural soft tissue at the site of surgery, irregular borders, early homogeneous enhancement and thecal retraction towards the soft tissue mass
- Disc: smooth borders and no central enhancement/delayed enhancement

DISCITIS

Involvement of two vertebrae and the intervertebral disc (i.e. one spinal segment) is nearly pathognomic of spondylodiscitis. Infection begins by haematogenous seeding or direct spread post-trauma/surgery/adjacent sepsis. A total of 85% of infections are in the lumbar and thoracic regions; up to 90% are due to *Staphylococcus aureus*. Back pain of gradual onset is the most common presenting feature (Figure 2.7).

MRI

- T1 (pre- and post-contrast), fat-saturated T2 or STIR sequences are most useful.
- Hypointense vertebral body signal on T1.
- Loss of endplate definition.
- Increased disc signal intensity on T2.
- Contrast enhancement of the disc and endplates.
- Enhancement of the epidural and paraspinal tissues.
- Homogeneous enhancement suggests phlegmon, ring enhancement favours abscess.
- Scoliosis/kyphosis as vertebral collapse ensues.
- Prominent bone sclerosis.
- Skip lesions and multiple levels (>3) suggest tuberculous discitis.

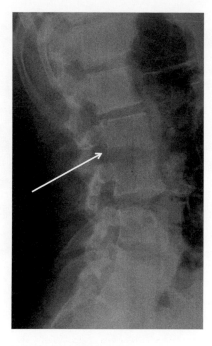

Figure 2.7 Discitis. Lateral lumbar spine x-ray demonstrating disc space narrowing and endplate destruction/loss of definition at L3/4 (white arrow).

X-RAY (FIGURE 2.7)

- Disc space narrowing
- Endplate irregularity/definition
- Paraspinal calcification suggests a tuberculosis (TB) spondylodiscitis

DRILLER WRIST

Vibratory arthropathy due to recurrent use of vibrating tools. Presents with Raynaud syndrome with or without bone changes. Bone changes are thought to be due to microfractures filling with synovial fluid to form cysts.

PLAIN FILM

- Mild cystic change in the carpal bones (occasionally other areas)
- Carpal bone fragmentation with continued exposure to vibration

EROSIVE OSTEOARTHRITIS

Also known as inflammatory osteoarthritis, this is a variant of osteoarthritis characteristically involving the interphalangeal joints of the hand.

PLAIN FILM (FIGURE 2.8)

- Interphalangeal joint space loss.
- Prominent marginal osteophytes.
- Central erosions give a 'gullwing' appearance.
- Proliferative synovitis may cause ankyloses.

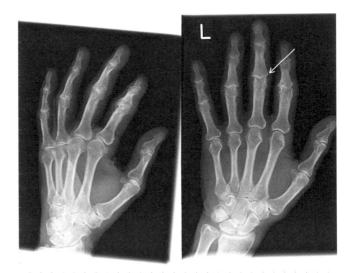

Figure 2.8 Erosive osteoarthritis. X-ray of the left hand demonstrating an arthropathy of the interphalangeal joints with joint space loss and central erosions ('gullwing' appearance [white arrow]).

FEMOROACETABULAR IMPINGEMENT (FAI)

Caused by abnormal hip morphology leading to repetitive contact of the femoral neck with the acetabular rim. This damages acetabular cartilage and eventually leads to labral tears, hip pain and early osteoarthritis. There is a 'cam' type and a 'pincer' type.

CAM FAI

Cam lesions are more common in active young men and are due to a non-spherical part of the femoral head impacting against the acetabular rim. Presents as chronic groin pain that is worse during exercise; clicking/locking suggests a labral tear.

Plain film
- Flattening of the femoral head–neck junction ('pistol grip' deformity)
- Osseous bump (either lateral or anterosuperior)
- Degenerative change

MRI
- Arthrography is preferred when labral tears are suspected, femoral neck is best assessed with axial oblique (angled along the axis of the femoral neck) and sagittal reformats.
- Classic triad: abnormal α angle ($>65°$), anterior–superior acetabular cartilage lesion and anterior superior labral tear.

PINCER FAI

Pincer lesions are more common in middle-aged active women and are due to abnormal contact between the femoral head–neck junction and an overhanging acetabulum.

Plain film
- Abnormally deep acetabulum
- Normal proximal femur

MRI
- Circumferential pattern of chondral injury

FONG DISEASE

Also known as nail patella syndrome, it is inherited in an autosomal dominant pattern. Associated with muscular hypoplasia, renal abnormalities and hypertension.

PLAIN FILM (FIGURE 2.9)

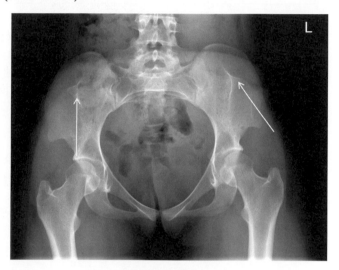

Figure 2.9 Fong disease. Pelvis x-ray demonstrating bilateral posterior iliac horns, pathognomonic for Fong disease (white arrows).

- Posterior iliac horns are pathognomonic
- Hypoplastic patella
- Scoliosis
- Large parietal foramina of the skull
- Hypoplastic radial head
- 11 rib pairs
- Madelung deformity

FREIBERG INFARCTION

AVN affecting the metatarsal heads, more common in females between the ages of 10 and 18 years.

PLAIN FILM
- Second metatarsal head most commonly affected (third or fourth also).
- Initial flattening and cystic lesions in the metatarsal head with widening of the metatarsophalangeal joint.

- Sclerosis and cortical thickening are late features.
- Osteochondral fragment.

GAUCHER DISEASE

Box 2.6 CAUSES OF AN ERLENMEYER FLASK DEFORMITY
Lead poisoning **G**aucher disease **N**iemann–Pick disease **O**steopetrosis **M**etaphyseal dysplasia (Pyle disease) '**E**ematological' (i.e. haematological causes—thalassaemia major [first 2 years of life])

Rare autosomal recessive disorder due to accumulation of glycolipids in the bone marrow, liver, spleen and lungs. More common amongst Ashkenazi Jews. The non-neuropathic form is most common and is associated with prominent skeletal abnormalities. Patients may be asymptomatic or present with anaemia, splenomegaly, large joint stiffness and bone pain.

PLAIN FILM (FIGURE 2.10)

- Modelling abnormalities (e.g. Erlenmeyer flask deformity), typically of the distal femur or proximal tibia, due to marrow infiltration during bone growth.
- Osteopenia.
- Osteonecrosis (AVN/bone infarct)—the combination of osteonecrosis and an Erlenmeyer flask deformity is pathognomic.

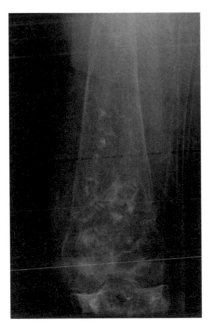

Figure 2.10 Gaucher disease. Femur x-ray demonstrating osteopenia, bone infarcts and Erlenmeyer flask deformity pathognomic for Gaucher disease. Also note the distal femoral fracture.

GOUT

Box 2.7 STAGES OF GOUT
1. Asymptomatic hyperuricaemia
2. Acute gouty arthritis
3. Intercritical gout
4. Chronic gout

More common in men aged 30–60 years. Dysfunction in urate metabolism leads to an accumulation of urate in the tissues, where it crystallises. Monosodium urate crystals are negatively birefringent on polarised light microscopy. A total of 40% of patients with gout also have concomitant CPPD.

US

- Joint effusion with debris (crystals)—first metatarsophalangeal joint is classic (also ankle, knee, elbow and hands).
- 'Double contour' sign—hyperechoic line (crystal infiltration) lying on the hypoechoic cartilage.
- Synovitis.
- Bone erosions (often next to tophi) in chronic disease.

PLAIN FILM (FIGURE 2.11)

- 45% have radiological features, not seen until 6–12 years after the initial attack.
- The distribution is asymmetrical and polyarticular.

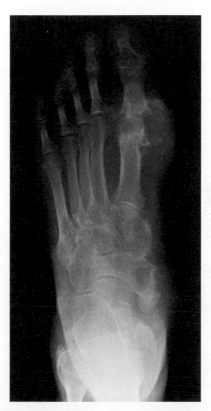

Figure 2.11 Gout. Foot x-ray demonstrating juxta-articular erosions affecting the first MTP joint with overhanging edges, preservation of bone density and marked surrounding soft tissue swelling and increased density/calcification in keeping with tophi.

- Look for soft tissue masses, preservation of joint space and bone density.
- Effusion is the earliest sign.
- Erosions are 'punched out', intra-articular/peri-articular, sclerotic and overhanging edges, often at the bases of the metacarpals.
- Chondrocalcinosis (5%).

MRI

- Tophi are low signal on T1 and heterogeneous signal on T2.
- Tophi may enhance.
- Bone oedema adjacent to erosions.

HAGLUND SYNDROME

This is a common cause of heel pain that is characterised by a calcaneal deformity (Haglund deformity), retrocalcaneal and superficial calcaneal bursitis and Achilles tendinitis.

PLAIN FILM

- Lateral calcaneal view shows a bump on the posterosuperior aspect of the calcaneus (Haglund deformity).

MRI

- Sagittal T1 may show the calcaneal bump.
- T2 hyperintensity in the retrocalcaneal/retroachilles bursae.

HAEMOCHROMATOSIS

Box 2.8 CAUSES OF CHONDROCALCINOSIS
5 H's + A + C **H**yperparathyroidism **H**ypothyroidism **H**aemochromatosis **H**ypomagnesaemia **H**aemosiderosis **A**lkaptonuria **C**alcium pyrophosphate deposition

Due to excess iron deposition in the tissues, either primary (autosomal recessive) or secondary to ineffective erythropoiesis (myelofibrosis), ineffective absorption or iron overload. The brain, heart (heart failure is the leading cause of death), liver (increased risk of hepatoma) and pancreas are also affected.

PLAIN FILM

- Osteoporosis (proportional to the extent of iron deposition)
- Small subchondral cysts in the metacarpal heads
- Enlargement and flattening of the metacarpal heads
- Joint space narrowing

- Chrondrocalcinosis (60%)
- Characteristic hooked osteophytes (differentiates from pseudogout) on the radial aspect of the metacarpal heads, index and middle fingers especially

MRI

- Bone marrow is low signal on T1- and T2-weighted imaging.

HIP PROSTHESIS LOOSENING

PLAIN FILM/CT

- Radiography only for surveillance, CT for further assessment.
- 1–2-mm lucent line at the cement interface, periosteal reaction and sclerosis are normal findings.
- Definite loosening is implied by lucency >3 mm.
- Check for migration of components and new malalignment.

HYPERTROPHIC OSTEOARTHOPATHY (HOA)

Box 2.9 CAUSES OF TIBIAL PERIOSTITIS
Bilateral Hypertrophic osteoarthopathy Venous stasis Pachydermoperiositis
Unilateral Trauma

This is a painful syndrome of proliferative periostitis of the long bones, arthritis and digital clubbing of the fingers and toes. In total, 90% of cases are associated with malignancy (mostly lung); other causes include cystic fibrosis, chronic pneumonia, pleural fibroma, congenital heart disease, inflammatory bowel disease, cirrhosis, etc.

PACHYDERMOPERIOSTOSIS

This is an autosomal dominant primary form of HOA. It causes a thick, symmetrical periostitis of the distal long bones, typically in young men, which arrests in adulthood. It is painless.

Plain film (Figure 2.12)

- Symmetrical smooth lamellar periosteal reaction affecting the diametaphyseal regions of the long bones, particularly the dorsal and medial aspects.

Bone scan

- 'Parallel track' sign, increased tracer uptake along the cortical margins of the metaphysis and diaphysis of the affected bones

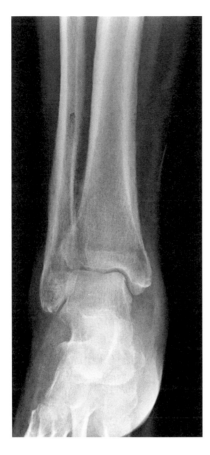

Figure 2.12 Hypertrophic osteoarthropathy (HOA). Ankle x ray demonstrating a lamellar solid periosteal reaction of the tibia and fibula.

HYPERPARATHYROIDISM

Box 2.10 CAUSES OF DIFFUSE OSTEOSCLEROSIS
• Metastases
• Mastocytosis
• Tuberous sclerosis
• Myelofibrosis
• Renal osteodystrophy
• Fluorosis
• Osteopetrosis

Causes are primary (parathyroid tumour), secondary (most commonly renal failure) or tertiary (autonomous hypersecretion of parathyroid hormone [PTH] from longstanding secondary disease). The presence of increased PTH results in increased osteoclast action, bone resorption, increased plasma calcium and thence increased bone formation.

PLAIN FILM
- Osteopenia is the hallmark (may include sacroiliac joints, symphysis pubis and distal clavicles).
- Chrondrocalcinosis.
- Soft tissue calcification including visceral, muscular, etc.

- Vertebral osteosclerosis may cause a 'rugger jersey' spine appearance where endplate sclerosis alternates with osteopenia—this is characteristic of secondary hyperparathyroidism due to renal failure (i.e. renal osteodystrophy).
- Bone softening: basilar invagination, vertebral collapse.
- Brown tumours are seen in primary hyperparathyroidism—these are lytic, expansile lesions that mimic metastases or myeloma, typically in the mandible, ribs or pelvis.
- Osteitis fibrosa cystica was a term historically used to describe advanced skeletal disease in primary hyperparathyroidism.

HAND X-RAY

- Subperiosteal erosion along the radial aspect of the phalanges of the middle and index fingers

IDIOPATHIC TUMOURAL CALCINOSIS

Rare disease due to a hereditary dysfunction of phosphate metabolism. The end result is prominent periarticular calcified masses, especially around large joints. The masses are painless and occur most frequently in children and adolescents of African descent.

PLAIN FILM

- Densely calcified, amorphous, loculated and lobulated peri-articular masses.
- Most commonly around the extensor surface of the shoulders, hips and elbows.
- Masses are extra-articular and so do not usually affect joint movement (unless very large).
- Initially, however, only faint calcification may be seen within the multiloculated lesions.
- A periosteal reaction may be present due to bone marrow involvement.

IMPACTION SYNDROMES

Ulnar-sided wrist pain caused by a spectrum of conditions: ulnar impaction syndrome, ulnar impingement syndrome, ulnocarpal impaction syndrome (secondary to non-union of the ulnar styloid process), ulnar styloid impaction syndrome and hamatolunate impingement syndrome.

ULNAR IMPACTION SYNDROME (MOST COMMON)

This is a degenerative condition secondary to excessive loading across the wrist. There is characteristically positive ulnar variance, accentuated in pronation and during firm grip.

MRI

- Used to identify complications (e.g. triangular fibrocartilage complex tear or bone marrow oedema)

IRON-DEFICIENCY ANAEMIA

Occurs where there is insufficient iron to support erythropoiesis.

PLAIN FILM

- Widening of diploe
- Hair-on-end appearance of the skull
- Osteoporosis in long bones
- Absence of facial bone involvement

KIENBOCK MALACIA

AVN of the lunate with associated negative ulnar variance. More common in the dominant hand and 20–40-year age group.

PLAIN FILM

- Lunate sclerosis
- Ulnar ≥ 2 mm shorter than the radius (negative variance)

MRI

- Low T1 signal, high T2 signal (marrow oedema in early disease)

MADELUNG DEFORMITY

A Madelung deformity is a non-specific dysplasia of the radius. Causes are idiopathic, post-traumatic, dysplastic (e.g. osteochondromatosis) and genetic (e.g. Turner syndrome). Other associated syndromes include nail patella syndrome, Ollier disease, epiphyseal dysplasias and dyschondrosteosis.

PLAIN FILM

- Lateral and dorsal radial curvature
- Short radius with a triangularised distal epiphysis
- Articular surface of the distal radius angled in an ulnar and volar direction
- Dorsal dislocation of the ulnar head
- 'V'-shaped proximal carpal row, 'carpal wedging'

MELORHEOSTOSIS

Rare, spontaneous mesodermal disease of unknown aetiology, often asymptomatic initially. It follows a slow course in adults and a more rapid course in children. It mostly affects one or more long bones of the upper or lower limbs, may be in a dermatome distribution and may cause thickening/fibrosis of the overlying skin.

PLAIN FILM

- Progressive cortical hyperostosis along one side of the affected bone in a 'sclerotome' (skeletal zones supplied by individual spinal sensory nerves).
- The appearance is of dripping candle wax, centred on the diaphysis.
- Can cross joints, leading to flexion contractures or fusion.
- Look for genu varus, genu valgus and leg length discrepancy.

MILWAUKEE SHOULDER

This predominantly affects elderly women and consists of a triad of a rotator cuff tear, osteoarthritis and joint effusion containing crystals (calcium hydroxyapatite and calcium pyrophosphate dehydrate). It results in a dysfunctional shoulder from the rotator cuff injury, is often bilateral (dominant side always involved) and may also affect the knee.

PLAIN FILM

- Superior subluxation of the humerus due to complete cuff tear.
- Osteoarthritis (loss of joint space, subchondral cysts and sclerosis).
- Loose bodies in the joint.
- Look for changes in the lateral compartment when the knee is affected.

MODIC ENDPLATE CHANGES

These are signal changes seen in the endplates and subchondral bone of the vertebral bodies in the context of degenerative disease. They may be associated with lower back pain. The pathogenesis is thought to be partly biomechanical and biochemical. The lumbar spine is more commonly affected (especially L4–5 and L5–S1). Type II is the most common type; type I is more symptomatic. Antibiotics may have a role in treating Modic I change (Table 2.1).

Table 2.1 Gross pathology and magnetic resonance imaging (MRI) characteristics of Modic change

Modic type	Pathology	MRI
I	Fluid	T1 low
		T2 high
II	Fat (due to red marrow replacement)	T1 high
		T2 high
III	Sclerosis	T1 low
		T2 low

MORTON NEUROMA

This is a benign lesion consisting of perineural fibrosis that entraps a plantar digital nerve; 80% of those affected are women. There is a strong predilection for the third common digital nerve. It presents with foot pain exacerbated by walking.

US

- Hypoechoic, rounded lesion found between the metatarsals.
- Larger in the axial than sagittal plane.
- Treated effectively with a steroid/local anaesthetic injection in 75% at 1 week's follow-up.

MRI

- Intermediate T1 signal (i.e. isointense to muscle) with enhancement post-gadolinium.

- Low T2 signal.
- It is often associated with metatarsal bursitis, which is high signal on STIR.

MAGNETIC RESONANCE IMAGING

GENERAL RULES

- STIR sequences are the best for evaluating for bone oedema/bruising and occult fractures.
- T2 or proton density fat-saturated sequences to investigate cartilage thickness.
- T1 post-contrast to assess the synovium and synovial inflammation.
- High signal on T2:
  – Osteoporotic vertebral collapse
  – Radiotherapy change
  – Haemangiomas
  – Type 1 and 2 Modic changes
  – Lytic metastases
- Isointense signal on T2:
  – Lymphoma
  – Gaucher disease
- Low signal on T2:
  – Sclerotic metastases
  – Myeloma after treatment
- Low signal on T1:
  – Lytic metastases
  – Sclerotic metastases

HIP

- Dilute solution of 0.2 mmol/L gadopentetate dimeglumine for direct arthrography.
- Normal labrum is low signal on T1.
- 10%–15% have a communication between the joint capsule and the iliopsoas bursa.

WRIST

- Best sequence for imaging tears is T2 or T2* in coronal plane.
- The coronal plane is angled parallel to the volar surface of the radius.
- Magnetic resonance arthrography of the wrist performed with a gradient echo in coronal plane.

KNEE

- Sagittal images are obtained at an angle of 10° anteromedially to a line drawn perpendicular to a line drawn through the posterior femoral condyles.
- Normal findings:
  – Bowing of the posterior cruciate ligament (PCL) on sagittal imaging (knee extended)
  – Low signal anterior cruciate ligament (ACL) on T1
  – Low signal menisci on T1 and T2
  – Medial patellar plica

SHOULDER

- Axial, coronal, sagittal oblique fat-suppressed T1 and axial oblique T1.
- Labrum is low signal on T1.
- Abduction, external rotation position preferred for assessing the anterior–inferior labrum, where most tears occur.

MYELOID HYPERPLASIA (RED MARROW RECONVERSION)

Box 2.11 NORMAL BONE MARROW CONVERSION
At birth, red (haematopoietic) marrow is present throughout the entire skeleton. Conversion of red to yellow (fatty) marrow occurs over a period of about 20 years, beginning distally in the hands and feet and migrating proximally until red marrow remains only in the: - Axial skeleton - Skull - Vertebral column - Thoracic cage - Pelvic girdle - Humeral and femoral metaphyses Normal haematopoietic bone marrow may appear similar to malignant infiltration—location is a major discriminator.

Myeloid hyperplasia is the repopulation of yellow (fatty) marrow with red marrow (haematopoietic cells). It occurs when the haematopoietic capacity of the existing red marrow in an adult is insufficient. This could be due to an increased physiological requirement (e.g. long-distance running), chronic anaemia (e.g. sickle cell disease) or treatment with chemotherapy containing granulocyte-macrophage colony-stimulating factor.

MRI

- Yellow marrow is high signal on T1, mildly hyperintense on T2.
- Red marrow is mildly T1, T2 and STIR hyperintense.
- Features suggesting malignant marrow infiltration: random distribution, enhancement with gadolinium, destruction of the bone cortex or a soft tissue mass.
- Haemochromatosis and Gaucher disease may cause bone marrow to be low signal on both T1 and T2.

MYOSITIS OSSIFICANS

Also known as heterotopic ossification, this is a benign, self-limiting inflammatory process characterised by mixed bone (mature lamellar bone)/cartilaginous masses within skeletal muscle. There are three forms: traumatic (75%, any injury leading to severe rhabdomyolysis), neurogenic (brain injuries, cord trauma, etc.) and congenital (myositis ossificans progressiva). New bone is surrounded by fibrotic connective tissue. Masses are painful.

PLAIN FILM

- Soft tissue swelling initially.
- Floccular calcification begins to form after about 3 weeks.
- Lamellar bone begins to form after 6–8 weeks.
- Mature lesions may show a dense periphery (bone cortex) with a more lucent centre (medulla).
- Difficult to distinguish from malignancy (e.g. parosteal osteosarcoma, tends to have dense calcification centrally).

CT

- More sensitive than plain films

OSTEITIS CONDENSANS ILII

Benign condition mostly seen after pregnancy in young women; presents with back pain persistent after delivery. May also occur in nulliparous women and men.

PLAIN FILM

- Bilateral, symmetrical, triangular-shaped subchondral sclerosis.
- Found at the inferior aspect of the iliac side of the sacroliliac joint.
- Joint space normal.
- Joint margin well defined.

OSTEOMALACIA

Due to a failure of bone mineralisation (osteomalacia means bone softening). The most common causes are dietary vitamin D deficiency and renal osteodystrophy, less commonly gastrointestinal/chronic liver disease, phosphate deficiency, biliary disease, etc.

Box 2.12 LOOSER ZONES
• Classically seen in osteomalacia.   • Other causes include osteogenesis imperfecta, Paget disease and fibrous dysplasia.

PLAIN FILM

- Diffusely reduced bone density suggests osteopenia.
- 'Cortical tunnelling' are foci of cortical lucency due to accumulation of osteoid in the cortex.
- Coarsened, fuzzy and fewer trabeculae.
- Deformities—bowing, protrusion, basilar invagination.
- Bilateral vertebral endplate collapse giving a 'fish' appearance to the disc space.
- 'Looser zones' are small lucent lines with sclerotic margins—they represent insufficiency fractures healing with un-mineralised osteoid.
  - Bilateral, symmetrical and do not extend across the whole bone.
- Typical sites for looser zones: medial femora, pubic rami, ribs, lateral borders of the scapulae, distal third of the radius, proximal third of the ulna, lesser trochanter and clavicle.

OSTEOMYELITIS

Underlying pathogen varies with age (e.g. *S. aureus*, *Streptococcus pneumoniae* and *Haemophilus influenzae* in the elderly) and other disease (e.g. *Salmonella* and *S. aureus* in patients with sickle cell disease).

PLAIN FILM
- Acute: soft tissue swelling, focal bone lucency and periostitis (periostium lifts in paediatric patients).
- The location of disease in the bone depends on patient age (i.e. area with richest blood supply): multifocal in neonates; epiphysis in infants/adults; metaphysis in children from ages 1 to 16 years.
- The following are seen in chronic infection:
  - Sequestrum: A focus of necrotic bone that is separated from living bone by granulation tissue.
  - Involucrum: A layer of living bone that forms around the necrotic bone focus.
  - Cloaca: An opening into the involucrum through which exudate may escape.
  - Sinus tracts may be seen leading to the skin surface.
- Cortical thickening and focal cortical lysis may also occur with chronic infection.

MRI
- Most sensitive and most useful for surgical planning.
- First sign is loss of normal marrow signal on T1 and T2/STIR hyperintensity.
- Sequestrum is low signal on T1/STIR, surrounding granulation tissue enhances with contrast.
- Look for tram track enhancement of a sinus tract and rim enhancement with an abscess.

BONE SCAN
- Three- and four-phase bone scans are used to assess infection (overall sensitivity 88%, specificity 36%)

OSTEOPATHIA STRIATA

Also known as Voorhoeve disease, it is rare and usually asymptomatic.

PLAIN FILM
- Fine, dense linear striations ('celery stalk') typically found in the metaphysis or diaphysis of the long bones
- Typically bilateral

OSTEOPOIKILOSIS

Rare, asymptomatic and inherited (autosomal dominant) or sporadic. A total of 25% have dermatofibrosis lenticularis dissemina (cutaneous lesions).

PLAIN FILM
- 'Spotted bone disease'
- 2–10-mm rounded densities similar to cortical bone throughout cancellous bone
- Diffuse symmetrical pattern

OSTEOPOROSIS

Defined as a bone mineral density ('T-score') >2.5 standard deviations below the young adult reference mean. Assessed with a dual-energy x-ray absorptiometry scan. T-score predicts the risk of fracture—osteoporotic wedge fractures double the risk of a subsequent femoral neck fracture, and there is five-fold greater risk of a further vertebral fracture.

PAGET DISEASE

Box 2.13 CAUSES OF AN IVORY VERTEBRA

Increase in opacity of a vertebral body whilst retaining size and contours.
- Osteoblastic metastases with sclerotic response
- Sclerotic osteosarcoma
- Paget disease
- Lymphoma
- Tuberculosis

Also known as 'osteitis deformans', this is a common disorder of osteoclasts and osteoblasts that results in disordered and excessive bone remodelling. Bone marrow is replaced by fibrous tissue with vascular channels. A total of 10% of Paget disease cases are seen in those aged >80 years. The spine and pelvis (75%) and skull (up to 65%) are most commonly affected.

The stages of disease are the active osteolysis (osteoclasts dominate), mixed active phase (osteoclastic and blastic action) and late inactive phase (osteoblasts dominate).

Box 2.14 COMPLICATIONS OF PAGET DISEASE

1. *Malignant transformation*
   a. Sarcoma
   b. Multicentric giant cell tumour
   c. Lymphoma
2. *Insufficiency fractures*
   a. Typically on convex side of a long bone, 'banana fracture' (e.g. tibia and femur)
3. *Nerve entrapment*
   a. Basilar impression compressing brainstem
   b. Spinal stenosis
4. *Early-onset arthritis*

PLAIN FILM (FIGURE 2.13)
- Typically polyostotic and asymmetrical pattern.
- Flame/grass-shaped metadiaphyseal lucencies in active phase—large lucencies may appear in the skull, known as 'osteoporosis circumscripta'.

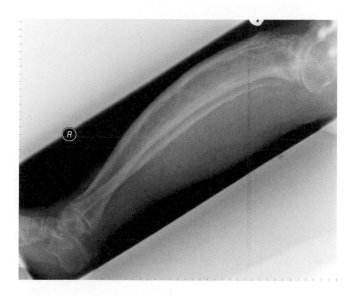

Figure 2.13 Paget disease. Lateral tibia x-ray demonstrating a sabre tibia with cortical thickening, coarsening of the trabeculae and bowing of the tibia.

- Key features of inactive disease are bone expansion, thickening of the cortex and coarsening of the trabecular pattern.
- Cotton wool sclerosis in the skull.

SPINE X-RAY
- Picture frame appearance (due to cortical thickening)
- Ivory vertebra
- Coarsening of the vertical trabeculations

BONE SCAN
- 90% sensitive.
- Typically, there is markedly increased uptake in the bone lesion in all phases of disease, particularly during active disease.
- Uptake at the margins is seen with osteoporosis circumscripta.
- Decreased uptake of technetium-99m sulphur colloid by bone marrow.

MRI
- Appearance varies according to disease phase.
- Chronic Pagetic bone has similar signal characteristics to fat.

PANNER DISEASE

This is AVN of the capitellum ('little leaguer's elbow') and is more common in athletic boys aged 5–10 years. Thought to be due to microtrauma.

PLAIN FILM
- Radiolucent band may appear at the capitellum, similar to hip osteonecrosis.
- Irregular contour.

- Increased density.
- Widening of the radiohumeral space.

MRI
- Low signal on T1, high signal on T2.
- No loose body (otherwise osteochondritis dissecans should be considered)

PATELLA BAJA

Meaning 'low patella', associated with previous trauma, polio, juvenile chronic arthritis and achondroplasia.

PLAIN FILM
- Insall–Salvati ratio (tendon length/patella length): measured on lateral film (or sagittal reformat), ideally with the knee at 30° of flexion; ratio <0.74 indicates 'baja' and >1.5 represents 'alta'.

PIGMENTED VILLONODULAR SYNOVITIS (PVNS)

This is a benign, proliferative disorder of the synovium and is more common between ages 20 and 40 years. Onset is insidious; 50% have a history of trauma. Presentation is typically increasing stiffness and soft tissue swelling affecting a single joint; the knee is most commonly affected (80%). In the hands and feet, it is known as a giant cell tumour (GCT).

PLAIN FILM
- Early—soft tissue swelling and effusion.
- Soft tissues appear dense due to haemosiderin deposits.
- Multiple sites of cystic radiolucencies/articular erosions due to bone invasion.
- Scalloping of pre-femoral fat pad.
- Soft tissue mass around the joint (if there is calcification, PVNS is excluded).
- Bone density is preserved.
- Preservation of joint space.

MRI
- Large lobular intra-articular mass, low signal on both T1 and T2 (due to haemosidcrin).
- Haemorrhage is relatively common and causes blooming artefact on gradient echo.
- Low signal effusion on all sequences is characteristic.
- Other joint lesions low on T1 and T2: haemophilia, synovial haemangioma and neuropathic osteoarthritis.

Box 2.15 PIGMENTED VILLONODULAR SYNOVITIS CHARACTERISTICS
• Low T2 signal mass + no calcification/ossification or gas in the mass on x-ray

POST-ARTHROGRAPHY PAIN

Direct contrast-enhanced MRI arthrography is useful for evaluating labral tears, cuff tears, loose bodies and cartilage defects. Imaging is performed after an injection of contrast medium into the joint.

- Pain is the most common complication, which begins at 4 hours and peaks by 12 hours, due to a chemical synovitis.
- Other complications: infection, vasovagal reaction and contrast reaction.

POTT DISEASE

The eponym for tuberculous spondylitis with vertebral collapse, this is a destructive process more commonly affecting multiple levels of lower thoracic/upper lumbar vertebrae (L1 most common). It occurs in <1% of patients with TB. Patterns of spinal TB infection include spondylodiscitis (centred on the disc) and spondylitis (Pott disease), where the disc is spared until later.

PLAIN FILM

- Loss of endplate margins.
- Anterior scalloping of the vertebral bodies by paravertebral (Pott) abscess—if this contains calcification, it is almost pathognomic.
- Wedge vertebral collapse, focal kyphosis and gibbus.
- Ivory vertebra.

MRI

- Most sensitive—infection starts at the anterior corner of the vertebral body and spreads under the anterior longitudinal ligament (disc spared until later).
- Anterior vertebral bodies scalloped ('gouge defect').
- Wedge vertebral collapse.
- Subligamentous, rim-enhancing abscess.

PSORIATIC ARTHRITIS

Box 2.16 FEATURES DIFFERENTIATING PSORIATIC ARTHRITIS FROM RHEUMATOID ARTHRITIS
• Periosteal reaction (periostitis)   • Preservation of bone density (juxta-articular osteopenia is seen in rheumatoid)   • New bone formation   • Enthesopathy   • Parasyndesmophytes   • Periarticular erosions are seen in rheumatoid

About 20% of those with psoriasis develop psoriatic arthropathy; the onset of arthritis often precedes the skin rash. Types of psoriatic arthritis include true psoriatic, rheumatoid-like, concomitant rheumatoid and psoriatic type. The overall distribution is variable and asymmetrical.

HAND X-RAY (FIGURE 2.14)

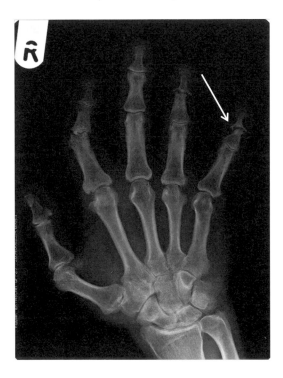

Figure 2.14 Psoriatic arthritis. Right hand x-ray demonstrating marginal erosions affecting the interphalangeal joints, with a 'pencil in a cup' deformity (white arrow), and preservation of bone density.

- Interphalangeal joints typically involved
- Marginal erosions, which may progress to a 'pencil in cup' deformity
- Soft tissue swelling, 'sausage digit'
- Resorption of the terminal phalangeal tufts (acro-osteolysis)
- Ivory phalynx
- Periosteal reaction (periostitis)

SPINE X-RAY

- Squaring of the vertebrae
- Atlantoaxial subluxation
- Joint space loss and ankylosis
- Preservation of bone density and new bone formation
- Enthesopathy (e.g. parasyndesmophytes—asymmetrical/unilateral paravertebral ossification with sparing of the annulus fibrosus)

MRI

- Bone marrow oedema can involve the whole vertebral body—distinguishing feature.
- Bilateral sacroiliitis in up to 40%.

REITER SYNDROME

The clinical triad is urethritis, conjunctivitis and mucocutaneous lesions. Plantar fasciitis is characteristic but not pathognomonic.

PLAIN FILM

- Sacroiliitis is usually bilateral and asymmetrical, and it often persists.
- Periarticular osteoporosis, reduced joint space, erosions and new bone formation.
- Hallux and metatarsophalangeal joints particularly.
- Subluxation and deformity of metatarsophalangeal joints.
- Enthesopathy.

RHEUMATOID ARTHRITIS

Box 2.17 RHEUMATOID ARTHRITIS VERSUS OSTEOARTHRITIS OF THE HIP

Both
- Cartilage loss

Osteoarthritis (OA)
- Subchondral sclerosis
- Cysts
- Osteophytes
- Femoral head migrates superolaterally
- Migrates medially with rheumatoid arthritis

Common systemic disease, seen in up to three-times more women and most often occurring between ages 45 and 65 years. It is regarded as an autoimmune disease and is associated with the *HLA-DR4* gene. A total of 60% of patients present with bilateral, symmetrical arthritis of joints in the hands. Felty syndrome is the combination of RA with splenomegaly and neutropenia.

PLAIN FILM (FIGURE 2.15)

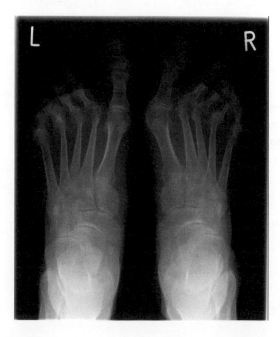

Figure 2.15 Rheumatoid arthritis. Foot x-ray demonstrating bilateral symmetrical polyarthritis, particularly affecting the MTP joints, with periarticular erosions and para-articular osteoporosis.

- Bilateral, symmetrical polyarthritis (three or more joints)
- Early signs: swelling and para-articular osteoporosis
- Soft tissue swelling + effusion = active disease
- Premature loss of joint space
- Periarticular erosions and loss of cartilage
- Subcortical cysts
- Late signs: ankylosis, subluxation and deformity
- Distribution: hands, feet, cervical spine, ribs, shoulders, hips and knees

HAND X-RAY

- Metacarpophalangeal (MCP) joints typically involved, distal interphalangeal (DIP) joints spared (if DIP joints involved, consider alternative diagnosis).
- Boutonnière deformity (fixed flexion of the proximal interphalangeal [PIP] joint with hyperextension at the DIP joint), most commonly affects the index fingers.

CERVICAL SPINE X-RAY

- 80% develop atlantoaxial subluxation after 2 years (due to erosive synovitis).
- Protrusion of the odontoid peg.

CHEST/SHOULDER X-RAY

- Scalloped erosion on underneath of clavicle
- Tapered margin of the distal clavicle

RIB NOTCHING (TABLE 2.2)

Table 2.2 Causes of rib notching by location

Superior	Both	Inferior
Connective tissue disorders	Neurofibromatosis	Vascular (enlarged collaterals,
Rheumatoid arthritis	Hyperparathyroidism	interrupted arch, subclavian
Scleroderma		stenosis, superior vena
Systemic lupus erythematosus		cava [SVC] obstruction)
Marfan syndrome		Neurofibromatosis

SAPHO SYNDROME

Rare combination of synovitis, acne, palmoplantar pustulosis, hyperostosis and osteitis/osteomyelitis. There may be a delay of several years between the onset of osseous symptoms and cutaneous manifestations. Similar to chronic, recurrent multifocal osteomyelitis in children.

PLAIN FILM

- Dominant feature is new and bizarre bone proliferation.
- The sternoclavicular joint is affected most commonly (70%–90%), then flat bones, then medial clavicles.

BONE SCAN

- Buffalo sign caused by increased activity in the manubrium sternum and medial clavicles.

SARCOIDOSIS

Multisystem granulomatous disorder that is more common in those of African descent. Osseous involvement is uncommon (5%); small bones of the hands and feet are affected most often. Lofgren syndrome is an acute form of sarcoidosis composed of arthralgia, erythema nodusum and bilateral hilar lymph node enlargement.

PLAIN FILM

- Lace-like, reticulated trabecular pattern
- Destruction and sclerosis of the terminal phalanges
- Periarticular calcification
- Subperiosteal bone resorption
- Periosteal reaction
- Diffuse sclerosis of vertebral bodies
- Well defined lucencies with a sclerotic margin—nasal bones, mandible and cranium (mimics metastases)

SCLERODERMA

Autoimmune disorder of unknown aetiology characterised by small-vessel disease and fibrosis. It more commonly affects females and peaks from 20 to 50 years of age. CREST syndrome is a limited cutaneous form of scleroderma characterised by calcinosis, Raynaud syndrome, oesophageal dysmotility, sclerodactyly and telangiectasia.

HAND X-RAY (FIGURE 2.16)

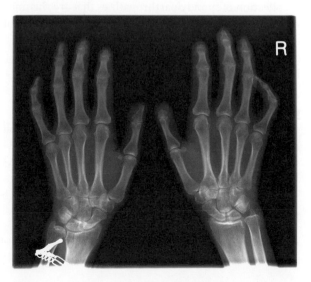

Figure 2.16 Scleroderma. Hand x-ray demonstrating resorption of the terminal phalanges (acro-osteolysis) with pencilling or sharpening of the terminal phalynx.

- Resorption of the terminal phalanges (acro-osteolysis) leading to pencilling or sharpening of the terminal phalynx.
- Subcutaneous/joint calcifications in 25%.
- Severe resorption of the first carpometacarpal joint with radial subluxation of the first metacarpal bone is nearly pathognomonic.

SEPTIC ARTHRITIS

Usually acquired through haematogenous spread (e.g. remote wound infection, intravenous drug use (IVDU), pneumonia, etc.). It usually affects the hip, knee, shoulder, elbow or ankle. *S. aureus* is the most common pathogen, then group A *Streptococcus* and *Gonococcus*. Septic arthritis in the setting of IVDU tends to occur in unusual locations and involves unusual organisms (e.g. *Pseudomonas* and *Klebsiella*).

PLAIN FILM

- The hallmark is a joint effusion in a patient with signs of infection.
- Blurring of the periarticular fat planes is common.
- Periarticular soft tissue swelling.
- Periarticular osteopenia.
- Later, there is irregular joint space narrowing.

MRI

- Synovial enhancement post-contrast
- Joint effusion
- Soft tissue and bone marrow oedema

SERONEGATIVE SPONDYLOARTHRITIS

A collection of spondyloarthropathies that are rheumatoid factor negative: anklyosing spondylitis, psoriatic arthritis, arthritis in the setting of inflammatory bowel disease, reactive (Reiter syndrome) and undifferentiated.

PLAIN FILM

- Joint space narrowing.
- Polyarticular involvement.
- Distal joints of the hands and feet with bone proliferation.
- Syndesmophytes, asymmetrical sacroiliitis, ankylosis and patchy bone marrow oedema are features of ankylosing spondylitis (AS) and psoriatic arthritis.

SEVER DISEASE

Also known as calcaneal apophysitis, this is the result of mechanical trauma to an immature skeleton. It is a cause of heel pain.

MRI

- Oedema within the calcaneal apophysis (may extend into the calcaneal tuberosity)

SHIN SPLINTS

Also known as medial tibial stress syndrome, this is a common cause of chronic shin pain in athletes. It is the result of repetitive stress to a normal bone.

NUCLEAR MEDICINE

- Linear symmetrical cortical uptake on bone scan, seen most avidly along the posterior aspects of the distal two-thirds of the tibia.
- Hot patella sign is non-specific.

MRI

- Spectrum of findings from marrow oedema to frank stress fracture

SINUS TARSI SYNDROME

This is a common complication of ankle sprains, but may also result from an inflammatory arthropathy. The sinus tarsi is the lateral space between the talus and calcaneus containing fat, nerves and the talocalcaneal interosseous ligaments. Ligamentous injury in the sinus tarsi causes lateral foot pain and hind-foot instability that typically presents between ages 30 and 40 years.

MRI

- Alteration of the fat signal (e.g. to low T1 and T2) in the sinus is the most specific sign (replaced with either fluid or scar tissue).
- Subtalar joint osteoarthritis.
- Synovial thickening.
- Diffuse enhancement of the tarsal sinus post-gadolinium.

SPINAL EXTRADURAL ABSCESS

Unusual diagnosis most often presenting with localized back pain. It is associated with diabetes, IVDU, trauma, surgery, immunosuppression and renal failure. Most is seeded haematogeneously; direct spread is usually from vertebral osteomyelitis or psoas abscess.

MRI

- Intermediate T1 signal in the epidural space posterior to the vertebral body (T1 signal is iso-slightly hyperintense to the adjacent cord).
- Focal T2 hyperintense epidural signal, which is difficult to separate from cerebrospinal fluid (CSF).
- The solid component enhances following intravenous gadolinium.
- Check for cord compression.
- Bone marrow/soft tissue oedema on fat-suppressed images.

SPONDYLOLYSIS

Refers to a common defect in the pars interarticularis causing lower back pain in about 25% of cases. A total of 50% of cases develop spondylolisthesis. It is thought to arise from repeated microfractures and elongation of a congenitally weakened pars. The pars defect is usually held together by fibrocartilage and may heal (which may account for a unilateral pars defect).

PLAIN FILM

- Visible abnormality in late childhood/adolescence.
- Scottie dog appearance on oblique radiographs (the dog's collar is the defect).
- 95% occur at L5.

CT

- Defect in the pars interarticularis—most clearly demonstrated on sagittal reconstructions.

SPONTANEOUS OSTEONECROSIS OF THE KNEE

This is actually an insufficiency fracture and not a true osteonecrosis. It is most common in women in their 70s and is associated with a sudden onset of pain. It is thought to be associated with a meniscal tear and microfractures.

PLAIN FILM

- Flattening of the medial femoral condyle.
- Radiolucent focus in the subchondral bone.
- Later, there is subchondral fracture and periosteal reaction

SYNOVIAL OSTEOCHONDROMATOSIS

Due to benign synovial neoplasia, which forms nodules that often calcify. It is more common in men aged 30–50 years and most commonly affects a single joint, usually the knee. It is self-limiting, but may recur following resection, and rarely transforms to chondrosarcoma.

PLAIN FILM/CT

- Intra-articular chondroid ('ring and arc') calcification—pathognomic
- Extrinsic erosion of the bone on both sides of the joint

MRI

- Lobulated, homogeneous intra-articular signal, which is intermediate on T1 and high on T2.
- May contain low T1/T2 foci (calcification), more obvious on gradient echo (susceptibility artefact).
- No haemorrhage, unlike PVNS.

SYSTEMIC LUPUS ERYTHEMATOSUS (SLE)

Common autoimmune disease causing inflammation, vasculitis and deposition of immune complexes. The musculoskeletal system is affected in 80% of SLE patients, typically the hands, wrists, knees and shoulders.

HAND X-RAY

- Peri-articular soft tissue swelling.
- Juxta-articular osteopenia.
- Ulnar deviation at the metacarpophalangeal joints without erosions or joint space loss, Boutonièrre deformity is known as 'Jaccoud arthropathy'.
- Carpal instability (scapholunate subluxation, distance >3 mm).

PELVIS X-RAY

- AVN of the femoral head (due to the disease or steroid use)

TARSAL COALITION

Abnormal union of the bones of the mid-foot or hind-foot; union is either cartilaginous, fibrous or bony. The site of union is commonly either the calcaneonavicular joint (45%) or the subtalar joint (45%). Coalitions restrict movement of the mid-foot and cause pain and pes planus.

PLAIN FILM

- With fibrous/cartilaginous coalition, look for joint space narrowing, indistinct articular margins and reactive sclerosis.
- Calcaneonavicular coalition best seen on an oblique, look for:
  - Elongated tubular extension of the anterior calcaneus, which fuses with the dorsolateral margin of the navicular.
  - Elongated calcaneus known as the 'anteater sign'.
- Talocalcaneal coalition:
  - Difficult to assess on standard views.
  - Look for a 'talar beak'.
  - 'C-sign' (lateral view) is a c-shaped sclerotic line extending between the posterior surface of the talus and the sustentaculum tali.

MRI

- Sagittal/axial best for calcaneonavicular coalition, coronal for talocalcaneal.
- More sensitive than CT for non-osseus coalition.

THYROID ACROPACHY

Rare complication of Grave disease; typically occurs in patients with thyroid eye disease.

PLAIN FILM

- Smooth, symmetrical periostitis affecting metacarpals, metatarsals and the phalanges of the hands and feet.
- Soft tissue swelling.

TEMPOROMANDIBULAR JOINT (TMJ) SYNDROME

Common, mostly arising due to trauma or arthritis; >80% of patients with pain and TMJ dysfunction have evidence of TMJ disc displacement on MRI. It is more common in females.

MRI

- Gold standard for assessing internal derangement.
- Coronal and sagittal reformats with the jaw open and closed are optimal.
- Disc displacement is most commonly anterior or anteromedial/lateral.
- Look for evidence of osteoarthritis.

TRANSIENT OSTEOPOROSIS OF THE HIP

First described as transient demineralisation of the femoral head in women in the third trimester of pregnancy, it is also known to affect middle-aged men. It causes hip pain and resolves without treatment after weeks to months. Related syndromes include migratory regional osteoporosis and transient bone marrow oedema.

PLAIN FILM (FIGURE 2.17)

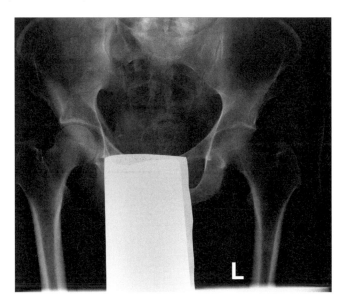

Figure 2.17 Transient osteoporosis of the hip. Pelvic x-ray demonstrating osteopenia of the left femoral head with no joint space narrowing.

- Radiographic features lag behind clinical features.
- Osteopenia of the femoral head seen 4–8 weeks after symptom onset.
- Loss of subchondral cortex of the femoral head is the hallmark.
- No joint space narrowing or subchondral bone collapse.
- Joint effusion.

NUCLEAR MEDICINE

- Homogeneously increased uptake on bone scan.

MRI (FIGURE 2.18)

- Bone marrow oedema (i.e. low T1, high T2), which is most intense in the subchondral bone of the femoral head and which fades as it extends down the femoral neck.

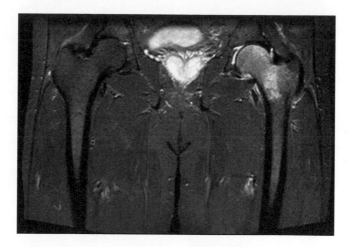

Figure 2.18 Transient osteoporosis of the hip. STIR coronal magnetic resonance image demonstrating bone marrow of the left femoral head and neck.

- Diffuse enhancement of the abnormal marrow post-contrast.
- Small effusion.

VERTEBRAL BODY COLLAPSE

Non-traumatic collapse commonly affects elderly patients, mostly in the thoracic or lumbar spine and mostly due to osteoporosis. However, up to 40% of bone metastases are to the vertebral bodies and may result in pathological fracture. Differentiating benign from malignant collapse is important for directing treatment.

MRI

- Acute fractures are low T1 regardless of cause—the low T1 signal normalises in benign fractures after about 6 weeks, enhancement is non-specific.
- Findings suggesting malignancy:
  - Convex posterior bulge of the vertebral body.
  - Abnormal signal extends to the pedicles/posterior elements.
  - Epidural mass.
  - Metastases elsewhere in the spine.
- Findings suggesting osteoporotic fracture:
  - Retropulsion of bone fragments.
  - Multiple fractures.
  - Intervertebral vacuum phenomenon.
  - Spared bone has normal signal intensity.
  - Fracture line band parallel to endplate.

VERTEBRA PLANA

Generic term for a completely collapsed vertebral body so that it resembles a very thin disc. Kummel disease is post-traumatic osteonecrosis, which may result in vertebra

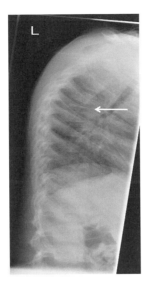

Figure 2.19 Vertebra plana. Lateral thoracic spine x-ray demonstrating complete flattening of a thoracic vertebra (white arrow).

plana. In young patients, the most common causes are eosinophilic granuloma (i.e. Langerhans histiocytosis); in adults, the most common causes are tumour or osteoporosis. See Table 2.3.

Table 2.3 Causes of vertebra plana

Young patients	Elderly
Eosinophilic granuloma	Osteoporosis
Infection (including tuberculosis)	Metastasis
Neuroblastoma metastasis	Myeloma
Trauma	Trauma
Ewing sarcoma	Infection (including
Lymphoma	tuberculosis)
Leukaemia	

PLAIN FILM (FIGURE 2.19)

- Complete loss of height of the vertebral body
- Normal intervertebral discs
- Can recover in children

CT

- Look for intravertebral fluid or gas ('vacuum cleft sign')—pathognomic for osteonecrosis and at risk of further collapse (malignancy, infection and acute injury are excluded).

VERTEBROPLASTY

Percutaneous fluoroscopic-guided procedure involving the injection of radiopaque cement into a partially collapsed vertebral body in order to stabilise the fracture, relieve pain and restore body height (kyphoplasty uses a balloon to achieve this). The indications are painful partial osteoporotic fractures (<70%) and painful bone tumours (benign and malignant).

MRI

- All patients assessed with MRI prior to vertebroplasty.
- Fractures should be low on T1, high on T2 and STIR (if there is no oedema, then vertebroplasty is not indicated).
- Contraindications include cord compression, infection and fracture of the posterior vertebral body wall.

PAEDIATRICS

ACHONDROPLASIA

Box 2.18 CAUSES OF POSTERIOR VERTEBRAL BODY SCALLOPING
• Ehlers–Danlos syndrome
• Neurofibromatosis
• Marfan syndrome
• Morquio syndrome
• Acromegaly
• Achondroplasia
• Ankylosing spondylitis
• Tumours in the canal (e.g. ependymoma, dermoid or lipoma)

This is the most common rhizomelic dwarfism and is inherited in an autosomal dominant pattern. The most significant complication is brain stem/cord compression due to spinal stenosis caused by abnormal alignment and a congenitally narrow canal (short pedicles and a reduced inter-pedicular distance contribute to this).

SKULL X-RAY/HEAD CT
- Flat nasal bridge
- Broad mandible
- Large skull
- Frontal bossing
- Narrow, anteriorly displaced foramen magnum
- Hydrocephalus

CHEST X-RAY
- Decreased AP distance
- Short, anteriorly flared, concave ribs

PELVIS X-RAY
- Tombstone iliac bones from squaring
- Champagne glass pelvic inlet
- Horizontal acetabular roof
- Short sacrosciatic notches
- Horizontal sacrum

APPENDICULAR X-RAY
- Trident hand (divergent middle and ring fingers)
- Short femoral necks
- Patella baja

SPINE X-RAY (FIGURE 2.20)

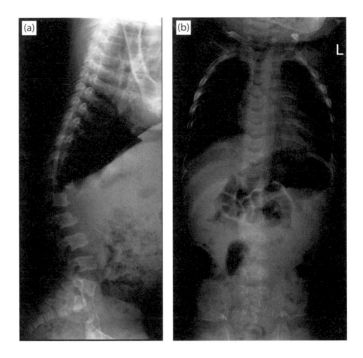

Figure 2.20 Achondroplasia. Lateral thoracic spine x-rays (a) demonstrating posterior vertebral scalloping, anterior inferior beaking and shortened pedicles. (b) is the AP view showing decreased interpedicular distance, tombstone iliac bones and horizontal acetabular roofs.

- Posterior vertebral body scalloping
- Anterior inferior beaking
- Bullet-shaped vertebrae
- Shortened pedicles
- Decreased inter-pedicular distance

AVULSION FRACTURES

More common in children due to growing apophyses being weaker than the soft tissue structures that attach to them. See Table 2.4.

PLAIN FILM
- Sharply defined bone fragment
- Mixed lytic/sclerotic appearance if old

MRI
- Bone injury best appreciated on T1.
- Look for a haematoma on T1 also.

Table 2.4 Avulsion fractures and the tendons responsible

Site	Tendon attachment
Anterior superior iliac spine	Sartorius
Anterior inferior iliac spine	Rectus femoris
Inferior pubic ramus	Gracilis
Ischial tuberosity (most common) (Figure 2.21)	Adductor magnus
Lateral tibial plateau (Segond fracture)	Lateral collateral ligament
Medial epicondyle (little leaguer's elbow)	Flexor–pronator muscles

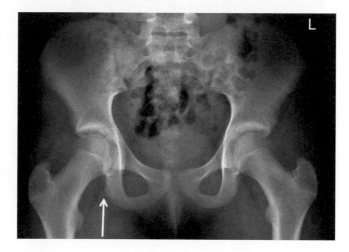

Figure 2.21 Avulsion fracture of the right ischial tuberosity.

BLOUNT DISEASE

Deformity arising from an insult occurring to the medial aspect of the proximal tibial epiphysis during development, also known as tibia vara. Two types are described.

INFANTILE

- Eight-times more common
- First few years of life
- Mostly bilateral (80%) and painless
- Obese early walkers

ADOLESCENT

- Children aged 8–15 years
- Mostly unilateral (90%)

Plain film (Figure 2.22)

- Varus deformity of the tibia owing to angulation of the metaphysis.
- Depressed medial tibial metaphysis.
- Beaking and irregularity of the tibial proximal medial metaphysis.
- Tibial shaft is adducted without intrinsic curvature.

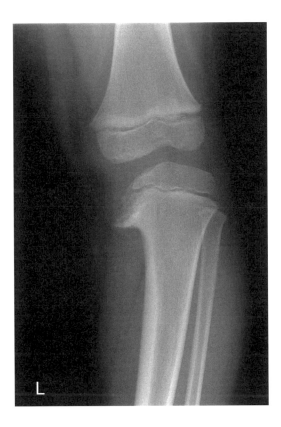

Figure 2.22 Blount disease. Frontal knee radiograph demonstrating a fragmented epiphysis with a depressed medial tibial metaphysis and associated beaking and irregularity. There is a varus deformity of the tibia.

BRODIE ABSCESS

Refers to the most common appearance of subacute osteomyelitis, typically occurs from ages 2 to 15 years and is mostly due to *S. aureus*.

PLAIN FILM (FIGURE 2.23)

- Lucency most commonly seen in the distal metaphysis, typically tibia or femur.
- Classic appearance for a Brodie abscess is a lucency with dense surrounding sclerosis.
- Thin, lucent channel extending towards the growth plate, 'serpentine sign'.

MRI

- Double line effect—high signal intensity granulation tissue surrounded by low signal intensity due to marked sclerosis.
- 'Penumbra sign'—hyperintense rim on non-gadolinium-enhanced axial T1-weighted image, due to protein-rich granulation tissue at the abscess margin.

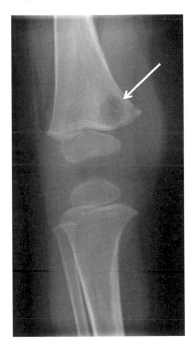

Figure 2.23 Brodie abscess. Frontal knee radiograph demonstrating a lytic lesion within the proximal femoral metaphysis.

CAFFEY DISEASE

This is a rare, benign, self-limiting condition also known as infantile cortical hyperostosis. It occurs in those aged <6 months and is associated with fever, soft tissue swelling and irritability combined with a characteristic x-ray appearance.

PLAIN FILM

- Soft tissue swelling.
- Marked cortical hyperostosis (mandible affected in 80%).
- Cortex appears lamellated.
- Diaphyseal—the epiphyses are spared.

CERVICAL SPINE

The cervical spine reaches adult proportions by age 8–10 years; beyond 12 years, the effects of cervical spine trauma are similar to those of adults.

PLAIN FILM

- Traumatic cervical spine injuries occur most between the skull base and C3 in children.
- Normal findings in children:
  - Pre-dentate space ≤5 mm.
  - Anterior wedging at C3.
  - Soft tissues thicker between C2 and C4 than a half-vertebral body.
  - Pseudosubluxation at C2–3 and C3–4.
- Pseudosubluxation is common in children aged <8 years due to ligament laxity and horizontal facet alignment; it reduces on extension (>2 mm displacement from the posterior cervical line is pathological).

CLEIDOCRANIAL DYSOSTOSIS

Box 2.19 CAUSES OF LATERAL CLAVICULAR OSTEOLYSIS

Bilateral clavicular osteolysis is associated with cleidocranial dysplasia, rheumatoid arthritis and hyperparathyroidism. It is the most common location for post-traumatic osteolysis that is preceded by a fairly severe injury to the shoulder, typically a dislocation or subluxation of the acromioclavicular joint. Changes may be evident after 1 month. Widespread idiopathic osteolysis is termed Gorham's or vanishing bone disease.

Other causes

- **C**leidocranial dysplasia
- **R**heumatoid arthritis
- **A**nkylosing spondylitis
- **S**cleroderma
- **H**yperparathyroidism
- **M**etastases and myeloma
- **G**out
- **L**ymphoma
- **O**steomyelitis (e.g. *Pseudomonas* or *Klebsiella*)

This is a rare, autosomal dominant condition that affects membranous bone formation and causes delayed ossification of midline structures. It is associated with short stature, delayed closure of cranial sutures, clavicular dysplasia and dental abnormalities. The clavicles and pubic symphysis are formed from membranous bone.

CHEST X-RAY (FIGURE 2.24)

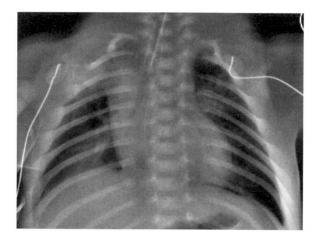

Figure 2.24 Cleidocranial dysostosis. Frontal chest radiograph demonstrating absent clavicles.

- Absent or hypoplastic lateral clavicles
- Supernumerary ribs (e.g. 13 ribs)
- Narrowed thorax

PELVIS X-RAY
- Hemivertebrae
- Widened pubic symphysis

APPENDICULAR X-RAYS
- Absent or short radius
- Elongated second metatarsals and metacarpals and large MCP/metatarsophalangeal (MTP) pseudoepiphyses

SKULL X-RAY
- Multiple wormian bones
- Delayed closure of sutures, widened anterior fontanelle and cranial enlargement
- Large mandible
- Small paranasal sinuses
- Hypertelorism

DEVELOPMENTAL DYSPLASIA OF THE HIP

This is more common in girls and is often undetected until adulthood. It is associated with a breech delivery, positive family history, prune belly syndrome and oligohydramnios. Early intervention reduces the risk of teenage-onset osteoarthritis.

US

- Performed at 1/12 of age (indicated if the hips feel unstable on examination or if there is a family history of hip dysplasia, breech delivery, premature or multiple birth).
- In the coronal plane, the α angle represents the angle between the iliac bone ('baseline') and the acetabular roof ('inclination line'); >60° is normal, <50° represents poor acetabular concavity seen in dysplasia.
- The β angle lies between the acetabular labrum and iliac bone and is a measure of roof coverage; <55° is normal and indicates adequate bony coverage (Table 2.5).

Table 2.5 Imaging characteristics of developmental dysplasia of the hip

Classification	α angle	Description
1	>60°	Mature hip
2A	50–59°	Physiological <3 months
2B	43–49°	Concentric but unstable
3	<43°	Dislocated

DOWN SYNDROME

Trisomy 21 is the most common chromosomal abnormality; diagnosis may be prenatal or postnatal. Characteristic features include typical facies (e.g. hypotelorism), congenital heart disease (40%, mostly ventricular or atrial septal defects), duodenal atresia (50%) and musculoskeletal findings.

CHEST X-RAY

- 90% have a hypersegmented manubrium
- Supernumerary ribs (11 pairs in 25%)
- Bell-shaped thorax
- Scoliosis

CERVICAL SPINE X-RAY

- Atlantoaxial subluxation
- Hypoplastic posterior arch of C1
- Odontoid hypoplasia/os odontoideum

PELVIC X-RAY

- Iliac index (sum of the acetabular and iliac angles) decreased
- Flattening of the acetabular roof
- Metaphyseal flaring
- Elongation and tapering of the ischia
- Iliac blades rotated in the coronal plane, flared 'Mickey Mouse' or elephant ear appearance typical
- Slipped upper femoral epiphysis
- Perthe disease

HAND/FOOT X-RAY

- Hypoplasia of the middle phalanx of the fifth digit of the hand
- Sandal gap sign—widening of the first metatarsal web space

DWARFISM (TABLE 2.6)

Table 2.6 Characteristics and syndromic associations in dwarfism

Type	Description	Syndrome association
Rhizomelic	Proximal limb shortening relative to distal	Achondroplasia
Mesomelic	Distal limb shortening relative to proximal	Dyschondrosteosis
Micromelic	Proximal and distal shortening	Thanatophoric dwarfism
		Osteogenesis imperfect
Acromelic	Distal extremity shortening	Pyknodysostosis

FRACTURES

The paediatric skeleton is more prone to fracture than an adult's due to a greater proportion of collagen and cartilage (though it is more elastic). The paediatric bone cortex is thicker and well vascularised, which leads to rapid healing and remodelling. Fractures of the distal radius are the most common childhood fractures (Table 2.7).

Table 2.7 Imaging characteristics of childhood fractures

Type	Description
Torus, 'buckle'	Cortex buckles due to compression injury (e.g. fall on outstretched hand). Usually stable
Greenstick	Cortical break due to tensile force and due to angulation. The compression side of the cortex remains intact. Often unstable
Plastic bowing	Intact cortex. Thought to be due to longitudinal stress causing microfractures. Most commonly affects the ulna with a radial fracture
Physeal, 'Salter–Harris' (see page 124)	Injury to the growth plate, more common in pre-adolescents due to the level of bone growth occurring
Lead pipe	Characterised by a torus fracture on one side of the bone and a greenstick fracture on the other

HAEMOPHILIA

An X-linked disease (therefore only males are affected) due to a deficiency of either factor VIII or IX. Haemophilia arthopathy arises from repeated bleeds, leading to the formation of pannus that erodes cartilage and leads to loss of subchondral bone and subarticular cyst formation. Intra-articular haemorrhage causes a chronic synovitis, synovial proliferation and periarticular osteopenia. Typically presents in affected patients aged 10–20 years with a tense, warm joint, fever and leucocytosis.

PLAIN FILM
- Accelerated maturation and enlargement of the epiphysis
- Soft tissue swelling

- Juxta-articular osteoporosis
- Erosion of the articular surface with subchondral cysts
- Preservation of joint space
- Squared patella with widening of the intercondylar notch
- Medial slanting of the tibiotalar joint and flattening of the condylar surface

MRI

- Low signal returned from hypertrophied synovium due to magnetic susceptibility of haemosiderin.
- Articular surfaces are devoid of cartilage.
- Joint effusion.

HIP EFFUSION

Causes include septic arthritis, transient synovitis and juvenile idiopathic arthritis.

US

- Bulging of the anterior joint capsule
- >3 mm distance between the bony femoral neck and joint capsule
- >2 mm difference from the contralateral side

PLAIN FILM

- Joint space widening—look for asymmetry.

HOLT–ORAM SYNDROME

Rare autosomal dominant syndrome, also known as heart–hand syndrome as it causes upper limb and cardiac abnormalities (arrhythmia and atrial septal defects).

PLAIN FILM

- Radial ray limb abnormalities: triphalangeal thumb and hypoplasia/aplasia of the radius
- Carpal bone abnormalities

HOMOCYSTEINURIA

Autosomal recessive inherited defect in methionine metabolism leading to a build-up of homocysteine in the blood and urine. There is a defect in collagen and elastin structure, which causes Marfanoid features and lax ligaments. There is an increased risk of stroke.

PLAIN FILM

- Generalised osteoporosis (75%)
- Carpal bone abnormalities: enlarged epiphyses, epiphyseal calcification, metaphyseal cupping and delayed ossification
- Scoliosis
- Biconcave vertebrae

JUVENILE IDIOPATHIC ARTHRITIS

Box 2.20 CAUSES OF A PERIOSTEAL REACTION IN A CHILD
Leukaemia is the important diagnosis of exclusion
●   Syphilis
●   Physiological
●   Caffey disease
●   Rickets
●   Juvenile idiopathic arthritis
●   Rheumatoid arthritis
●   Leukaemia
●   Scurvy

Defined as any idiopathic arthritis presenting at <16 years of age and of >6 weeks' duration; 80% of patients present by 7 years. The monoarticular variant is most common and most often affects the knee. Joint pain and stiffness along with fever, malaise, weight loss and hepatosplenomegaly are commonly demonstrated. Most are seronegative; anaemia and elevated erythrocyte sedimentation rate (ESR) may be found. Associated with a salmon-coloured rash and palpable lymph node enlargement.

US

● More sensitive than x-ray for detecting effusions and synovitis

CHEST X-RAY

● Pleural effusion
● Hepatosplenomegaly

APPENDICULAR X-RAY

● Soft tissue swelling.
● Joint space widening (due to joint effusion and synovial hypertrophy).
● Periarticular osteopenia (thickened synovium causes hyperaemia in the adjacent bone and radiolucency).
● Periostitis is typical and most common in the metacarpal/metatarsal bones, where it gives the bones a more rectangular appearance.
● Premature closure of growth plates/accelerated skeletal maturation.
● Ankylosis and growth disturbance in chronic disease.
● Widened intercondylar notch/squared patella (classic).
● Other typical findings include balloon epiphyses, gracile tubular bones and ribbon ribs.
● Unlike rheumatoid arthritis (RA), bone changes occur late and there is more ankylosis and widening of the metaphyses.

KLIPPEL–FEIL SYNDROME

Congenital abnormality of vertebral segmentation. Fusion of the vertebral bodies and posterior columns at C2/3 is the most common variant and causes a restriction of movement. Associated features include a short neck and a low posterior hairline.

Other associations are the Sprengel deformity (25%–40%), syndactyly, clubbed foot, hypoplastic lumbar vertebrae and congenital heart disease (5%, mostly atrial septal defects or coarctation).

US

- 50% have a renal anomaly, commonly ectopia, agenesis or horseshoe kidney.

PLAIN FILM

- Partial fusion of C2 and C3.
- Partial or complete fusion of C1 with the occiput ('occipitalisation of the atlas') and hypoplastic C1.
- Scoliosis.
- Hemivertebrae.
- Spinal stenosis.
- Rib fusion.
- Thumb anomalies are common: triphalangeal thumb, hypoplasia and polydactyly.
- Sprengel deformity—look for medial rotation and elevation of the scapula, hypoplastic scapula or an omovertebral bone (connects scapula to the spine).

LANGERHANS CELL HISTIOCYTOSIS (LCH)

Formerly known as histiocytosis X, this is a disease of immune regulation resulting in excessive histiocytes and granuloma formation. It is more common in children and causes varying effects from eosinophilic granuloma (single/few bones affected), Hand–Schüller–Christian disease (children aged 1–5 years, multiple bones and extra-skeletal involvement) and the most severe Letterer–Siwe disease (multisystem disease, children aged <2 years and often fatal).

PLAIN FILM

- 50% of bone lesions occur in the skull, mandible, ribs or pelvis.
- Lucent lesion with periostitis (appear aggressive early on).
- Look for endosteal scalloping and soft tissue nodules.
- Vertebra plana (Figure 2.19)—LCH is the most common cause in children.
- Lesions may resolve completely or appear sclerotic.

LEAD POISONING

Children are more susceptible to poisoning from lead found in the environment and industry. Lead deposition occurs in high concentrations in the metaphyses. It presents with loss of appetite, anaemia, vomiting, constipation and abdominal pain. Affected patients are short for their age.

PLAIN FILM

- Delayed skeletal maturity.
- Bands of increased density at metaphyses of tubular bones (femur, tibia and radius, particularly).
- Metaphyseal bands may be normal in a child aged <3 years.

- 'Bone in bone' appearance.
- Differential: healed rickets, leukaemia or scurvy.

MACRODYSTROPHIA LIPOMATOSA

This is a rare, localised form of gigantism due to overgrowth of fibroadipose tissue. Associated hyperaemia results in bone and soft tissue enlargement. It usually affects the hands and feet, where it follows the distribution of the median nerve or plantar nerve, respectively.

PLAIN FILM

- Bone and soft tissue hypertrophy.
- Cortical thickening and overgrowth of the articular margins.
- Lucencies in the soft tissues characteristic of fat.
- The bone trabecular pattern is normal.

MARFAN SYNDROME

Box 2.21 CAUSES OF A PECTUS EXCAVATUM
<ul><li>Prematurity</li><li>Down syndrome</li><li>Marfan syndrome</li><li>Homocysteinuria</li><li>Foetal alcohol syndrome</li></ul>

Multisystem connective tissue disorder with a 70% autosomal dominant inheritance. Cardiac disease is the cause of death in 90%. There are numerous musculoskeletal manifestations.

SPINE X-RAY

- Progressive scoliosis (about 60% affected)
- Scalloping of the posterior lumbosacral vertebral bodies (due to dural ectasia)
- Spondylolisthesis

HANDS/FEET X-RAY

- Arachnodactyly (i.e. elongated metacarpals) is non-specific.
- Pes planus.
- Hallux valgus.

PELVIS X-RAY

- Acetabular protrusion

MORQUIO SYNDROME

This is the most common mucopolysaccharidosis, and it is inherited in an autosomal recessive pattern. It is associated with multiple skeletal manifestations occurring in the first 18 months of life.

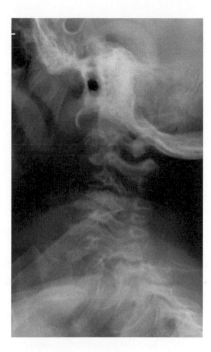

Figure 2.25 Morquio syndrome. Lateral cervical spine x-ray demonstrating atlantoaxial subluxation and platyspondyly.

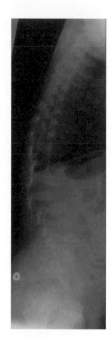

Figure 2.26 Morquio syndrome. Lateral thoracic spine x-ray demonstrating ovoid vertebral bodies, posterior vertebral body scalloping and anterior central beaking.

SPINE X-RAY (FIGURES 2.25 AND 2.26)

- Anterior central beak is relatively specific.
- Atlantoaxial subluxation due to odontoid hypoplasia.
- Platyspondyly (i.e. diffuse flattening of the vertebral bodies, which reduces distance between the endplates).
- Ovoid vertebral bodies.
- Posterior vertebral body scalloping and central beaking.
- Widened intervertebral disc space.
- Exaggeration of the lumbar lordosis.

Box 2.22 CAUSES OF ANTERIOR VERTEBRAL BODY BEAKING

Central
Morquio syndrome

Inferior
Hurler syndrome
Achondroplasia
Down syndrome

PELVIS X-RAY

- Fragmentation and flattening of the femoral heads
- Flared iliac wings

KNEE X-RAY

- Lateral sloping of the tibial plateaux
- Genu valgus deformity

HANDS AND FEET X-RAY

- Bullet-shaped metacarpals
- Short, wide tubular bones with metaphyseal irregularity

NEUROFIBROMATOSIS TYPE 1

Type 1 accounts for 90% of neurofibromatosis, due to a chromosome 17 long arm mutation that is inherited in an autosomal dominant fashion. It is associated with multiple abnormalities of the central nervous system. Up to 60% have musculoskeletal abnormalities either due to pressure from adjacent neurofibromas or a mesenchymal abnormality.

CHEST X-RAY

- Ribbon ribs/inferior rib notching (due to pressure from neurofibromas arising from intercostal nerves)

APPENDICULAR X-RAY

- Pseudarthrosis of the wrist, tibia, fibula and clavicle
- Anterolateral bowing centred at the junction of the middle-distal thirds of the tibia (associated with cystic and sclerotic change)

SPINE X-RAY

- Scoliosis—this is the most common skeletal abnormality (affects up to 40%).
- Posterior vertebral scalloping (due to dural ectasia).
- Kyphosis.
- Cystic osteolytic lesions with a sclerotic margin (most commonly affects the mandible).

SPINE CT

- Low-attenuation masses (neurofibroma), dumbbell-shaped along the exiting nerve
- Hypoplasia of the pedicles/transverse processes/spinous processes (due to lateral thoracic meningocele/neurofibroma)

SPINE MRI

- Neurofibromas are low signal on pre-contrast T1; they enhance centrally.
- Neurofibromas may have central low T2 intensity with peripheral high signal ('target sign') and high signal on T2.

> **Box 2.23 CAUSES OF PSEUDARTHROSIS**
>
> - Neurofibromatosis
> - Fibrous dysplasia
> - Osteogenesis imperfecta
> - Non-united fracture
> - Congenital

OSGOOD–SCHLATTER DISEASE

Microtrauma to the patella tendon at its insertion causes osteochondritis of the tibial tuberosity. It affects vigorously active children aged 10–15 years and presents with pain and swelling at the tibial tuberosity.

PLAIN FILM

- Increased radiodensity of the infrapatellar fat pad due to oedema
- Fragmentation of the tibial tubercle
- Anterior swelling

MRI

- Bone marrow oedema on STIR imaging
- Thickening of the distal patellar tendon
- Oedema in the soft tissues and the Hoffa fat pad
- Distension and fluid in the deep infrapatellar bursa

OSTEOPETROSIS

Rare disease of abnormal osteoclast activity where there is failure of resorption and remodelling, leading to thickened, sclerotic bone that is weak and brittle. The autosomal recessive subtype causes stillbirth or death in infancy. The autosomal dominant type is commonly asymptomatic or may cause mild anaemia or cranial nerve palsies due to narrowing of the cranial foramina.

APPENDICULAR X-RAY (FIGURE 2.27)

- Increased density of the bone medulla.
- 'Bone within bone' appearance.
- Alternating sclerotic and lucent bands in the metaphysis (striations).
- Metaphyseal widening and remodelling (Erlenmeyer flask deformity).
- Bony sclerosis + Erlenmeyer flask deformity = osteopetrosis.
- Patients are at increased risk of fractures, mal-union and non-union.

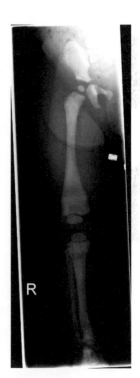

Figure 2.27
Osteopetrosis. Frontal x-ray of the right lower limb demonstrating diffuse bony sclerosis and Erlenmeyer flask deformity of the distal femoral metaphysis.

> **Box 2.24 THE 'BONE WITHIN BONE' APPEARANCE**
>
> Used to describe a radiographic appearance in which one bone appears to arise within another, 'endobone'. It is best seen in the vertebrae.
>
> **Physiological**
> - May be seen in infants and neonates due to new bone formation
>
> **Pathological**
> - Altered bone growth (e.g. nutritional disturbance)
> - Impairment of osteoclastic activity
> - Altered bone metabolism (e.g. sickle cell disease)

SPINE X-RAY (FIGURE 2.28)

- Vertebral endplate sclerosis, 'sandwich sign' (similar to renal osteodystrophy, but sacroiliac joints are spared).

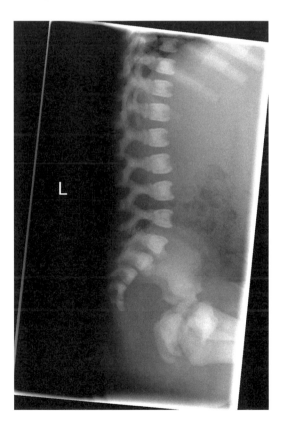

Figure 2.28 Osteopetrosis. Lateral lumbar spine x-ray demonstrating vertebral endplate sclerosis.

CHEST X-RAY

- Check proximal humeri for the Erlenmeyer flask deformity.

BONE MRI

● Bone medulla is low signal on T1 and T2 as normal marrow is replaced by bone.

HEAD CT

● Sclerosis of the skull vault, which may cause hydrocephalus
● Optic nerve atrophy
● Subarachnoid haemorrhage
● Obliteration of the sinuses

OSSIFICATION CENTRES (TABLE 2.8)

Table 2.8 Approximate age of appearance of the elbow ossification centres[a]

Ossification centre	Approximate age of appearance
Capitellum	1 year
Radial head	3 years
Internal epicondyle	5 years
Trochlear	7 years
Olecranon	9 years
External epicondyle	11 years

[a] This is helpful to differentiate normal from a fracture fragment.

OSTEOCHONDRITIS DISSECANS

This is an osteochondral fracture affecting the articular epiphysis that is thought to be due to a combination of trauma and ischaemia. It is more common in males with a mean age of onset of 15 years. It occurs most commonly in the knee (75% medial femoral condyle), talar dome, tibia, patella and femoral head. It is bilateral in up to 25%.

KNEE X-RAY

● Normal initially or joint effusion
● Flattening and cortical irregularity of the lateral surface of the medial femoral condyles
● Detached loose osteochondral fragment (50%)

KNEE MRI

● Useful to determine stability of the lesion and indication for surgical management
● Four features of instability:
    1. High T2 signal between fragment and parent bone
    2. Cartilaginous defect on T1
    3. High signal in the articular cartilage
    4. Cystic lesion between fragment and parent bone (needs to be 5 mm or larger)

OSTEOGENESIS IMPERFECTA

Box 2.25   WORMIAN BONES AND THEIR ASSOCIATION

These are intra-sutural ossicles that give the skull a 'crazy paving' appearance. They are most common in the lambdoid suture. They may be normal up to 6 months of age.

Causes
Pyknodysostosis
Osteogenesis imperfecta (OI)
Rickets (healing phase)
Kinky hair syndrome
Cleidocranial dysostosis
Hypothyroidism/hypophosphatasia
Otopalatodigital syndrome
Pachydermoperiostosis
(Syndrome) of Down

Rare inherited disorder due to a defect in type-1 collagen formation. The result is poor bone density and brittle bones prone to fracture. There are four subtypes of varying severity; type II is the most severe and is frequently fatal *in utero*. Type I is mild, type IV moderate and type III severe (manifest at birth).

APPENDICULAR X-RAY (FIGURE 2.29)

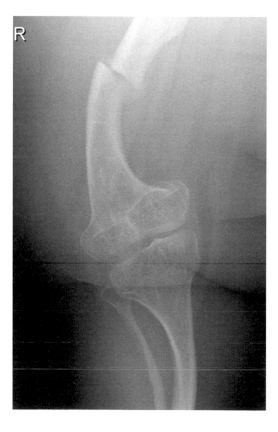

Figure 2.29 Osteogenesis imperfecta. Frontal knee radiograph demonstrating osteopenia, femoral fracture with callus formation and bone deformity with bending and thinning.

- Multiple, repeated, unexplained fractures with minor/no trauma.
- Exuberant callus.
- Fractures typically affect the long bones, spine and apophyses.
- Pseudarthroses.
- Poor bone density.
- Bone deformity—bending and thinning of the long bone diaphysis; may be marked and cause e.g. 'shepherd's crook' deformity of the femur

SKULL X-RAY

- Deformity of the skull (e.g. platybasia, prominent occiput, 'Darth Vader skull')
- Wormian bones (>10)
- Basilar invagination
- Enlarged sinuses and abnormal teeth

SPINE X-RAY

- Compression fractures at multiple levels
- Spondylolysis
- Lumbar hyperlordosis

Box 2.26 OSTEOGENESIS IMPERFECTA OR NON-ACCIDENTAL INJURY (NAI)?

It may be difficult to differentiate NAI from OI. However:
- Fracture location may be atypical for NAI
- Impaired hearing in OI
- Wormian bones
- Blue sclera in OI

PERTHES DISEASE

Legg–Calvé–Perthes disease is a common idiopathic AVN of the capital femoral epiphysis that is more common in boys between 4 and 8 years of age. It is bilateral in up to 20%.

PLAIN FILM (FIGURE 2.30)

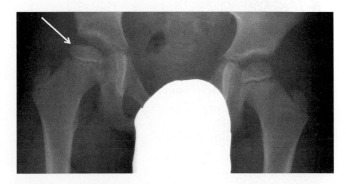

Figure 2.30 Perthes disease. Frontal pelvis radiograph demonstrating subchondral lucency within the right femoral epiphysis (white arrow).

- Subchondral lucency is the earliest sign; the 'crescent sign'.
- In early disease, also look for widening of the medial joint space, a small femoral epiphysis, sclerosis of the femoral head and localised bone demineralisation.
- In late disease, there is fragmentation of the femoral head, subchondral fracture on the anterolateral epiphysis and cysts in the femoral neck.
- Staging:
  - 1—normal radiograph
  - 2—sclerosis and cyst formation
  - 3—loss of structural integrity
  - 4—acetabular involvement

NUCLEAR MEDICINE

- Reduced uptake in early disease.
- Uptake is increased in late disease.

PROGERIA

Very rare autosomal recessive disease, it presents with absence of the adolescent growth spurt and beginning of premature ageing. There is short stature, skin and muscle atrophy and diabetes.

PLAIN FILM

- Resorption of the lateral clavicles
- Narrow chest with thin ribs

PYKNODYSOSTOSIS

This is an autosomal recessive disease that is often diagnosed early in childhood. Patients present with growth retardation/dwarfism, micrognathia, dystrophic nails and characteristic facies (beaked nose, receding jaw and yellowed teeth).

APPENDICULAR X-RAY

- Generalised increased density to the long bones (but medullary cavity is spare, unlike in osteopetrosis).
- Thickened bone cortex.
- Multiple healing fractures of varying ages.
- Short distal phalanges.

FACIAL BONES X-RAY

- Hypoplastic facial bones and sinuses
- Wormian bones
- Brachycephaly
- Widened sutures

CHEST X-RAY

- Resorption of the lateral ends of the clavicles

RADIAL RAY ABSENCE

Absence of the radius with or without absence of the thumb. Causes include:

- VACTERL (vertebral defects, anal atresia, cardiac defects, trachea-oesophogeal fistula, renal abnormalities, and limb abnormalities)
- Holt–Oram syndrome (atrial septal defect and radial ray absence)
- Fanconi anaemia (pancytopenia and radial ray absence)
- Thrombocytopaenia absent radius syndrome
- Trisomies 13 and 18
- Cleidocranial dysostosis

RICKETS

Box 2.27 IMAGING FEATURES OF RICKETS
Reriosteal reaction **I**ndistinct cortex **C**oarse trabeculation **K**nees, wrists and ankles most affected **E**piphyseal plates are widened, epiphyses osteopenic and irregular **T**remendous metaphysis (cupping, splaying and fraying) **S**pur (metaphyseal)

Rickets is essentially osteomalacia occurring in an immature skeleton—by definition, the growth plates must not have fused. The most common underlying cause is a dietary deficiency of vitamin D, which results in a failure of bone mineralisation during bone growth.

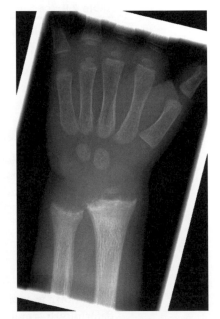

- Hypophosphatasia is a rare inherited metabolic disorder that has similar radiographic features to rickets (see below for an important exception)—it is also associated with craniosynostosis.

APPENDICULAR X-RAY (FIGURE 2.31)
- Widened growth plate in a child is due to rickets until proven otherwise.
- Changes are best seen at the ends of growing bones, particularly the wrists and knees.
- Metaphyses are cupped or splayed.
- Bowing deformity due to softening.
- Coarsened trabeculae.
- Poorly defined epiphysis, which is poorly mineralised.
- Delayed bone age.
- Lucent expansions into the metaphyses (uncalcified bone matrix) suggest hypophosphatasia.

Figure 2.31 Rickets. Frontal wrist radiograph demonstrating metaphyseal cupping and splaying of the ulnar and radius.

SKULL X-RAY

- Delayed closure of the fontanelles
- Craniotabes
- Basilar invagination

PELVIS X-RAY

- Triradiate appearance due to protrusion

CHEST X-RAY

- Enlargement, cupping and fraying of the costochondral junction ('rachitic rosary')

RUBELLA

Patients with postnatal rubella do not generally require imaging. Congenital rubella infection is associated with impaired intra-uterine development and profound malformation and may result in spontaneous abortion or stillbirth.

PLAIN FILM

- Celery stalk appearance—dense femoral diaphysis with alternating lucent/dense lines extending longitudinally through the metaphysis
- No periosteal reaction (distinguishes it from syphilis)

SALTER–HARRIS CLASSIFICATION (TABLE 2.9)

Table 2.9 The Salter–Harris classification of growth plate fractures

Type	Frequency	Description	Mnemonic
I	6%–8%	Slip along the axis of the growth plate	**S**lip
II	75%	Fracture line extends proximally into the metaphysis from the physis	**A**bove growth plate
III	6%–8%	Fracture line extends distally into the epiphysis from the physis (involves articular surface)	**L**ower than growth plate
IV	10%–12%	Fracture line extends from the metaphysis, across the physis and epiphysis	**T**hrough growth plate
V	1%	Crush injury	**R**ammed

Note: Types I and II usually heal without limitation of function; Types III and IV involve the articular surface and so may cause a joint deformity; Type V injuries are likely to affect function of the joint adversely.

SCHEUERMANN DISEASE

Also known as adolescent kyphosis, this is the second most common paediatric spinal deformity. It is more common in boys aged 13–17 years.

PLAIN FILM

- Most common finding is Schmorl nodes and anterior vertebral wedging with disc space narrowing.

- Mostly thoracic (75%).
- Usually three to five vertebral bodies are affected.
- Kyphosis must be >35°.

Box 2.28 SCHMORL NODES
These represent extrusions of the nucleus pulposus through the vertebral body endplate.

SCOLIOSIS

This is an abnormal lateral curvature of the spine of >10°; it is mostly idiopathic and painless (80%). Congenital scoliosis accounts for another 10%. Causes of painful scoliosis include tumour (e.g. osteoid osteoma or GCT), infection, degeneration and trauma. Lateral curvature <10° that is asymptomatic and does not progress is known as spinal asymmetry.

X-RAY

- Mainstay for diagnosis and monitoring is the Cobb angle—the angle made by intersecting lines drawn parallel to the endplate of the superior end vertebra and another drawn parallel to the endplate of the inferior end vertebra.
- The angle is measured in increments of 5°; an increase of ≥5° between radiographs indicates progression.

SCURVY

Box 2.29 DENSE METAPHYSEAL BANDS, 'SCCRROLL'
- **S**curvy - **C**hronic disease - **C**hemotherapy - **R**adiation - **R**ickets - **O**steopetrosis - **L**eukaemia - **L**ead poisoning

Vitamin C deficiency causes abnormal collagen and bone development and bleeding diathesis. Vitamin C is required by osteoblasts to lay down bone matrix; without it, osteoclast resorption stops, although chondrocytes continue to lay down calcification. It does not develop before 4 months of age due to maternal vitamin C levels.

PLAIN FILM

- Earliest signs seen at the knees.
- Ground-glass osteoporosis is characteristic of scurvy (it is often the only sign in adults).
- Sclerosis of the margins of the epiphysis (Wimberger sign) with loss of epiphyseal density.

- Metaphyseal spurs (Pelcan spurs).
- Dense metaphyseal lines (white lines of Frankel) due to a dense zone of provisional calcification.
- Trummerfield zone is a radiolucent zone on the diaphyseal side of the Frankel line.
- 'Pencil point' cortical thinning.
- Corner fractures (Parkes corner sign).
- Exuberant periosteal reaction (secondary to recurrent periosteal bleeding).
- Haemarthorosis.
- 'Hair on end' appearance of the skull vault.

SICKLE CELL DISEASE

This is a haemolytic anaemia resulting from the presence of abnormal β-globin chains within haemoglobin. Musculoskeletal abnormalities may be due to the effects of chronic anaemia (e.g. marrow proliferation/reconversion, extramedullary haematopoiesis or bone softening/infarction) or infection (up to 70% due to *Salmonella*).

APPENDICULAR X-RAY

- Osteopenia and coarsening of the trabeculae
- 'Bone in bone' appearance due to infarctions
- AVN

CHEST X-RAY

- Rib thinning with notching.
- Check the humeral heads for AVN.
- H-shaped ('cod fish') vertebrae due to central vertebral endplate infarction.

SKULL X-RAY

- Skull—widening of the diploe with 'hair on end' striations

NUCLEAR MEDICINE

- Decreased uptake on bone marrow scan, although uptake is increased after collateralisation.

Box 2.30 CAUSES OF AVASCULAR NECROSIS, 'PATCHIS'

- **P**ancreatitis and pregnancy
- **A**lcohol
- **T**rauma
- **C**ushing syndrome
- **H**aematological (sickle and Gaucher)
- **I**diopathic
- **S**teroids (most common cause of shoulder avascular necrosis) and systemic lupus erythematosus

---

SINDING–LARSEN–JOHANSSON DISEASE

Also known as 'jumper's knee', the mechanism of injury is as for Osgood–Schlatter disease, except the abnormality is focused on the site of insertion of the patella tendon to the patella. It is a cause of anterior knee pain in adolescents.

PLAIN FILM

- Calcification in the patella tendon
- Unfused skeleton

MRI

- Focal thickening of the proximal third of the patella tendon (look for thickening >7 mm on sagittal images).
- Prepatellar oedema and increased T2 signal in the proximal tendon.

SLIPPED UPPER FEMORAL EPIPHYSIS (SUFE)

This is the most common hip abnormality affecting adolescents aged 10–16 years. It is more common in boys, obesity, trauma, hypothyroidism, rapid growth spurts, renal osteodystrophy and poor nutrition. It is bilateral in 50%.

PLAIN FILM

- Early slippage best seen on lateral or frog lateral views.
- Femoral head often slips posteriorly first, then medially.
- Line of Klein (drawn along the lateral aspect of the femoral neck should intersect the lateral aspect of the superior femoral epiphysis).
- Look for a widened physis with indistinct margins or reduced epiphyseal height (due to slipping).
- Ill-defined areas of increased opacification (metaphyseal blanch sign) may be seen in the proximal metaphysis, which is thought to represent a healing response.

THALASSAEMIA MAJOR

This is an inherited disorder of haemoglobin synthesis. There is decreased/absent production of β-chains, resulting in marrow hyperactivity and excess production of foetal haemoglobin. Marrow hyperactivity causes marrow hypertrophy, resulting in skull/facial deformities, pathological fractures and retarded growth. Haemoglobinopathy results in extramedullary haematopoiesis and hepatosplenomegaly. See Figure 2.32.

Box 2.31 CAUSES OF A 'HAIR ON END' SKULL
<ul><li>Thalassaemia (look for rodent facies)</li><li>Sickle</li><li>Polycythaemia</li><li>Myelofibrosis</li><li>Spherocytosis</li><li>Leukaemia</li></ul>

CHEST X-RAY

- Posterior mediastinal mass in the mid-lower thorax (i.e. paraspinal mass from extramedullary haematopoiesis)

SKULL X-RAY

- Maxillary hypertrophy and forward placement of the incisors producing 'rodent facies' appearance (considered pathognomic)
- Hypoplastic paranasal sinuses and mastoid air cells
- 'Hair on end' appearance with widening of diplopic spaces in the skull
- Thinned outer skull table

APPENDICULAR X-RAYS

- Osteopenia with thinned cortices and coarse trabeculation
- Mild expansion of the medullary cavities
- Erlenmeyer flask deformity of the femora
- 'Bone within bone' appearance
- Premature fusion of the epiphyses

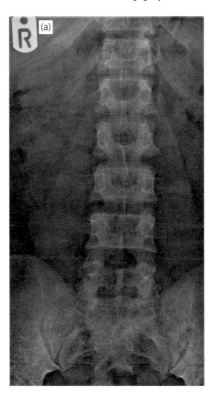 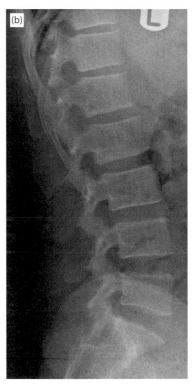

Figure 2.32 Thalassaemia. AP (a) and lateral (b) lumbar spine radiographs demonstrating osteopenia, medullary expansion, thinned cortices and coarsening of the trabeculae.

THANATROPHIC DWARFISM

This is the most common, lethal micromelic dwarfism. It is inherited in an autosomal dominant pattern. X-rays are post-mortem.

SKULL X-RAY

- Premature fusion of the sutures—'cloverleaf skull' (Kleeblattschädel)
- Large skull
- Small foramen magnum
- Small face
- Depressed nasal bridge

CHEST X-RAY

- Short, horizontal ribs and narrowed thorax.
- Costochondral junctions are widened and cupped.

SPINE X-RAY

- Severe platyspondyly, 'wafer thin' on lateral
- 'H-shaped' vertebral bodies on AP radiograph

PELVIS X-RAY

- Short iliac bones
- Horizontal acetabular roofs
- Short and broad ischial bones

LIMB X-RAY

- Marked micromelia
- Irregular flared metaphyses
- Bowed 'telephone receiver' femora (in some)

TRANSIENT SYNOVITIS OF THE HIP

This is the most common cause of a limp in children aged 5–10 years. It is a self-limiting inflammation of the hip synovium. The aetiology is unclear, but may be related to viral infection, previous trauma or allergy. It is important to exclude septic arthritis and juvenile rheumatoid arthritis (RA).

US

- Joint effusion in the anterior recess (capsular distension >2 mm).
- No synovial thickening.
- Effusion resolves after 10–15 days.

TUBEROUS SCLEROSIS

Autosomal dominant inherited syndrome characterised by multi-organ hamartomas. Particularly affects the lungs, central nervous system, heart and kidneys.

PLAIN FILM

- Multiple bone islands—calvarium, vertebrae and long bones
- Thickening of the diploe
- Periosteal thickening in the long bones
- Expansion and sclerosis of the ribs

TURNER SYNDROME

Common chromosomal abnormality due to the absence of genes from the short arm of an X chromosome (i.e. monosomy 45 or X0); only occurs in females. There are numerous associated anomalies; cardiovascular anomalies (e.g. hypoplastic left heart and aortic coarctation) are most serious in early life. Renal anomalies (e.g. ectopia and horseshoe kidney) make patients prone to urinary infections and hypertension.

HAND X-RAY

- Shortened third and fourth metacarpal.
- Shortened second and fifth middle phalanges.
- Madelung deformity; ulna is shortened and the ulna styloid is absent (unlike Down syndrome).
- Positive carpal sign (scaphoid–lunate–triquetrum <117°).
- Osteoporosis (due to gonadal failure).

SPINE X-RAY

- Squared lumbar vertebrae
- Kyphoscoliosis

LIMB X-RAY

- Enlarged medial femoral condyle

CHEST X-RAY

- Thinned ribs

MSK TUMOURS

ANEURYSMAL BONE CYST (ABC)

This is a benign lesion, more common in men aged <30 years (peak age is 16 years). It is a lucent, expansile lesion containing multiple thin-walled, blood-filled cavities. It presents with pain. Giant cell tumours (GCT) are a common differential, but are found in the third or fourth decade.

APPENDICULAR X-RAY (FIGURE 2.33)

- May occur anywhere, but the femur is most commonly affected (then ulna and tibia).
- Lytic, expansile metaphyseal lesion with a thinned cortex and fine internal trabeculation ('soap bubble' appearance).
- Lesion is eccentric and expansion asymmetrical.
- Check for pathological fractures.

SPINE X-RAY

- May be found anywhere in the spine, but more common in the posterior elements (especially the spinous processes).
- May cross intervertebral disc or facet joints.
- Vertebral collapse.

MRI

- Multiple cysts of different signal intensity (i.e. blood products) with a low signal rim and heterogenous enhancement post-gadolinium.
- Fluid-fluid levels within the cysts—non-specific, but if they occupy >70% of the lesion, then ABC is favoured.
- Hyperintense to muscle on T1.
- Heterogenous with areas of low signal intensity on T2.
- Marrow oedema is not typical.

CT

- Check for fluid-fluid levels (also seen in GCTs and teleangiectatic osteosarcoma)
- Assess soft tissue extent of the lesion and internal matrix

BONE DESTRUCTION

The most important distinction is between probably benign versus probably malignant lesions.

GEOGRAPHIC

- Term used to describe marginated or solitary area of bone lucency.
- Margins of the lesion could be traced easily with a pencil line.
- More likely benign.

MOTH-EATEN

- Caused by numerous smaller osteolytic lesions.
- Endosteal excavations.
- Likely malignant.

PERMEATIVE

- Aggressive infiltrative process that causes cortical tunnelling.
- Numerous tiny and indistinct osteolytic lesions with poor margination between abnormal and normal bone.
- Likely malignant.

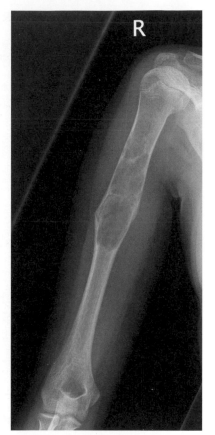

Figure 2.33 Aneurysmal bone cyst. Frontal radiograph of the right humerus demonstrating osteopenia, medullary expansion, thinned cortices and coarsening of the trabeculae.

BONE TUMOUR LOCATION (TABLE 2.10)

Table 2.10 Bone tumours organised by their typical location

Location	Tumour
Epiphysis (including the patella, calcaneum, tarsal and carpal bones)	Chondroblastoma
	Giant cell tumour
	Infection in <2–year-old children and adults
Epiphysis/metaphysis	Giant cell tumour
Metaphysis	Osteosarcoma
	Fibrous cortical defect
	Aneurysmal bone cyst
	Simple bone cyst
	Enchondroma
	Infection aged 2–16 years
Metaphysis/diaphysis	Ewing sarcoma
Diaphysis	Lymphoma
	Metastases
	Enchondroma
	Fibrous dysplasia
	Eosinophilic granuloma
	Chondrosarcoma
	Osteoid osteoma

BROWN TUMOUR

Also known as an osteoclastoma, they are seen in both primary (more commonly) and secondary hyperparathyroidism. The brown tumour is a focus of bone resorption replaced by vascular fibrous tissue. It mimics metastases and myeloma.

PLAIN FILM

- Well-defined, often solitary cortical lesion.
- Lytic and expansile.
- Commonly found in the jaw, rib or pelvis.
- No periosteal reaction.
- After treatment, brown tumours may disappear, be persistently lucent or become sclerotic/calcified.

CHONDROBLASTOMA

This is a rare, benign cartilaginous tumour occurring before growth plate closure. Presentation is with a long history of pain. It may become locally aggressive and rarely metastasises.

PLAIN FILM

- Hallmark is a well-defined osteolytic lesion that is centrally or eccentrically located within the epiphysis or apophysis of a long bone.
- Most common in the femur (33%), then humerus and proximal tibia (20% each).
- Thin sclerotic rim.
- Usually internal matrix is chondroid (i.e. rings and arcs) of calcification.

MRI
- Useful for assessing extension into the metaphysis.
- Lobulated margin of low signal intensity corresponding to the sclerotic margin on the x-ray.
- Low signal lesion on T1, variable on T2 and high on STIR.
- Lesion may contain fluid–fluid levels.
- Florid marrow oedema.

CHONDROMYXOID FIBROMA

This is a rare, benign cartilaginous tumour typically affecting those aged between 30 and 40 years. It presents with pain.

PLAIN FILM
- Well-defined lucent lesion in the metaphysis with a prominent sclerotic rim
- Most common in the proximal tibia
- Geographic bone destruction
- Contains trabeculations and stippled calcification (about 10%)
- No periosteal reaction

MRI
- Useful to demonstrate true tumour extent prior to surgery
- Non-specific low T1 signal, high T2 signal and heterogeneous enhancement with contrast

CHONDROSARCOMA

Most common primary bone tumour in adults; more common in males, with a median age of onset of 45 years. Broad range of behaviour from very slow growing to highly aggressive and metastasising. In total, 90% of cases are 'conventional' chondrosarcomas (other types include dedifferentiated chondrosarcoma, secondary chondrosarcoma, etc.). Hyperglycaemia paraneoplastic syndrome is common (up to 85%).

PLAIN FILM
- Pelvis and femur (40%), spine and ribs (25%), shoulder and proximal humerus (15%).
- Outside the hands and feet chondrosarcoma is five-times more common than enchondroma.
- Central location most common, begins in the metaphysis and extends to diaphysis.
- Well-defined lytic lesion, endosteal scalloping and thinning/destruction of the cortex.
- Internal matrix is chondroid.
- Large lesion (>5 cm).
- Periositis (fluffy or lamellated).
- Soft tissue mass.

MRI

- Gold standard for pre-operative planning and post-operative surveillance.
- Defines extent of the bone and soft tissue lesion.
- Non-specific low signal on T1, high on T2 with enhancement post-contrast.

CHORDOMA

Box 2.32 A DIFFERENTIAL DIAGNOSIS OF SACRAL TUMOURS
Malignant Metastases (most common) Chordoma (most common primary) Myeloma Ewing sarcoma Lymphoma
Benign Giant cell tumour Aneurysmal bone cyst

Excluding lymphoproliferative disorders, this is the most common primary malignant tumour of the spine in adults. It is the most common primary tumour to affect the sacrum. It typically affects men aged 60–70 years and originates from embryonic remnants of the notochord (therefore it is a midline tumour; i.e. sacrum, spine, clivus and coccyx). Rarely metastasises (to the lung).

PLAIN FILM (FIGURE 2.34a)

- Large (average 10 cm) lytic, expansile lesion in the sacrum with moderate internal calcification.
- Sacrum affected most (up to 60%), then clivus/spheno-occipital region (35%).
- Narrow zone of transition.
- Large soft tissue component.
- May extend across the intervertebral disc space or SI joint.

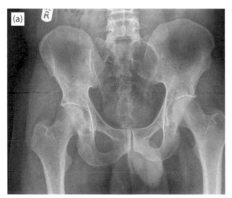
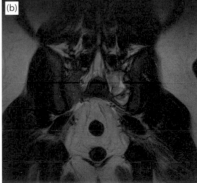

Figure 2.34 (a) Chordoma. Frontal radiograph of the pelvis demonstrating a lytic expansile lesion of the left sacrum. (b) Chordoma. Coronal T2-weighted magnetic resonance image of the pelvis demonstrating a lobulated high-signal mass involving the left sacrum.

CT

- Bone destruction with lobulated soft tissue mass.
- Mass is mixed density with areas of low attenuation (myxoid) and calcifications.
- Enhances modestly with contrast.

MRI (FIGURE 2.34b)

- Lobulated sacral mass high signal on T2 with foci of T1 high signal (internal haemorrhage and calcification)—this is relatively specific.

NUCLEAR MEDICINE

- Poor uptake of technetium-99m–DTPA (diethylenetriaminepentacetate)

ENCHONDROMA

This is a common, benign cystic cartilaginous lesion of the medullary cavity. It is found most commonly in the metacarpals and also long bones. Rarely becomes malignant (chondrosarcoma).

OLLIER DISEASE

Numerous enchondromas, particularly in the hands, this is often unilateral and monomelic (affects one limb only). It causes pain and deformity (including Madelung) and there is an increased risk of malignant transformation (osteosarcoma for young adults, chondrosarcoma or fibrosarcoma for older adults). It is associated with juvenile granulosa cell ovarian tumours.

MAFFUCCI SYNDROME

Numerous enchondromas with haemangiomas and lymphangiomas. It also tends to be unilateral. Complications are similar to those of Ollier disease. There is an increased risk of malignant transformation (mostly chondrosarcoma) compared to Ollier disease.

Plain film (Figure 2.35)

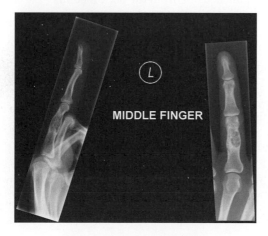

Figure 2.35 Enchondroma. Frontal and lateral radiographs of the left middle finger demonstrating a lytic expansile lesion within the proximal phalanx with a narrow zone of transition and a chondroid matrix.

- Originate in the metaphysis.
- Well-defined lucent lesion with ground-glass matrix (occasionally chondroid matrix).
- Thinning, expansion and occasionally disappearance of the cortex.

- Usually smaller than 3 cm.
- Pathological fracture.
- Outside the hands and feet, chondrosarcoma is five-time more common than enchondroma.
- Frank cortical destruction, a lesion >5 cm or a soft tissue mass suggests malignancy.

EOSINOPHILIC GRANULOMA

This is a disease of immune regulation resulting in excessive histiocytes and granuloma formation. Eosinophilic granuloma is the term given to Langerhans cell histiocytosis localised to either the bone or lung. It is a monostotic disease affecting young children (5–10 years of age). Patients present with pain and a mass, and back pain or scoliosis if there is spinal involvement.

SKULL X-RAY

- 50% involve the skull (25% axial skeleton).
- Well-defined lytic lesion, 'punched out' of the parietal or temporal bone.
- The edges of the lesion have a scalloped appearance.
- The lytic lesion is associated with a soft tissue mass.

SPINE X-RAY

- Complete collapse (vertebra plana) of a thoracic spine vertebral body.
- Posterior elements rarely involved.
- No kyphosis, disc spaces normal.
- Eosinophilic granuloma/Langerhans cell histiocytosis is the most common cause of vertebral collapse in children.

APPENDICULAR X-RAY

- Affects the diaphysis.
- Well-defined lucency 'punched out' from the bone medulla.
- Surrounded by dense sclerosis and mature periosteal new bone.

CT

- Shows a soft tissue mass enhancing within the area of bone lysis.

MRI

- Soft tissue mass is high signal on T1 due to histiocyte content.

EPIDERMOID CYST

Intraosseous epidermoid cysts are rare, benign and slow growing. Radiographic features are non-specific.

PLAIN FILM

- Well-defined lucent lesion with mild expansion, thinned cortex and a thin rim of sclerosis.
- The skull and terminal phalynx are the preferred sites.

EWING SARCOMA

Second most common primary bone tumour of children and adolescents (after osteosarcoma). It accounts for 10% of primary bone tumours, and 95% occur between 4 and 25 years of age (peak 10–15 years of age). Patients commonly present with a >6–month history of pain and swelling with or without fever.

PLAIN FILM (FIGURE 2.36)

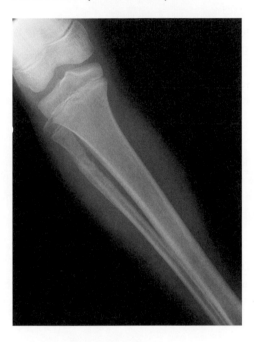

Figure 2.36 Ewing sarcoma. Frontal radiograph of the tibia/fibula demonstrating a lesion within the metadiaphyseal region of the fibula with a permeative appearance, wide zone of transition and periostitis.

- 75% are found in the pelvis and long bones (if the spine is involved, it is usually the sacrum, 6% overall).
- Overall most common is the metadiaphyseal region of the femur.
- Permeative or moth-eaten osteolysis.
- Poor margination (wide zone of transition).
- Cortical erosion.
- Exuberant periostitis (lamellated or sunburst).
- Soft tissue mass.

MRI

- Marrow replacement, cortical destruction and soft tissue mass.
- Lesion is intermediate on T1 and T2 and there is diffuse or peripheral enhancement with contrast.

NUCLEAR MEDICINE

- Increased tracer uptake on scintigraphy, gallium scan and positron emission tomography (PET).
- PET/CT is highly sensitive (88%) for staging and restaging.

FIBROUS CORTICAL DEFECTS

These are found in up to 40% of children aged <2 years; 95% are seen in those aged under 20 years of age. After 30 years of age, they are rare. They are benign, asymptomatic and regress spontaneously. Lesions >2 cm are known as non-ossifying fibroma. Most affect a single bone, 25% are polyostotic (associated with neurofibromatosis, fibrous dysplasia or Jaffe–Campanacci syndrome).

PLAIN FILM

- Well-defined lytic lesion with a thin sclerotic border in the metaphysis of a long bone.
- 80% lower extremity (particularly around the knee).
- May be expansile.
- Aligned along the axis of the bone.
- If >3.3 cm and occupying more than half of the bone diameter, they should be follow-up.

FIBROUS DYSPLASIA

Relatively common idiopathic skeletal disorder (sometimes called Lichtenstein–Jeffe disease), it typically presents in adolescents and young adults. Caused by fibroblast proliferation and maturation in the bone medulla. May be monostotic (affects a single bone most commonly) or polyostotic.

PLAIN FILM

- Wide range of appearances.
- Typically a well-defined lesion centred on the bone medulla, which has a uniform ground-glass internal density and may be surrounded by a thick sclerotic margin ('rind').
- Diaphyseal location.
- May contain internal calcification 'popcorn'.
- Bone cortex may be scalloped.
- Bone expansion.
- Pathological fractures and bone deformity are common (e.g. Shepherd's crook deformity of the proximal femur).
- Lesions may increase in size with pregnancy.

MRI

- T1—isointense with areas of hypointensity, patchy enhancement post-contrast
- T2—heterogeneously hyperintense

MONOSTOTIC

Accounts for up to 80% of fibrous dysplasia, it presents at between 5 and 15 years of age (75% by <30 years of age). It presents with pain or pathological fracture and rarely becomes malignant (<1%).

FEATURES

- Most commonly affects the ribs (most common benign rib tumour).
- Femur (proximal most), tibia and craniofacial bones are next most common.
- Commonly affects the proximal femur, then distal femur.

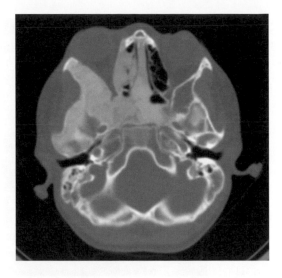

Figure 2.37 Leontiasis ossea. Axial CT image of the facial bones demonstrating asymmetrical cortical thickening/ground-glass appearance of the right facial bones with obliteration/ involvement of the sphenoid and ethmoid sinuses.

- Craniofacial fibrous dysplasia may give the leontiasis ossea appearance (Figure 2.37).
- Obliteration of the paranasal sinuses.

Box 2.33 FIBROUS DYSPLASIA IN THE SKULL

Features distinguishing fibrous dysplasia in the skull from Paget disease.
- Ground glass is characteristic of fibrous dysplasia.
- Asymmetrical distribution.
- Presence of a soft tissue mass.
- Cyst-like changes.
- Thickness of the cranial cortices.
- Involvement of the facial bones (maxilla, sphenoid, orbits and nasal cavity).
- Obliteration of paranasal sinuses.

POLYOSTOTIC

Accounts for up to 30% of fibrous dysplasia; 90% affect one limb only. Symptoms are pain, limp and fracture. See Figure 2.38.

FEATURES

- Presents early in life (mean 8 years of age).
- McCune–Albright syndrome consists of two of polyostotic fibrous dysplasia, café au lait spots and endocrine dysfunction (particularly precocious puberty).

CHERUBISM

This is a familial form of fibrous dysplasia inherited by autosomal dominance.

- Characterised by bilateral expansile lesions in the mandible associated with multilocular cystic areas.

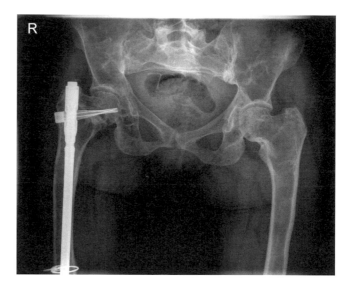

Figure 2.38 Polyostotic fibrous dysplasia (McCune–Albright syndrome). Frontal radiograph of the pelvis demonstrating a right intramedullary femoral nail and multiple lytic expansile lesions with a ground-glass appearance and cortical scalloping.

MAZABRAUD SYNDROME

Rare association of fibrous dysplasia with soft tissue myxoma. It is non familial and more common in women.

MRI

- Myxoma most commonly found in the thigh.
- Appears as a well-defined lesion with signal intensity similar to water, often has a fat rind.
- Adjacent muscle high signal on T2 images.
- Moderately intense heterogeneous enhancement.
- Reported cases of malignant change to osteosarcoma.

GANGLION CYSTS

Benign bone lesion containing mucous material. May be intra-articular, extra-articular, intra-osseous and periosteal.

PLAIN FILM

- Intra-osseous ganglia are well-defined lucent lesions near a joint, sclerotic margin, most <5 cm in size.

MRI

- T1—low to intermediate signal.
- T2—high signal.
- With or without communication to a joint.
- Internal septations.
- Periosteal new bone formation occurs with periosteal ganglia.

GIANT CELL TUMOUR (GCT)

Relatively common benign tumour (accounts for 20% of all benign bone tumours) composed of stromal cells and multinucleated giant cells that behave like osteoclasts. Slightly more common in females; 80% occur between 20 and 50 years of age. May occur with Paget disease. They are locally aggressive in behaviour, and recurrence is up to 30% after resection. GCTs can metastasise to the lungs in up to 6% (may not require treatment). Rarely (<1%) GCTs undergo malignant transformation (usually to high-grade sarcoma).

PLAIN FILM (FIGURE 2.39)

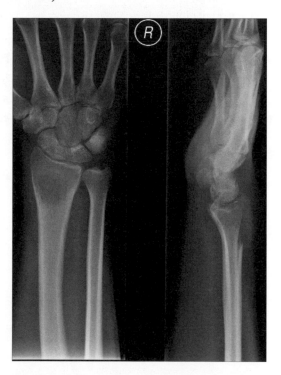

Figure 2.39 Giant cell tumour. Frontal and lateral radiographs of the wrist demonstrating a lucent expansile lesion with a narrow zone of transition within the distal radius. The dorsal cortex is involved, but there is no perisoteal reaction and no associated soft tissue mass.

- Up to 90% are seen in long bones (most commonly distal femur, proximal tibia and distal radius).
- More common in the spine when there is Paget disease—usually the sacrum or a vertebral body are affected.
- Lucent lesion with a well-defined non-sclerotic margin, eccentric location.
- Extends to the subchondral (i.e. subarticular) bone.
- Mild expansion of the affected bone.
- No internal matrix calcification.
- With or without pathological fracture.
- Can have aggressive features: wide zone of transition, cortical destruction, soft tissue mass.

MRI

- Non-specific features: mainly low signal on T1 and T2, enhancement with contrast.
- Heterogeneous low signal on T2 in a whorled or uniform pattern from cellularity and deposition of haemosiderin and collagen.
- Sharp low signal rim due to haemosiderin.
- Fluid–fluid levels are seen in up to 14% from formation of a secondary ABC.

NUCLEAR MEDICINE

- Increased uptake of technetium-99m methylene diphosphonate at the periphery of the lesion.
- Central photopoenia due to lysis/necrosis.

GIANT CELL TUMOUR OF THE TENDON SHEATH

Painless, benign extra-articular proliferation of synovial tissue, considered to be an extra-articular PVNS. More common in females aged 40–50 years and commonly affects the hands and feet (most commonly a soft tissue mass here after a ganglion).

US

- Solid hypoechoic mass with vascularity typically adjacent to the flexor tendons of the hands.

MRI

- Mass is low signal on T1 and T2 due to haemosiderin (relatively specific).
- Homogeneous enhancement of the mass.

PLAIN FILM

- Bone erosion is associated with the mass in up to 15%.
- Mass is usually not calcified.

HAEMANGIOMA

Common, benign vascular malformation; may arise in any organ. The vertebral bodies and skull are the most commonly affected bones. Usually asymptomatic, but a rare cause of cord compression from haemorrhage or soft tissue extension.

PLAIN FILM

- Mildly expansile.
- Thoracic spine is typical.
- Coarse vertical trabeculations, 'corduroy appearance'.
- Paget disease has a similar appearance, but the cortex is spared with a haemangioma.

CT

- 'Polka dot' appearance on axial slices

MRI

- Vertical trabecular thickening
- High signal on T1 and T2 from intratumoural fat (variable)

INTRAOSSEOUS LIPOMA

Rare (<0.5% of bone tumours) lesions more common from 40–50 years of age; commonly present with pain. Typically found in the metadiaphyses of the long bones, particularly the intertrochanteric/subtrochanteric femur. Rarely become malignant.

PLAIN FILM

- Lucent lesion with a thin sclerotic margin
- Occasionally lobular or intraosseous ridge
- Lucent lesion + thin sclerotic margin + central calcified nidus = intraosseous lipoma

CT

- Lesion is fat dense (-60 to -100 HU).
- Resorption of trabeculae.

MRI

- Signal characteristics of fat differentiate it from a simple bone cyst (lipoma high T1 signal, cyst high T2 signal).
- Cystic centre.
- Low signal intensity rim (sclerosis).

MALIGNANT FIBROUS HISTIOCYTOMA (MFH)

Also known as pleomorphic sarcoma, this is the most common primary malignant soft tissue tumour of adulthood (>40 years of age). It is aggressive and presents with an enlarging, painless intramuscular thigh mass. Treatment is with excision. MFH may metastasise to the lungs.

MRI

- Intramuscular mass with non-specific signal characteristics.
- Foci of calcification are low signal on T1 and T2.
- Foci of haemorrhage (may be high signal on T1) and necrosis (high signal on T2).
- Peripheral/nodular enhancement with contrast.

NUCLEAR MEDICINE

- Bone scans are sensitive for detecting bone metastases.

METASTASES

Bone metastases tend to involve the axial skeleton rather than the appendicular skeleton as it is richer in red marrow. Carcinoma of the bronchus is the tumour most associated with bone metastases (accounts for 50% of all bone metastases).

PLAIN FILM/CT

- Lytic or sclerotic.
- Diaphyseal location favours metastases over primary bone tumour.
- Sites especially prone to malignant pathological fracture are the subtrochanteric femur and lesser trochanter.

MRI

- Non-specific signal characteristics, low on T1 and high on T2.
- Differential includes metastases, myeloma and lymphoma.
- Involvement of the posterior elements (i.e. pedicles) of a vertebral body suggests metastases.
- Soft tissue masses are non-specific for metastases and myeloma.

NUCLEAR MEDICINE

- Overall, the most common site for metastatic bone disease is the anterior aspect of the vertebral body (Table 2.11).

Table 2.11 The typical characteristics of bone metastases; lytic lesions may sclerose in response to treatment

Lytic	Lytic expansile	Lytic/sclerotic	Sclerotic
Colon	Renal	Breast	Prostate
Lung	Thyroid		Breast
	Pheochromocytoma		Bladder
	Melanoma		Carcinoid

MULTIPLE MYELOMA

Multiple myeloma is a cancer of the plasma cells found in bone marrow. It accounts for 10% of haematological malignancy with peak age of 65 years. Plasma cell proliferation destroys the bone, causing pain and releasing calcium. Infiltration may be focal, diffuse or variegated.

PLAIN FILM (FIGURE 2.40)

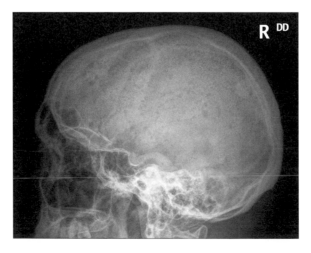

Figure 2.40 Multiple myeloma. Lateral skull radiograph demonstrating multiple well-defined, 'punched out' lucent lesions in keeping with the so-called pepperpot skull.

- Well-demarcated, radiolucent lesions of uniform size without a sclerotic border.
- May be symmetrical and associated with osteopenia.
- Endosteal cortical scalloping.
- Bones involved in haematopoiesis are more commonly affected: spine, skull, ribs, pelvis and femoral and humeral shafts.
- The shoulders, elbows, distal clavicles, acromion, glenoid and ulnar olecranon are also often affected.
- Mandibular involvement favours myeloma over metastases.
- Associated with plasmacytomas—these are solitary bone lesions found in the spine (spares posterior elements), pelvis and ribs that may be expansile.

MRI

- Lesions appear similar to marrow oedema, but enhance with gadolinium.
- Lesions restrict on diffusion-weighted imaging.
- Whole-body diffusion-weighted imaging is now used for diagnosis and response to treatment assessment.

NUCLEAR MEDICINE

- Radionuclide examinations are often negative in myeloma due to the lack of osteoblastic activity.

OSTEOBLASTOMA

This is a rare, benign bone tumour, with 90% occurring between 20 and 30 years of age. It is similar histologically to osteoid osteoma. The central nidus is typically >1.5 cm and of variable appearance, ranging from lytic to densely sclerotic. Up to 40% are found in the spine, mostly the posterior elements.

PLAIN FILM

- Well-defined expansile lesion in the posterior elements of the spine is typical.
- Matrix calcification.
- Frequently associated with an extra-cortical mass.

MRI

- Non-specific low signal on T1 and high signal on T2 with mild marrow oedema

NUCLEAR MEDICINE

- Intense uptake on bone scan

OSTEOCHONDROMA

Most common benign bone tumour (up to 50% of benign lesions) and constitutes up to 15% of all bone tumours. It is composed of cortical and medullary bone with an overlying hyaline cartilage cap. The pathognomic feature is continuity of the lesion ('exostosis') with the native bone cortex and medulla. The lower limb is most commonly affected, typically the distal femur. Fractures, neurological and vascular compromise and malignant transformation are complications.

SOLITARY OSTEOCHONDROMA

Usually incidental, may present with a painless, enlarging deformity. About 1% become malignant.

Plain film

- Cortical and medullary bone protruding from a bone (more difficult to appreciate if arising from a flat bone).
- Tends to be directed away from the joint (due to tendon/muscle forces).
- Cartilaginous cap that may contain chondroid calcification.
- Benign lesions can reach 10 cm in size.
- Continued lesion growth, particularly of the cartilage cap, is suggestive of malignancy.
- Cartilage cap should not exceed 1.5 cm after skeletal maturation.

CT

- Gold standard for demonstrating the characteristic cortical and medullary continuity of the lesion.
- Also sensitive for demonstrating the cartilaginous cap.

DIAPHYSEAL ACLASIS

Rare, also known as hereditary multiple osteochondromatosis; it is inherited by autosomal dominance. Most patients are diagnosed by 5 years of age. There is short stature in 40%. About 5% become malignant.

Plain film

- Humerus and knees involved in nearly all cases
- May be bilateral and symmetrical

DYSPLASIA EPIPHYSEALIS HEMIMELICA

Very rare autosomal dominant disease, also known as Trevor disease, it is an osteochondroma arising from an epiphysis. It presents in young children (up to 4 years of age) due to gait disturbance.

Plain film

- Premature appearance of an ossification centre that is enlarged, asymmetrical and contains stippled calcification.
- Physis may close early and the lesion then appears like any other exostosis.
- Usually affects multiple epiphyses in the same limb, most commonly the ankle region.
- Often restricted to either the medial or lateral side of the limb (hence hemimelic).

BIZARRE PAROSTEAL OSTEOCHONDROMATOUS PROLIFERATION

Osteochondroma-like lesion (also known as a Nora lesion) that is more common from 30–40 years of age. It is characterised by the presence of heterotopic ossification arising from but not disrupting the cortical bone. Unlike an exostosis, there is no medullary continuity.

Plain film
- Soft tissue swelling then florid periostitis (aggressive pattern).
- Similar appearance to a broad-based exostosis, but not angulated away from the joint and no medullary continuity.

OSTEOID OSTEOMA

Common benign bone lesion composed of a central core of vascular osteoid tissue and peripheral sclerosis. It classically presents with pain that is worse at night and effectively relieved by salicylates (i.e. aspirin). More common in males (three-fold) and between 10 and 30 years of age. Responds well to thermal ablation.

PLAIN FILM (FIGURE 2.41)

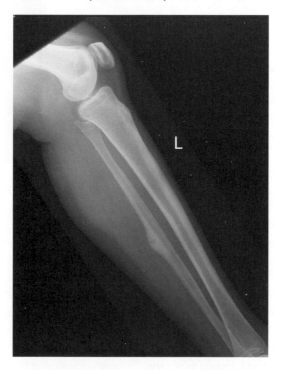

Figure 2.41 Osteoid osteoma. Lateral radiograph of the tibia/fibula demonstrating a small focal lucent lesion within the mid-left fibula cortex with surrounding sclerosis.

- Small lucent lesion (<1.5 cm) surrounded by reactive sclerosis, most commonly found in the bone cortex.
- Femoral neck is the most common location (also typically tibia, humerus, hands, feet and spine).
- The posterior elements (e.g. pedicle) of the spine are affected more commonly, and it causes a painful scoliosis.

CT
- Well-demarcated, low-attenuation lesion surrounded by sclerosis

MRI
- Prompt arterial enhancement
- Intermediate signal intensity nidus with marked enhancement post-contrast

NUCLEAR MEDICINE

- 'Double density' sign: focus of very high tracer uptake surrounded by a diffuse area of more modest tracer uptake

OSTEOSARCOMA

Most common primary bone tumour in children and adolescents; overall, second most common primary bone tumour after myeloma. There is a second peak between 70 and 80 years of age due to malignant transformation of Paget disease (i.e. secondary osteosarcoma). 'Conventional' primary osteosarcoma is most common; other subtypes include small cell, telangiectatic, low-grade central osteosarcoma and surface types (parosteal, periosteal, etc.). Treatment is a combination of surgery and chemotherapy.

CHEST X-RAY

- Check for lung metastases (may be dense).

APPENDICULAR X-RAY (FIGURE 2.42)

- Ill-defined lytic/sclerotic metaphyseal lesion in the distal femur or anteromedial tibia.
- Internal osteoid matrix (characteristic and needed for a histological diagnosis).
- Florid, aggressive periostitis—sunburst, 'hair on end' or Codman's triangle.
- Soft tissue mass containing speckles of calcification.
- Telangiectatic osteosarcoma mimics an ABC or GCT.

MRI

- Lesion is high signal on T2 and contains foci of high signal on T1 (haemorrhage).

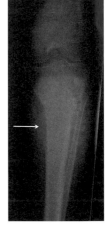

Figure 2.42 Osteosarcoma. Frontal radiograph of the left knee demonstrating an ill-defined lytic/sclerotic lesion within the metaphyseal region of the proximal tibia. There is a florid periostitis with Codman's triangle identified (white arrow).

PERIOSTEAL REACTION (TABLE 2.12)

Table 2.12 Characteristics of benign and malignant periostitis

Benign (never malignant)	Aggressive (may not be malignant)
Soap bubble	Codman's triangle (periosteum elevated)
Thick/dense	Lamellated
Wavy	Multi-layered, 'onion skin'
	Sunray
	Spiculated, 'hair on end'

Note: The periosteum has time to form new periosteum in benign processes, hence the periosteum is thickened and dense. There is no time for the periosteum to consolidate in aggressive disease.

SACROCOCCYGEAL TERATOMA

This is the most common solid tumour in newborns. It is more common in girls (however, it is rare) and is generally benign. There is an association with other congenital abnormalities: spinal dysraphism, sacral agenesis, hydronephrosis, imperforate anus and gastroschisis. The majority present in the first few days of life.

CT

- Mostly cystic, may contain foci of bone, calcification and fat
- Coccyx always involved

MRI

- High signal on T2 (cystic components), foci of high signal on T1 (fat), bone/calcification usually signal void.
- Malignant lesions extend into the adjacent soft tissues and may metastasise.

SCLEROTIC VERSUS NON-SCLEROTIC RIM LESIONS (TABLE 2.13)

Table 2.13 Lucent bone lesions with and without sclerotic margination

Sclerotic rim	Non-sclerotic rim
Simple bone cyst	Giant cell tumour
Chondroblastoma	Aneurysmal bone cyst
Chondromyxoid fibroma	Brown tumour
Fibrous dysplasia	
Fibrous cortical defect	
Epidermoid cyst	

SIMPLE BONE CYST

Also known as a unicameral bone cyst, it is more common in males and most common from 4–10 years of age (70%).

PLAIN FILM (FIGURE 2.43)

- Central metaphyseal/diaphyseal lesion in a long tubular bone (especially proximal humerus, proximal femur and tibia).
- It is a well-defined lucency lying in the long axis of the bone and marginated by a thin sclerotic rim.
- The bone is typically mildly expanded (symmetrical).
- Look for a fracture and subsequent 'fallen fragment'.

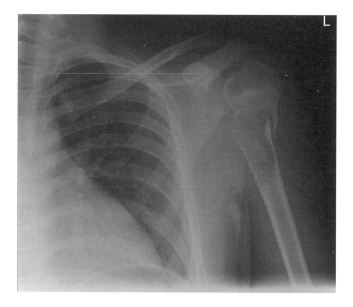

Figure 2.43 Simple bone cyst. Frontal radiograph of the left shoulder demonstrating a lucent expansile lesion with a narrow zone of transition centred on the metadiaphyseal region. There is an associated fracture with a fragment at the inferior aspect of the lesion in keeping with a 'fallen fragment' sign that is pathognomonic of a simple bone cyst.

SYNOVIAL CELL CARCINOMA

Relatively common primary soft tissue malignancy; the typical age at presentation is 15–35 years. Patients present with a slow-growing soft tissue mass, most commonly at the knee.

PLAIN FILM

- Often normal, especially with small lesions.
- 30% of lesions contain calcification.
- Periostitis (non-aggressive appearance) of the underlying bone indicates bone involvement.

MRI

- Multi-lobulated soft tissue mass, heterogeneous T1 and T2 signal
- May contain fluid–fluid levels
- Prominent heterogeneous enhancement with contrast

CHAPTER 3

Gastrointestinal

GASTROINTESTINAL (GI) TRACT

ACHALASIA

The myenteric plexus (of Auerbach) at the gastro-oesophageal junction (GOJ) degenerates, resulting in failure of GOJ relaxation. However, the whole oesophagus is abnormal. The GOJ only opens when pressure in the distal oesophagus exceeds that in the stomach. Causes are primary (e.g. idiopathic, affects young patients) or secondary (e.g. tumour infiltration of the myenteric plexus). Malignancy occurs in about 5% of patients with primary achalasia.

BARIUM SWALLOW (FIGURE 3.1)

- Starts with defective peristalsis and mild narrowing at GOJ.
- Then 'bird's beak' at GOJ coupled with a dilated, aperistaltic oesophagus. Warm water provokes the GOJ to open.
- Food residue builds up in the oesophagus → risk of aspiration and malignancy.

AMOEBIC COLITIS

Only causes colitis when it is invasive. An amoeboma is a mass of granulation tissue that mimics cancer and causes an irregular luminal stricture. It forms in about 10%.

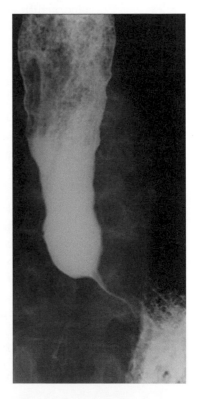

Figure 3.1 Achalasia. Barium swallow demonstrating a dilated oesophagus with a smooth stricture at the gastro-oesophageal junction with a 'bird's beak' appearance.

CT

- The classic appearance is a coned caecum.
- The terminal ileum is spared.

Box 3.1 CAUSES OF A 'CONED' CAECUM

- Tuberculosis
- Crohn disease
- Carcinoma
- Amoebiasis

ANNULAR PANCREAS

This is a relatively common congenital abnormality that is usually asymptomatic. It may present with abdominal pain, vomiting or pancreatitis. The problem is a ring of pancreatic tissue encircling the duodenum secondary to the abnormal migration of the ventral pancreas. It may result in duodenal obstruction, usually at the second part of the duodenum. It is commonly associated with congenital abnormalities including Down syndrome, tetralogy of Fallot, duodenal atresia and imperforate anus.

PLAIN FILM

- Double bubble appearance of duodenal obstruction

BARIUM FOLLOW-THROUGH

- Narrowing of the second part of the duodenum
- Prominent notching of the lateral wall of second part of the duodenum (D2)

MAGNETIC RESONANCE CHOLANGIOPANCREATOGRAPHY (MRCP)

- 'Crocodile jaw' of pancreatic tissue extending anterior and posterior to the duodenum (incomplete annular pancreas).
- If pancreatic tissue completely encircles the duodenum, it is a 'complete' annular pancreas.
- Check for pancreatitis and pancreas divisum.

AORTOENTERIC FISTULA

May be primary (e.g. due to abdominal aortic aneurysm) or more commonly secondary (e.g. post-aortic repair). The third to fourth part of the duodenum is commonly affected. A smaller 'herald' bleed tends to precede massive GI haemorrhage.

CT

- Periaortic/perigraft gas >3 months after surgery/intervention
- Disruption of the aortic wall
- Pseudoaneurysm
- Extravasation of contrast to the bowel lumen

APPENDICITIS

This is a common surgical emergency that is slightly more common in teenaged/young adult males.

PLAIN FILM

- Cecal wall thickening.
- Small bowel dilatation.
- Focal extraluminal gas.
- Rarely, a faecolith is visible.

US

- Frequently used to investigate complicated appendicitis (e.g. abscess) or alternative diagnoses (e.g. ovarian cyst).
- Look for an appendix with diameter of >6 mm and wall thickness >2 mm.
- Findings to suggest perforation: fluid collection adjacent to the appendix, gas bubbles near the appendix and loss of visualisation of the submucosal layer.

CT

- Dilated, thick-walled appendix.
- Inflammatory fat stranding.
- Rim-enhancing fluid collection (i.e. abscess).
- Peri-appendiceal gas locules (localised perforation).
- Small bowel dilatation.
- Note—in patients >50 years of age, consider appendix mucocele (can be benign or malignant); wall calcification is specific but not sensitive for this.

ATROPHIC GASTRITIS

This is atrophy of gastric glands and inflammatory change; 90% of cases are due to pernicious anaemia secondary to B12 deficiency.

BARIUM MEAL

- Tubular, narrowed, featureless stomach
- Loss of rugae
- Smooth greater curve

Box 3.2 CAUSES OF THICKENED GASTRIC FOLDS (DEFINED AS >3–5 MM IN THE DISTAL PREPYLORIC STOMACH AND >8–10 MM IN THE FUNDUS)

- Most common is alcoholic gastritis.
- Most common neoplasm is lymphoma.
- Inflammatory causes: Zollinger–Ellison syndrome, eosinophilic enteritis, Crohn disease, sarcoidosis, *Helicobacter pylori*, Menetrier disease.

BARRETT OESOPHAGUS

Chronic reflux causes metaplasia of the normal squamous epithelium so it becomes columnar. Diagnosis is made by endoscopy and biopsy; >2 cm of metaplasia is diagnostic. Barrett oesophagus is linked to a 40-fold increased risk of oesophageal cancer. The immediate precursor is high-grade dysplasia. See Table 3.1 for causes of benign oesophageal strictures.

Table 3.1 Causes of benign oesophageal strictures by site affected

Lower oesophagus	**Reflux stricture**
	Scleroderma
	Long-term nasogastric tube
	Zollinger–Ellison syndrome
Mid and upper oesophagus	**Barrett oesophagus**
	Caustic ingestion
	Mediastinal radiotherapy
	Skin disease (e.g. epidermolysis bullosa, pemphigoid, erythema multiforme)
Others	**Crohn disease**
	Candida oesophagitis
	Behçet disease

BARIUM SWALLOW

- Classic appearance is a wide, 'patulous' hiatal segment with an accompanying hiatus hernia.
- Long stricture in the mid or lower oesophagus.
- Large, deep, solitary ulcer (Barrett ulcer).
- Fine reticular pattern.
- Thickened, irregular mucosal folds.
- Fine granular mucosal pattern.

Box 3.3   CAUSES OF OESOPHAGEAL STRICTURE BY THE LENGTH OF THE STRICTURE

- Long
  - Caustic
  - Radiation
  - NG tube
- Short
  - Reflux/Barrett disease
  - Drug
  - Carcinoma

BEHÇET DISEASE

Rare, more common in those of Turkish descent. It mimics ileocecal tuberculosis (TB) and Crohn disease. It is a chronic granulomatous disease causing a lymphocytic vasculitis.

CT

- Oedematous terminal ileum with large penetrating ulcers.
- Check for perforation or fistulation.

BENIGN DUODENAL POLYPS

Unlike the stomach, duodenal polyps are usually adenomas and are precursors to adenocarcinoma. The more distal the polyp, the more likely it is to be an adenoma or villous adenoma. GI stromal tumour (GIST) and pancreatic rests can occur anywhere in the duodenum, but are more common in the proximal half of the duodenum. Patients with Gardner syndrome and familial adenomatous polyposis (FAP) are more likely to have duodenal polyps.

BARIUM FOLLOW-THROUGH

- Cauliflower/soap bubble filling defect (shouldering suggests malignancy).
- May be sessile.
- Multiple intraluminal polyps suggest a polyposis syndrome.
- The more distal the lesion, the greater the importance.

CT

- Check for lymph node enhancement—this would favour malignancy.

BENIGN GASTRIC ULCERATION

In total, 95% of cases are benign and most are secondary to *Helicobacter pylori* (alcohol and non-steroidal anti-inflammatory drugs [NSAIDs] are responsible for the remainder).

BARIUM MEAL

- Benign ulcers are mostly found on the lesser curve (NSAIDs and malignant ulcers tend to affect the greater curve, 'sump ulcer').
- Barium collects in a round/oval pit on the dependent wall.
- Penetration sign—ulcer projects beyond the gastric lumen when viewed in profile.
- Smooth gastric fold extending to the edge of the ulcer crater.
- Areae gastricae and rugae are seen within the oedema up to the ulcer crater (otherwise, malignancy is suggested).
- Hampton's line = narrow lucent line (1–2 mm) crossing the neck of the ulcer—indicates a benign ulcer.
- Aphthous ulcers are up to 2 mm in size, shallow and usually due to *H. pylori*.
- The most reliable sign of a benign ulcer is healing after treatment.
- Malignant ulcers rarely heal and are eccentric in a tumour mound—other signs include the 'Carman meniscus', absent Hampton line, etc.

BEZOARS

These are masses of accumulated ingested material, mostly seen as a complication of gastric surgery. Phytobezoars are most common—they are balls of partly digested fibre and vegetable matter. Trichobezoars are typically larger and made of hair.

BARIUM MEAL

- Mobile, intraluminal filling defects.
- Mottled appearance.
- Dilated bowel loops—bezoars can obstruct.

BOERHAAVE SYNDROME

About 15% of oesophageal perforations spontaneously arise from vigorous vomiting (Boerhaave syndrome). Such cases present with chest pain and dysphagia. A partial-thickness tear (Mallory–Weiss syndrome) is associated with blood-tinged vomiting and chest pain. Iatrogenic injury is the most common cause of oesophageal perforation.

PLAIN FILM/CT (FIGURES 3.2 AND 3.3)

- Pneumomediastinum and subcutaneous emphysema.
- Pleural effusion or hydropneumothorax.
- Left lower lobe atelectasis.
- Widening of the mediastinum may accompany the development of mediastinitis or mediastinal haematoma.

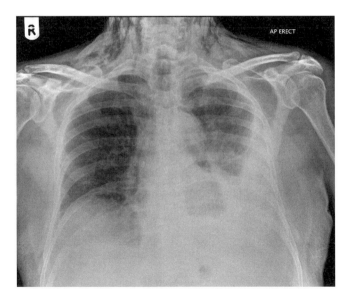

Figure 3.2 Boerhaave syndrome. Frontal chest radiograph demonstrating large volume pneumomediastinum and subcutaneous emphysema with a left pleural effusion.

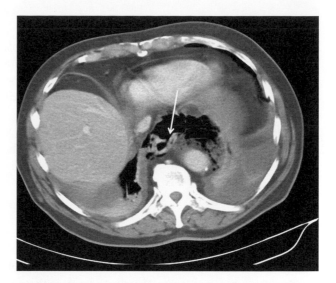

Figure 3.3 Boerhaave syndrome. Axial CT image of the chest with intravenous contrast demonstrating a perforation of the oesophagus (white arrow) with pneumomediastinum and bilateral pleural effusions.

WATER-SOLUBLE SWALLOW

- The leak is most often just above the diaphragm at the left posterolateral edge.

BOWEL OBSTRUCTION

Common mechanical causes of small bowel obstruction include adhesions, hernia, Crohn disease and malignancy. Mechanical causes of large bowel obstruction are commonly malignancy, diverticulitis and volvulus. Non-mechanical causes include neuropathy, myopathy and systemic sclerosis.

PLAIN FILM

- Small bowel loops >3 cm in diameter, large bowel loops >6 cm and caecum >9 cm ('3, 6, 9').
- Check for pneumoperitoneum.
- Review the hernia orifices—is there an obstructing hernia?

CT

- Dilated loops before obstruction and collapsed loops after—look for a transition point (this may be easier to identify on coronal reformats).
- Closed loop obstruction may give a U- or C-shaped configuration to the dilated loops and stretched mesenteric vessels converging to a torsion point—the end result is gut ischaemia; check for pneumatosis.

Box 3.4 CAUSES OF DILATED SMALL BOWEL, 'SOS'
• **S**cleroderma • **O**bstruction/ileus • **S**prue—coeliac disease

CANDIDA OESOPHAGITIS

This is the most common cause of infectious oesophagitis. There is dysmotility and atonia initially, then plaque-like filling defects reflecting ulceration and thickened mucosal folds. It is particularly seen in the immunosuppressed and also in patients with scleroderma and achalasia. It is frequently associated with oral candidiasis (thrush).

BARIUM SWALLOW

- Upper half of the oesophagus typically (though whole oesophagus can be affected).
- Linear, longitudinally orientated filling defects (plaques of necrotic debris and fungal colonies).

CARCINOID

This is the most common primary tumour of the small bowel; it is a low-grade malignancy. It mostly originates in the distal small bowel, outside the gut lumen, and rarely causes symptoms in itself. It may present with pain, obstruction or carcinoid syndrome (7%). Urine analysis shows 5-hydroxyindole-acetic acid (5-HIAA). Carcinoid syndrome is a clinical entity comprising flushing, wheezing and diarrhoea in the presence of lung and liver metastases.

CT (FIGURE 3.4)

- Mesenteric mass is the most typical feature, 70% contain calcification.
- Surrounding desmoplastic reaction—multiple linear strands that radiate out towards the adjacent bowel loops, giving a 'spoke-wheel' appearance.
- Appendix and distal small bowel most commonly.

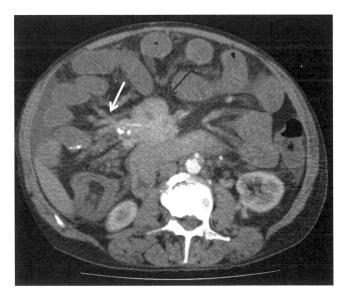

Figure 3.4 Carcinoid. Axial CT image of the abdomen with intravenous contrast demonstrating a calcified soft tissue mesenteric mass (red arrow) with a surrounding desmoplastic reaction (spoke-wheel appearance [white arrow]).

- Thickening of surrounding small bowel loops.
- Liver metastases enhance avidly—more common with ileal carcinoid.
- Associated with low-density lymphadenopathy due to necrosis.

NUCLEAR MEDICINE

- Indium-111-labelled octreotide study is specific for carcinoid and its liver metastases.

Box 3.5 CAUSES OF A MESENTERIC MASS ('CLAMM')
- **C**arcinoid
- **L**ymphoma
- **a**nd
- **M**elanoma
- **M**etastases

CAUSTIC OESOPHAGITIS

Due to ingestion of alkaline ('lye') or acidic substances. There is an increased risk of malignancy (squamous cell carcinoma).

BARIUM SWALLOW

- Most common acute finding is spasm, atony or dilation (i.e. motility disorder).
- Superficial mucosal irregularity and perforation.
- Chronically, there is fibrosis and stricturing (more common after alkali ingestion).

CHAGAS DISEASE

Due to *Trypanosoma cruzi*, this is endemic in Central and South America. Chronic disease can lead to myocarditis and left ventricular aneurysm formation.

BARIUM SWALLOW

- Diffuse oesophageal dilatation tapering at the GOJ—appearance similar to primary achalasia

PLAIN FILM

- Megacolon
- Cardiomegaly

CYTOMEGALOVIRUS (CMV) AND HIV OESOPHAGITIS

Both have similar appearances and are radiologically indistinguishable.

BARIUM SWALLOW

- The distal oesophagus is affected.
- Large solitary ulcer with a well-defined rim.
- One or more large, flat ulcers.

COELIAC DISEASE

This is a common, secondary reaction to gluten associated with an increased risk of lymphoma and other neoplasms. Diagnosis is made with duodenal biopsy. Imaging is performed only if there is a concern of malignancy or no response to a gluten-free diet. Patients with long-term coeliac disease may present with an acute ulcerative form of the disease called ulcerative jejuno-ileitis.

BARIUM FOLLOW-THROUGH

- Dilatation of the proximal small bowel.
- Thickening or loss of the jejunal folds—the ileum compensates by increasing its fold number, so-called 'jejunisation of the ileum'.
- Dilution of the barium column due to hypersecretion of fluid, 'barium segmentation and flocculation'.

CT

- Multiple mesenteric lymph nodes with central low attenuation or fat fluid levels— 'cavitating mesenteric lymph node syndrome' (a rare complication of Coeliac disease).
- Splenic atrophy.

COLORECTAL CANCER

This is the second most common cancer in the U.K.; the lifetime risk is about 1:20, which is doubled with a positive family history. Most tumours (90%) are in the rectosigmoid, and 60% are in the sigmoid itself. Overall, 5–year survival is >50%. Endorectal US is useful for distinguishing between T1 and T3 rectal tumours.

COLONOGRAPHY CT

- Overall sensitivity is about 95%.
- Nodes >1 cm or in clusters of more than three suggest malignancy.
- Check for peritoneal nodules or ascites.

Box 3.6 THE MALIGNANT POTENTIAL OF COLORECTAL ADENOMA INCREASES THE LARGER THEY ARE

- Adenoma >1 cm → 2.5% risk of cancer at 5 years and 25% at 20 years.
- Adenoma >2 cm → 50% risk of cancer.
- Flat adenomas are associated with more rapid malignant transformation (Tables 3.2 to 3.4).

MAGNETIC RESONANCE IMAGING (MRI)

- MRI is the gold standard for local staging of rectal malignancy.
- Tumour has intermediate signal intensity on T2.

Table 3.2 Staging colorectal cancer

UICC	TNM	Duke's	5–year survival
I	T1: invades submucosa	A	85%–95%
	T2: invades muscularis		
II	T3: beyond muscularis	B	60%–80%
	T4: adjacent organs		
III	N1: 1–3 nodes	C	30%–60%
	N2: >3 nodes		
IV	M1: distant metastases	D	<10%

Source: Union for International Cancer Control (UICC). 2011. TNM Classification for Malignant Tumours, 7th Edition. Wiley, Blackwell, Hoboken, New Jersey.

Table 3.3 Tubular adenoma versus villous adenoma

Tubular adenoma	Common
	Small
	Low risk of malignancy
	Can be on long stalk
Villous adenoma	10% of adenomatous polyps
	Broad based, 'sessile' over 2 cm
	Frond-like projections
	Associated with mucous production, which may cause diarrhoea or electrolyte depletion

Table 3.4 Benign versus malignant polyps

Feature	Benign	Malignant
Size	<1 cm	>2 cm
Stalk	Present (pedunculated, thin)	Absent (sessile)
Contour	Smooth	Irregular, lobulated
Number	Single	Multiple
Underlying colonic wall	Smooth	Indented, retracted

- The closer the tumour is to the circumferential resection margin (CRM), the poorer the outcome—1.6-times more likely to have died by 5 years with tumour ≤1 mm from the CRM compared to 10 mm from the CRM.
- If tumour is <5 mm from the CRM, evidence suggests a benefit from pre-operative ('neoadjuvant') chemotherapy.
- Extramural vascular invasion—associated with a significantly reduced disease-free survival time.

NUCLEAR MEDICINE

- Positron emission tomography (PET)/CT preferred for detecting disease recurrence.

Box 3.7 READ MORE

Kelly, S.B., Mills, S.J., Bradburn, D.M., Ratcliffe, A.A., Borowski, D.W.; Northern Region Colorectal Cancer Audit Group. 2011. Effect of the circumferential resection margin on survival following rectal cancer surgery. *British Journal of Surgery* 98:573–581.

CROHN DISEASE

Usually involves the small intestine, almost always the terminal ileum. The colon is also commonly involved. If the stomach is involved, typically the distal stomach is affected first (it can resemble a linitis plastica). The hallmark is skip lesions; these begin as superficial ulcers, progressing to full-thickness ulcers resulting in sinuses, fistulae and abscesses. Chronically, there is fibrofatty proliferation adjacent to the affected bowel, which causes a stricture with or without upstream obstruction.

BARIUM FOLLOW-THROUGH (FIGURE 3.5)

- Aphthous ulcers (small barium-filled pits surrounded by oedema).
- Linear ulcers on the mesenteric border are nearly pathognomonic.
- 'Cobblestone' appearance (a combination of longitudinal and transverse ulceration).
- Solitary strictures.
- Bowel wall thickening.
- Pseudodiverticula (islands of normal mucosa surrounded by ulceration).

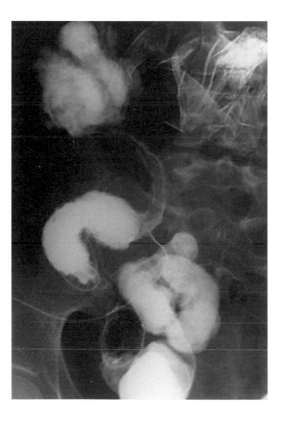

Figure 3.5 Crohn disease. Fistulogram demonstrating a long, ulcerated segment of terminal ileum with a stricture.

CT

- Especially useful to assess an acute Crohn presentation (e.g. obstruction, perforation, abscess).
- Bowel wall thickening (>10 mm) and vascular engorgement ('comb sign').
- Fat stranding.
- Circumferential submucosal hypoattenuation, surrounded by higher attenuation ('halo sign').
- Bones: spondylitis, sacroiliitis, complications of steroid use.
- Check for gallstones and renal stones.

MRI

- Very useful for monitoring disease activity (no radiation) and depicts Crohn pathology well—MRI is also specific in Crohn.
- Wall thickening (5–10 mm), enhancement and oedema.
- Fold thickening ('picket fence' appearance).
- Fistulae are best highlighted as high signal tracts on fat-suppressed axial/coronal T2, their origin is in an ulcer/fissure, sign of advanced Crohn.
- Fistulae enhance post-contrast.
- Strictures—these are considered significant if the upstream bowel is dilated (i.e. >3 cm for small bowel).
- Intramural fat—low signal in the bowel wall demonstrated on fat-suppressed images.
- Lymph node enhancement.

Box 3.8 THE BASIC ELEMENTS OF SMALL BOWEL MAGNETIC RESONANCE IMAGING

- Typically, the patient is scanned prone following oral mannitol to distend the bowel.
- Sequences include heavily T2-weighted imaging to highlight oedema, fistulae, etc.; rapidly acquired sequences to demonstrate motility; pre- and post-contrast imaging to highlight areas of disease activity and pathological lymph nodes.

Read more:
Tolan, D.J. et al. 2010. MR enterographic manifestations of small bowel Crohn disease. *Radiographics* 30:367–384.

US

- Limited role for monitoring disease activity in those not suitable for MRI/assessing for a fluid collection.
- Overview of the abdomen performed with a standard low-frequency probe, then focused scan of the right iliac fossa with a high-frequency linear probe to assess the terminal ileum.
- Look for bowel thickening, hyperaemia on Doppler or enhancement after contrast.

CYSTIC FIBROSIS (CF)

The GI tract is affected in the majority of patients. Paediatric manifestations include meconium plugging, meconium ileus, distal intestinal obstruction and microcolon.

BARIUM SWALLOW/FOLLOW-THROUGH

- Gastro-oesophageal reflux
- Duodenal fold thickening
- Small bowel dilatation

CT

- Colonic stricture
- Pneumatosis intestinalis

DIFFUSE OESOPHAGEAL SPASM

This presents with chest pain, which may come on with swallowing.

BARIUM SWALLOW

- Strong, non-propulsive waves of peristalsis.
- 'Corkscrew oesophagus' appearance.
- The oesophageal wall may become very thickened, associated with diverticula formation.

DIVERTICULA OF THE OESOPHAGUS

ZENKER/PHARYNGEAL POUCH

Herniation of the mucosa and submucosa through the midline of the posterior oesophageal wall at the cleavage plane between the oblique and transverse fibres at the level C5–6.

Barium swallow

- Posterior pouch arising at the junction of the pharynx and oesophagus
- May be transient

TRACTION DIVERTICULA

This is due to traction from adjacent mediastinal or pulmonary fibrosis.

Barium swallow

- Diverticulum arising from the mid-oesophagus

PULSION DIVERTICULA

These are false diverticula; they arise due to raised intra-oesophageal pressure.

Barium swallow

- More common in the distal oesophagus
- Associated with diffuse oesophageal spasm

DIVERTICULITIS

Mostly in the sigmoid (80%), rarely localises to the right colon (5%) or rectum; 10% of diverticulosis cases get diverticulitis. Complications include local perforation, abscess, generalised perforation, faecal peritonitis and bleeding (more likely with diverticula in the proximal colon). Other complications include long-segment strictures that may obstruct and fistulate.

Box 3.9 HINCHEY'S CLASSIFICATION FOR COMPLICATED DIVERTICULITIS
I. Small/localised pericolic or mesenteric abscess
II. Large (usually) pelvic abscess
III. Perforated diverticulitis
IV. Diverticulitis with perforation and faecal peritonitis

BARIUM ENEMA (FIGURE 3.6)

- Long, smooth stricture with diverticula disease (malignancy cannot be excluded— ulceration or abrupt calibre change suggests a tumour).

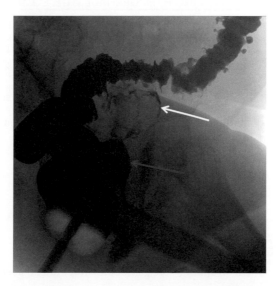

Figure 3.6 Diverticular abscess and colovaginal fistula. Water-soluble contrast enema demonstrating a perforation following an abscess cavity (white arrow) and subsequent fistula with contrast filling the vagina (red arrow).

CT

- Mural thickening and adjacent fat stranding (beware tumour!).
- Rim enhancing collection (i.e. abscess).
- Perforation.
- Fistulae—commonly to the bladder, look for bladder wall thickening or gas in the bladder lumen.

Box 3.10 CAUSES OF GASTROINTESTINAL FISTULATION
Diverticular disease
Crohn disease
Malignancy
Radiation
Infection (tuberculosis, actinomycosis)

DUODENAL TRAUMA

May arise due to penetrating or blunt trauma. Deceleration injury may cause rupture at D2–3 (these segments are retroperitoneal and fixed).

CT

- Retroperitoneal gas, duodenal oedema.
- Peripancreatic stranding.
- Active haemorrhage.
- Intramural haematoma (blunt trauma).
- Check the solid organs—pancreas, liver and spleen are commonly injured alongside the duodenum.

Box 3.11 IMAGING HAEMORRHAGE WITH COMPUTED TOMOGRAPHY
The rate of haemorrhage must exceed 0.5 mL/minute for detection of haemorrhage by computed tomography angiogram.

DUODENAL ULCERS

Mostly bulbar (95%) and on the anterior wall. They are a common cause of perforation. Healed ulcers may cause duodenal stenosis.

PLAIN FILM

- Check for pneumoperitoneum
- Subdiaphragmatic free gas, Rigler sign, outlining of the falciform ligament

CT

- Fat stranding, free gas locules and fluid adjacent to the proximal duodenum/ gallbladder.
- Check for free gas at the margin of the anterior liver.
- Posterior duodenal wall ulcers may invade the pancreas.

ECTOPIC PANCREAS

This is relatively common and usually found on the greater curvature of the antrum. It is at risk of pathology affecting the pancreas (e.g. inflammation and tumour).

BARIUM MEAL

- Well-defined sub-mucosal nodules (<2 cm).
- 50% have a pathognomic depressed central duct remnant.

EMPHYSEMATOUS GASTRITIS

Either benign (i.e. pneumatosis gastritis, like pneumatosis intestinalis) or a very serious infection with high mortality. Pathogens include *Escherichia coli* and *Clostridium*. It is more common in diabetic and immunocompromised patients.

CT

- Gas in the stomach wall
- Distension of the stomach
- With or without pneumoperitoneum

EOSINOPHILIC OESOPHAGITIS

Affects young patients; typically, there is a history of dysphagia to solids.

BARIUM SWALLOW

- Stepladder oesophagus similar to reflux with transverse folds or 'feline' oesophagus

EOSINOPHILIC ENTERITIS

Very rare infiltration of the GI tract by eosinophils. The stomach and small bowel are equally affected. Patients present with abdominal pain and diarrhoea. The disease may respond to steroid treatment.

BARIUM FOLLOW-THROUGH/CT

- Stomach/small bowel fold thickening/stenosis
- Ascites

EPIPLOIC APPENDAGITIS

Torsion of one of the fatty epiploic appendages arising from the serosal surface of the colon. Mostly occurring anterior to the sigmoid and caecum. Torted appendix epiploica may infarct, causing pain like diverticulitis/appendicitis. Most resolve in 2 weeks.

Box 3.12 EPIPLOIC APPENDAGITIS VERSUS OMENTAL INFARCTION
• Omental infarction lacks ring enhancement.   • Omental infarction is typically seen as an oval soft tissue mass in the right lower quadrant deep into the anterior abdominal muscles.

CT

- Small, focal, pedunculated, oval-shaped mass with a hypodense (fat, -60 HU) centre
- Peripheral enhancement
- Surrounding inflammatory fat stranding

FAMILIAL ADENOMATOUS POLYPOSIS (FAP)

This accounts for about 1% of colorectal cancers. It is inherited by autosomal dominance. Expect to find microadenoma in early adolescence and macroadenoma by late adolescence. Presents with diarrhoea, rectal bleeding and mucus per rectum. Colorectal cancer is considered inevitable, so panproctocolectomy is performed.

CT

- Colonic, gastric and duodenal polyps.
- >100 adenomas are needed to make the diagnosis.
- Hamartomas of the stomach (non-specific appearance).
- Colorectal tumour or periampullary mass.
- Desmoid tumours are common, especially post-surgery—look for small bowel tethering, mesenteric infiltration or a large mass causing colonic/ureteric obstruction.

GARDENER SYNDROME

Inherited by autosomal dominance; 100% of patients develop colonic polyps.

PLAIN FILM

- Review the bones—osteoma may develop; these are specific to Gardener syndrome and are more common in the mandible and calvarium.

CT

- Ill-defined mesenteric fibrosis or a focal enhancing mesenteric mass (i.e. desmoid tumour).
- Duodenal polyps are most common.
- Gastric hamartoma.
- Associated with periampullary carcinoma.

GASTRIC CARCINOMA

Box 3.13 TNM STAGING OF GASTRIC CANCER
T1—lamina propria/submucosa only (85% alive at 5 years) **T2**—muscularis propria (50% alive at 5 years) **T3**—penetrates subserosa **T4a**—invades serosal layer **T4b**—invades adjacent structures **N1**—1–2 regional nodes **N2**—3–6 regional nodes **N3a**—7–15 regional nodes **N3b**—>16 regional nodes
Source: Union for International Cancer Control. 2011. *TNM Classification for Malignant Tumours, 7th Edition.* Wiley, Blackwell, Hoboken, New Jersey.

This is the third most common GI malignancy and is more common in Japan. The risk of gastric cancer is increased with pernicious anaemia, adenomatous polyps, chronic atrophic gastritis and after Bilroth II surgery.

CT

- Early features are an irregular, flat and non-healing ulcer.
- 40% found in the fundus and cardia; atrum and gastric body 30% each.
- Stomach wall >1 cm thick is abnormal in a distended stomach.
- Large, irregular mass ± ulceration in advanced disease.
- Linitis plastica (diffuse infiltration of the stomach leading to fibrosis and a narrowed/rigid stomach).
- Local nodes that enlarge are found in the gastrohepatic ligament, gastrocolic ligament and around the stomach.
- Liver metastases are most common.

Box 3.14 CHARACTERISTICS AND CAUSES OF LINITIS PLASTICA

Barium meal features
- Mural thickening
- Irregularity
- Reduced distensibility
- Absent peristalsis

Causes
- Scirrhous cancer is most common.
- Tumours (lymphoma, breast and lung metastases, pancreatic).
- Inflammation (erosive gastritis, radiation therapy).
- Ingestion (corrosives, iron ingestion).
- Infiltrative disease (sarcoid, amyloid, Crohn disease, intramural haematoma).
- Infection (tuberculosis, syphilis).

GASTRIC LYMPHOMA

The stomach is the most common site for GI lymphoma, mostly non-Hodgkin (i.e. mucosa-associated lymphoid tissue [MALT] lymphoma). It accounts for about 3% of gastric malignancies, either as a primary or direct invasion from an adjacent tumour. *H. pylori* is a risk factor.

CT

- Thickened gastric folds or solitary mass, multiple masses or polyps.
- May cause linitis plastica.
- Gastric wall may be thicker than is seen with gastric carcinoma.
- Check for involvement of the duodenum (unlike gastric cancer).
- Tends to metastasise to the liver first, then the mesentery.
- Larger nodes than with gastric cancer.

PET/CT

● Useful for follow-up to assess response to treatment/disease recurrence.

GASTRIC METASTASES

Most commonly due to haematogenous spread of e.g. breast, lung or melanoma. There may be direct spread from the colon (via the gastrocolic ligament) or liver (gastrohepatic liver) or pancreas.

BARIUM MEAL

● Multiple submucosal nodules
● Target appearance (bull's eye lesion)—a sharply demarcated lesion with central ulceration

---

Box 3.15 CAUSES OF THE 'BULL'S EYE' LESION ON BARIUM MEAL

Metastatic melanoma is the most common neoplastic cause.

Other metastatic causes:
● Breast
● Lung

Other causes:
● Gastrointestinal stromal tumour
● Lymphoma
● Kaposi's sarcoma
● Neurofibromatosis (NF) (multiple lesions)
● Pancreatic rests

GASTRIC POLYPS

These are unusual overall; 90% are benign hyperplastic polyps that have no malignant potential. They arise in the body of the stomach against a background of chronic gastritis, as well as syndromes including FAP, Peutz–Jegher, Cronkhite–Canada, Cowden and Gardner, in addition to juvenile polyposis. Endoscopy is the preferred examination.

BARIUM MEAL

● Round, smooth and sessile
● Up to 1 cm in size
● Commonly multiple
● Note up to 25% have a synchronous gastric cancer
● If >2 cm, more likely an adenomatous polyp (malignant in 50%)

GASTRIC VOLVULUS

Comprises rotation of part/all of the stomach, leading to obstruction with or without ischaemia. The typical presentation is with the Borchadt triad: severe pain, retching and inability to pass an NG tube. There are two types:

1. Organoaxial—most common (Figure 3.7)
   - Rotation occurs around the long axis of the stomach so that the greater curvature ends lying cranially—'upside down' stomach.
   - Usually chronic and asymptomatic, complications are rare.
   - More common with large hiatus hernias.
2. Mesenteroaxial—rare (Figure 3.8)

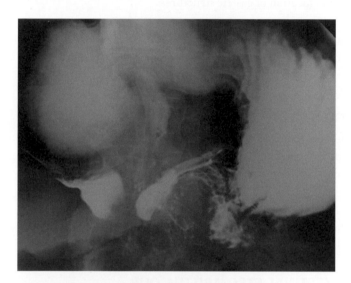

Figure 3.7 Organoaxial gastric volvulus. Barium meal demonstrating the stomach to have revolved around its long axis with the great curvature lying cranial.

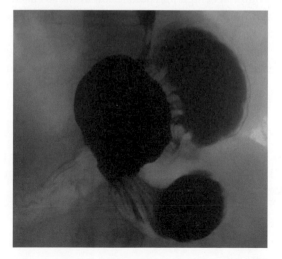

Figure 3.8 Mesenteroaxial gastric volvulus. Barium meal demonstrating the stomach to have revolved with the distal stomach projected above the fundus.

- Rotation occurs around the gastrohepatic ligament so the distal stomach may be projected over or above the fundus.
- Obstruction and ischaemia is common.
- Associated with traumatic diaphragmatic rupture.

PLAIN FILM

- Unexpected location of the gastric bubble
- Air–fluid levels in the mediastinum
- Distended, gas-filled stomach

CT

- Abnormal location of gastric structures

GASTROINTESTINAL AMYLOIDOSIS

The GI tract is most commonly affected in patients with primary amyloidosis, typically the colon.

BARIUM FOLLOW-THROUGH

- When seen, there can be uniform fold thickening or more focal nodular pattern of 5–10 mm nodules.
- Thickened valvulae and mucose.

CT

- Bowel dilatation
- Mural thickening

GASTROINTESTINAL STROMAL TUMOUR

GIST is the second most common benign polypoid lesion in the stomach (accounts for 70%). It is a mesenchymal tumour expressing a tyrosine kinase growth factor receptor. In total, 60% are found in the submucosal stomach, and growth may also be outside the stomach, being extra- or intra-luminal. A total of 30% of GISTs are seen in the small bowel and 7% are ano-rectal. Lesions <5 cm without evidence of invasion are most likely benign. Oesophageal, colonic and ano-rectal GISTs are usually malignant (i.e. leiomyosarcoma). GIST is more common in patients with neurofibromatosis type-1.

BARIUM MEAL

- Submucosal mass, forming an obtuse angle with the gastric wall in profile
- No change to the stomach's mucosal surface—areae gastricae maintained
- Focal areas of ulceration

CT

- Smooth, large (e.g. 30 cm) solid mass sometimes with cystic areas and a sizeable exophytic component.
- Peripheral enhancement—large vessels or a vascular blush are common.
- Central low attenuation representing necrosis, haemorrhage and cyst formation.

- Large GISTs show a crescent-shaped area of necrosis (Torricelli–Bernoulli sign).
- Large cavitating GISTs may fistulate to the gut lumen.
- Nodal involvement is rare—another primary is more likely!
- Malignant lesions commonly metastasise to the liver and peritoneum.

GRAFT-VERSUS-HOST DISEASE

Donor lymphoid tissue mounts a response to the recipient liver, skin and GI tract.

BARIUM FOLLOW-THROUGH

- Thickened folds and wall, followed by fold effacement, ulceration and then strictures.
- Strictures are usually confined to the jejunum/ileum.
- Resolution may follow, ileal thickening may remain.

CT

- Bowel wall thickening and fat stranding/mesenteric thickening
- 'Halo' appearance due to bowel oedema

HEREDITARY NON-POLYPOSIS COLORECTAL CANCER

Also known as Lynch syndrome, this accounts for about 5% of colorectal cancers and presents earlier than non-syndromic colorectal cancer.

CT

- 70% in the proximal colon.
- Synchronous tumours are common.
- Associated with breast, endometrial, ovarian and pancreatic cancer ('Lynch II').

Box 3.16 OTHER POLYPOSIS SYNDROMES

Turcot
Autosomal recessive. Associated with central nervous system tumours, especially supratentorial glioblastoma and occasionally medulloblastoma, which affect life expectancy.

Cowden
Hamartomatous polyps in the stomach and rectosigmoid. Skin lesions and oral disorders (gingival hyperplasia, oral papillomas and mucocutaneous pigmentation). Increased risk of breast and thyroid malignancy.

Muir–Torre
Associated with bowel polyps, cutaneous adenoma and keratoacanthoma.

Cronkhite–Canada
Non-familial polyposis associated with malabsorption, polyposis and skin disorders (alopecia, skin hyperpigmentation and onychodystrophy). No increased risk of malignancy.

HERNIAS

Superficial hernias are common and often asymptomatic, but are a common indication for emergency surgery. Common hernias are described in Table 3.5.

US

- Mass demonstrated protruding through a defect in the abdominal wall.
- Fluid within the hernia sac or bowel wall thickening suggest incarceration.

CT

- Useful for assessing large hernia or investigating complications.

Table 3.5 Deep and superficial abdominal hernia and their anatomical associations

Common name	Anatomical association
Femoral	Inferolateral to the pubic tubercle
Inguinal	Superomedial to the pubic tubercle
Spigelian (Figure 3.9)	Inferolateral abdominal wall
Obturator	Obturator foramen (between pectineus and obturator externus)
Paraduodenal	Left of D4, due to a defect in the descending mesocolon
Right paraduodenal	Passes behind the superior mesenteric artery, displaces the superior mesenteric vein superior to the superior mesenteric artery (associated with malrotation)
Foramen of Winslow	Between the portal vein and inferior vena cava

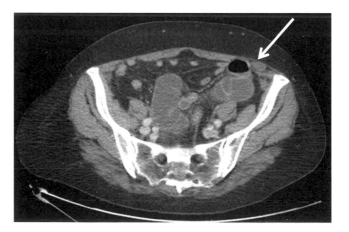

Figure 3.9 Obstructing Spigelian hernia. Axial CT image with intravenous contrast demonstrating a left Spigelian hernia with protrusion of the small bowel lateral to the rectus abdominis (white arrow) with dilatation of small bowel loops within the pelvis.

HERPES OESOPHAGITIS

Typically seen in the context of HIV infection. The oral cavity, rectum and anus are also affected. Behçet disease can appear similar.

BARIUM SWALLOW

- Multiple small (<1–cm) superficial ulcers in the upper and mid-oesophagus without plaque formation
- Punctuate configuration and surrounded by radiolucent mounds of oedema

HIATUS HERNIA

Most are sliding (95%), defined as a Z-line <40 cm from incisors. It is more likely to reflux than the rolling type.

BARIUM SWALLOW

- Look for gastric mucosa above the diaphragmatic hiatus.

INTESTINAL LYMPHANGIECTASIA

This is a rare abnormality of the lymphatic channels that become obstructed, dilated and then rupture. It tends to affect children and young adults and presents with malabsorption, hypoalbuminaemia and hypogammaglobulinaemia. It can be congenital or acquired (due to e.g. malignancy or amyloidosis).

BARIUM FOLLOW-THROUGH

- Thickened folds or micronodularity representing engorged villi

CT

- Mesenteric stranding
- Masses
- Lymph node enlargement

INTRAMURAL PSEUDODIVERTICULOSIS

This is a condition causing dilatation of the ducts of the submucosal glands of the oesophagus. It is associated with diabetes, chronic alcoholism and severe oesophagitis. In total, 90% have a history of reflux, and *Candida* may be cultured in about 50%.

BARIUM SWALLOW (FIGURE 3.10)

- Multiple tiny, flask-shaped collections of barium arranged in longitudinal rows.

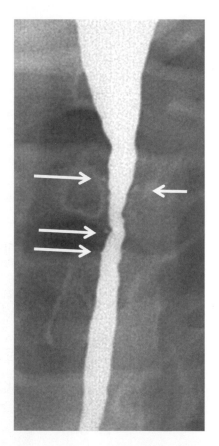

Figure 3.10 Intramural pseudodiverticulosis. Barium swallow demonstrating a strictured segment of oesophagus with small flask-shaped collections.

- These appear to 'float' outside the oesophagus, as the connection to the lumen may not be appreciated.
- Associated strictures in the distal oesophagus are common.

ISCHAEMIC BOWEL

Due to arterial or venous thromboembolism, hypoperfusion or extrinsic vascular compression. Ischaemia causes mucosal oedema and sloughing, which may repair itself completely or progress to fibrosis and stricture.

CT

- Dilated and thickened bowel—the splenic flexure is a typical location (watershed zone between superior mesenteric artery/inferior mesenteric artery [SMA/IMA]).
- Hypoenhancement of the affected bowel.
- Stranding of the adjacent fat suggests transmural infarction.
- Pneumatosis or portal venous gas indicates transmural necrosis.
- Engorged mesenteric veins and ascites.
- Follow-up for several months to monitor for stricture formation.

Box 3.17 PNEUMATOSIS COLI—MECHANISM AND AETIOLOGY

Pneumatosis coli represents small pockets of gas in the submucosal/subserosal layers of the gut.

There are four main mechanisms:
1. Bowel necrosis
2. Mucosal disruption
3. Increased mucosal permeability
4. Pulmonary disease (may also transgress to the mesenteric and portal veins)

The cause may be:

Ischaemic
Idiopathic
Infectious (e.g. necrotising enterocolitis, pseudomembranous colitis)
Inflammatory (e.g. Crohn disease)
Iatrogenic (e.g. endoscopy, surgery, steroids)
Traumatic
Respiratory (e.g. chronic obstructive pulmonary disease, asthma)

Box 3.18 PSEUDODIVERTICULA/SACCULATION

These are typical of ischaemic strictures. They also occur with scleroderma; sacculation also occurs in Crohn disease.

LIPOMA

The large bowel is the most common site for GI lipoma; 45% are found in the caecum. Lipomas >4 cm are likely to cause pain, bleeding or intussusception.

CT

- Ileocecal valve of >3 cm is suggestive.
- Fat density (HU −80 to −120) mass in the bowel lumen.

MALIGNANT DUODENAL TUMOURS

These are rare; the peak incidence is at 70 years of age. In total, 50% have metastases at diagnosis. The duodenum may also be involved through direct invasion from a pancreatic mass.

CT

- Polypoid or intramural mass.
- Paraganglionomas have a 'dumbbell' appearance.

MALIGNANT OESOPHAGEAL TUMOURS

Most (70%) are squamous cell carcinomas—typically affecting the mid-oesophagus. Alcohol, smoking, achalasia, head and neck cancer, caustic ingestion and tylosis are risk factors. The remaining 30% are mostly adenocarcinomas; typically they are distal and associated with reflux disease (i.e. Barrett disease and scleroderma). Endoscopic US (EUS) is preferred for local staging. Common sites for metastasis are the liver, lungs, bones and adrenal glands.

BARIUM SWALLOW

- Irregular, 'shouldering' stricture with nodular elements.
- The varicoid variant may appear as thickened folds.
- Check for secondary achalasia with low tumours (due to malignant infiltration of the myenteric plexus).

CT

- Asymmetric thickening of the oesophageal wall (>5 mm) and with dilated proximal oesophagus.
- Loss of perioesophageal fat plane implies local invasion.
- May be resectable if <90° of the aorta are encircled.

Box 3.19 STAGING OESOPHAGEAL CANCER

T1—submucosa only (EUS)
T2—invades muscularis (EUS)
T3—invades adventitia (EUS, PET/CT)
T4—adjacent structures
N1—1–2 nodes (EUS, PET/CT)
N2—3–6 nodes (EUS, PET/CT)
N3—>6 nodes (EUS, PET/CT)

Source: Union for International Cancer Control. 2011. *TNM Classification for Malignant Tumours, 7th Edition*. Wiley, Blackwell, Hoboken, New Jersey.

PET/CT

- For staging, the sensitivity and specificity of PET/CT are better than those of CT alone, as oesophageal cancer is very fluorodeoxyglucose (FDG) avid.
- PET/CT is especially useful for nodal assessment and tracking response.
- Useful for distinguishing fibrosis from malignancy post-treatment.
- >15% fall in standardized uptake value (SUV) is required for a partial response.

INTERVENTION

- Stenting is an option for symptom control (below C7).
- Stents are typically made of nitinol (nickel/titanium alloy) and covered.
- Complications are bleeding, perforation, migration and tumour in-growth.

MASTOCYTOSIS

Rare accumulation of mast cells in the skeletal, reticuloendothelial and abdominal systems.

US

- Hepatosplenomegaly
- Enlarged lymph nodes

BARIUM FOLLOW-THROUGH

- Distorted, thickened nodular folds.
- Tiny nodular mucosal deposits, especially in the jejunum.
- Always look at the vertebral bodies, as mastocytosis can involve the bone marrow and produce dense sclerotic vertebrae.

CT

- Irregular small bowel fold thickening
- Ileal wall thickening
- Lymph node enlargement

Box 3.20 CAUSES OF THICKENED MUCOSAL FOLDS IN THE SMALL BOWEL

Mastocytosis
Amyloidosis
Whipple disease
Radiotherapy
Graft-versus-host disease

MECKEL DIVERTICULUM

Rule of 2s: present in 2%, 2 ft from ileocecal valve, symptoms in 20%–40% and ectopic gastric mucosa in 20%. Due to failure in closure of the yolk sac. Complications include ulceration, bleeding, perforation, volvulus, intussusception, hernia, etc.

NUCLEAR MEDICINE

- Technetium-99m sodium pertechnetate scan is most sensitive in children, but only positive if there is ectopic gastric mucosa in the diverticulum.

INTERVENTION

- An angiogram may be performed to investigate or treat haemorrhage—it should show a persistent omphalomesenteric artery.

MÉNÉTRIERE DISEASE

This is a rare disease due to gastric gland hypertrophy, which sheds protein into the gut. In total, 10% of affected patients will get gastric cancer. Patients present with pain, weight loss, oedema, etc., due to protein loss.

BARIUM MEAL

- Marked thickening and tortuosity of the rugae, though the stomach distends normally (unlike with malignancy).
- The antrum is spared in 50%.
- Folds alter in size and position during the examination.
- Mucous hypersecretion causes dilution of contrast.
- Small bowel fold thickening.
- Ulceration due to achlorydia.

CT

- Thickened gastric folds project into the gastric lumen.
- The serosal contour is smooth.

OESOPHAGEAL LEIOMYOMA

This is the most common benign oesophageal tumour (accounts for 50% of benign oesophageal tumours)—others are fibrovascular polyps, papilloma and glycogenic acanthosis. Leiomyoma is a benign tumour of the smooth muscle; it is often asymptomatic, but can present with haematemesis. It is more common in men.

BARIUM SWALLOW

- Large, well-defined, lobulated intramural mass causing a luminal deformity.
- Lower or middle third of the oesophagus.
- It is the only oesophageal tumour to calcify.

OESOPHAGEAL LEIOMYOSARCOMA

This very rare tumour affects the smooth muscle of the distal oesophagus. It is the malignant counterpart of leiomyoma. Metastasises late, therefore is prognostically better than carcinoma.

CT

- Large, non-obstructing polypoid mass—extrinsic (like leiomyoma)

OESOPHAGEAL REFLUX

A small amount of reflux is considered normal and is cleared by the secondary wave of peristalsis. Reflux beyond the aortic knuckle is likely to be symptomatic. Most patients with reflux have a hiatus hernia (because this reduces lower oesophageal pressure) or a wide GOJ. Not all hernias cause reflux. In the long term, reflux causes oesophagitis and Barrett disease.

BARIUM SWALLOW
- Contrast refluxes above the GOJ—best demonstrated in the prone position.
- Fixed, thickened transverse folds with 'stepladder' appearance of the distal oesophagus.
- Granular appearance of the mucosa with or without ulceration.
- Luminal narrowing.
- Schatzki ring (thought to be due to reflux)—a slender, symmetrical narrowing at GOJ, usually only symptomatic if the narrowing is <12 mm.

OESOPHAGEAL SCLERODERMA

The oesophagus is the part of the GI tract most affected by scleroderma. The jejunum and proximal ileum are also commonly affected. There is fibrosis of the smooth muscle, resulting in a dilated oesophagus with absent or reduced peristalsis in the lower two-thirds. The upper oesophagus is composed of skeletal muscle and is therefore unaffected. Reflux, Barrett disease and distal strictures are the result.

BARIUM SWALLOW
- Dilated oesophagus.
- Aperistalsis of the distal oesophagus.
- Loss of primary and secondary contractions, tertiary contractions may be seen.
- Lower oesophagus is wide (patulous), in contrast to the tapered narrowing seen in achalasia.
- Gastro-oesophageal reflux.
- Distal stricture (e.g. 5 cm above the GOJ).
- Oesophageal shortening.

BARIUM FOLLOW-THROUGH
- Atrophy of the circular muscle causes stacking of the valvulae—the so-called 'hide bound' appearance.
- Sacculations/wide-mouthed diverticulae.
- Delayed transit, reduced peristalsis and pseudo-obstruction.

OESOPHAGEAL VARICES

These are dilated submucosal veins working as collateral drainage due to blockage elsewhere. Varices may be uphill (lower oesophagus, seen with portal hypertension or splenic/hepatic/portal vein obstruction) or downhill (either proximal or whole oesophagus, seen with e.g. SVC obstruction).

BARIUM SWALLOW (FIGURE 3.11)

- Best seen with the patient prone.
- Dilated, smooth, serpiginous filling defects.
- Varicose carcinoma of the oesophagus is the differential.

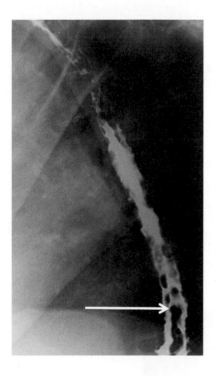

Figure 3.11 Oesophageal varices. Barium swallow demonstrating long serpiginous filling defects (white arrow).

CT

- Gastric varices are usually seen at the fundus/GOJ.
- If there are only gastric varices, check for a splenic vein thrombosis.

OESOPHAGEAL WEB

Seen near cricopharyngeus and arises at right angles from the anterior oesophageal wall. Plummer–Vinson syndrome is characterised by oesophageal webs, iron-deficiency anaemia, stomatitis, glossitis, dysphagia, thyroid disorders and spoon-shaped nails. Temporary symptom relief can be achieved with balloon angioplasty.

BARIUM SWALLOW

- Small, shelf-like filling defect arising from the anterior oesophageal wall

PEUTZ–JEGHER SYNDROME

Autosomal dominant syndrome that causes multiple benign hamartomatous polyps; more common in the stomach and small bowel. No malignant potential. It is the most common polyposis syndrome to involve the small intestine. It can also appear in the large bowel, where polyps are larger, pedunculated and bleed. There is a risk of malignant transformation in the bowel, as well as in the ovary, thyroid, testis, pancreas and breast.

CT

- Intussusception is a common presentation

PSEUDOMEMBRANOUS COLITIS

Diffuse colitis arising due to infection with *Clostridium difficile*. It tends to cause gross mural/haustral thickening, then ileus.

Box 3.21 **THE UNDERLYING ORGANISM IN INFECTIOUS COLITIS MAY BE PREDICTED BY THE SEGMENT OF BOWEL AFFECTED**

Salmonella—Ascending colon
Shigella—sigmoid colon
Cytomegalovirus—ileocolic
Herpes simplex virus—proctitis

CT (FIGURE 3.12)

- Gross mural thickening (>12 mm).
- Mucosal hyperenhancement and severe submucosal low attenuation oedema produces the 'accordion sign' in severe inflammation.
- Ascites.
- Large bowel dilatation.

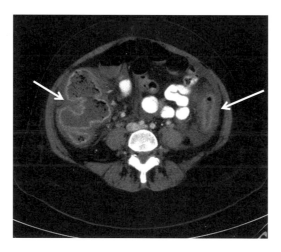

Figure 3.12 Pseudomembranous colitis. Axial CT image with intravenous contrast demonstrating gross mural thickening of the ascending and descending colon (white arrows) with mucosal hyperenhancement, severe submucosal low-attenuation oedema and small volume ascites.

Box 3.22 **PSEUDOMEMBRANOUS COLITIS VERSUS INFLAMMATORY BOWEL DISEASE**

- Small bowel is not thickened
- Ascites differentiates from Crohn disease and ulcerative colitis

---

RADIATION ENTERITIS

Radiotherapy damages gut vasculature and therefore causes ischaemia. It tends to occur with doses >45 Gy and presentation may be delayed by many years.

CT

- Mural and fold thickening (acute)
- Ulceration
- Increased attenuation of the associated mesentery
- Widening of the pre-sacral space
- Rarely strictures or fistulation (chronic)

SMALL BOWEL AIDS

In total, 50% of patients with AIDS have small bowel pathology; it is a common site for opportunistic infection. Causes include CMV, *Mycobacterium avium*, cryptosporidiosis, giardiasis and histoplasmosis.

CT

- Non-specific small bowel thickening and fat stranding.
- Ascites.
- Large ulcers are associated with CMV.
- Important differentials are lymphoma and Kaposi sarcoma.

Box 3.23 CAUSES OF DIFFUSE SMALL BOWEL THICKENING ('HAIL-WC')

- **H**aemorrhage
- **A**myloidosis
- **I**ntestinal lymphangiectasia
- **L**ymphoma
- **W**hipple disease
- **C**rohn disease

SMALL BOWEL INFECTIONS

TB

Commonly affects the ileocecal region (90% in the terminal ileum) and mimics Crohn disease.

Barium follow-through

- Deep fissures and large, shallow, linear ulcers with elevated margins are characteristic.
- Hourglass stricture of the caecum.
- Incompetent, thickened, rigid and gaping ileocecal valve.
- Nodular fold thickening leads to fold effacement and distortion in later stages—crosses into the cecal pole, which may show more obvious ulceration prior to fibrosis and the 'shrinking caecum'.

CT

- Low-attenuation lymph node enlargement
- TB peritonitis = diffuse mesenteric/omental nodules, dense ascites and peritoneal thickening

> **Box 3.24 DIFFERENTIATING TUBERCULOSIS FROM CROHN DISEASE**
>
> This may be difficult; however, tuberculosis:
> - Involves the caecum > terminal ileum
> - Causes caecal retraction
> - Is associated with low-attenuation mesenteric lymph node enlargement
> - Causes dense (high attenuation) ascites

> **Box 3.25 CAUSES OF HIGH-ATTENUATION ASCITES**
>
> - Tuberculosis
> - Unseen ovarian tumour
> - Appendiceal tumour
> - Meig syndrome

YERSINIOSIS

This may cause an acutely inflamed terminal ileum and mimics appendicitis.

CT

- Distal ileal thickening
- Lymph node enlargement

> **Box 3.26 CAUSES OF TERMINAL ILEITIS**
>
> - Crohn disease
> - Tuberculosis
> - *Yersinia*
> - Lymphoma

ACTINOMYCOSIS

Commonly affects the appendix and classically mimics an appendiceal abscess. The sigmoid colon is also commonly affected. It may appear similar to diverticulitis, cancer, TB and Crohn disease.

CT

- Mass compressing the caecum/ileum.
- Look for sinus tracts and fistulae.

GIARDIASIS AND STRONGYLOIDIASIS

Both are parasitic infections: giardiasis due to a protozoa (*Giardia lamblia*) and strongyloidiasis due to a tapeworm. Both cause diarrhoea.

Barium follow-through

- Non-specific fold thickening in the duodenum/proximal jejunum

ANISAKIASIS

Transmitted from raw and pickled fish. Most cases arise in The Netherlands and Japan. It presents with an acute abdomen.

CT
- Concentric narrowing of ileum with proximal dilatation.
- Imaging findings mimic Crohn disease.

ASCARIASIS

This is due to a tropical roundworm; if numerous, it may cause obstruction or appendicitis. It can migrate into the biliary system and cause cholangitis or pancreatitis.

Barium follow-through
- Filling defect caused by the worm.
- The hallmark is opacification of the worm's GI tract with contrast.

SMALL BOWEL LYMPHOMA

Non-Hodgkin lymphoma is the most common malignancy of the small bowel, often affecting the terminal ileum. Characteristically, lymphoma infiltrates the muscularis and myenteric plexus, leading to large masses with aneurysmal dilatations and no obstruction. If the oesophagus is affected, it is usually due to direct invasion from a gastric tumour.

CT (FIGURE 3.13)
- Aneurysmal dilatation—large, irregular, cavitatory lesion without obstruction
- Circumferential bowel wall thickening
- Multifocal
- Thickened folds
- Extraluminal mass
- Nodal proliferation and enlargement

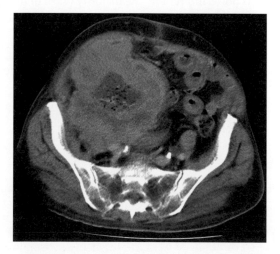

Figure 3.13 Lymphoma. Axial computed tomography image with intravenous contrast demonstrating gross circumferential mural thickening with aneurysmal dilatation of the bowel with mild thickening of further small bowel loops but without proximal obstruction.

SMALL BOWEL TRAUMA

In total, 95% of intestinal traumas occur in the duodenum and proximal jejunum. The anti-mesenteric border of the proximal jejunum is most commonly affected. The remaining 5% affect the large bowel (mostly the transverse colon).

CT

- Focal mural thickening.
- Free fluid.
- A focal haematoma (>60 HU) is a sensitive marker of the site of injury.

SUPERIOR MESENTERIC ARTERY (SMA) SYNDROME (WILKIE SYNDROME)

Rare—there is obstruction of the third part of the duodenum by its compression between the SMA and aorta. It is associated with severe weight loss (fat around the duodenum is reduced), lumbar lordosis and pregnancy. Patients present with intermittent abdominal pain and vomiting; this may be relieved when prone.

CT

- Sagittal reconstructions of a CT angiogram are required.
- Look for a tight angle between the SMA and aorta (between 6° and 22°).
- The distance between the aorta and SMA is reduced to 2–8 mm.
- Expect dilatation of the proximal duodenum and stomach.

SUPERIOR MESENTERIC VEIN (SMV) THROMBOSIS

This is an unusual cause of gut ischaemia. It presents with abdominal pain; peritonitis suggests bowel infarction. The majority (95%) of mesenteric venous thromboses occur in the SMV. Surgery, sepsis and malignancy are risk factors.

CT

- Enlarged SMV with rim enhancement surrounding central low-density thrombus
- Bowel thickening and adjacent fat stranding
- Ascites
- Check for pneumatosis (bowel infarction)

TAILGUT CYSTS

These are mucous-secreting, larger cysts that may cause rectal bleeding, constipation, anal fistulae or recurrent rectal abscess.

CT

- Presacral, multilocular, low-density cyst.
- Long, tail-like coccyx.
- Malignant transformation can occur.
- Duplication cysts are usually unilocular, dermoids contain fat.

TYPHILITIS

This is neutropenic colitis; it occurs in patients undergoing treatment for leukaemia, lymphoma and sometimes other malignancies. It typically affects the paediatric population.

CT

- Bowel wall thickening typically affecting the caecum, appendix or terminal ileum.
- 20% have pneumatosis.
- Inflammatory fat stranding.

ULCERATIVE COLITIS (UC)

This is three-times more common than Crohn disease. The peak is between 15 and 25 years of age. After 10 years of UC, there is an increased risk of malignancy (though most UC strictures are still benign). The hallmark of fulminant colitis is toxic megacolon (it can also occur in Crohn disease, ischaemic or infective colitis). Toxic megacolon arises due to deep ulceration causing bowel denervation and hence massive dilatation.

Box 3.27 CAUSES OF PANCOLITIS ('UCIC')
<ul><li>**U**lcerative colitis</li><li>**C**rohn disease</li><li>**I**schaemia</li><li>**C**ytomegalovirus and *Cryptosporidium* (in the context of immunosuppression)</li></ul>

BARIUM ENEMA

- Tends to affect the rectum first and extend proximally.
- May cause a pancolitis.
- Granular pattern.
- Shallow ulceration—deeper ulceration may cause the 'collar button' appearance as the submucosa is eroded.
- Reflux ileitis—typical of UC and resolves after colectomy.
- Severe ulceration causes multiple 'mucosal islands'.

PLAIN FILM

- Ahaustral, thickened and dilated large bowel (tendency to affect the transverse colon) suggests toxic megacolon (dilatation >5.5 cm is worrying).
- Toxic megacolon commonly perforates.

CT

- Non-specific bowel wall thickening and fat stranding.
- Look for lymph node enlargement in acute cases.
- In chronic UC, there is submucosal fat proliferation.
- Note: In the acute phase, the diagnosis may be masked; if it is not clear whether it is Crohn disease or UC, then the diagnosis is most likely Crohn disease (Table 3.6).

Table 3.6 Characteristics of Crohn disease versus ulcerative colitis

Crohn disease	Ulcerative colitis
Aphthous ulcers	Mesorectal fat proliferation
Deep/fissuring ulcers	Perforation (especially in the first year)
Asymmetric/skip lesions	Toxic megacolon
Pseudodiverticula/sacculation	Granular mucosa
Enteroenteric fistulae	
Multiple anal fistulae	

VOLVULUS

SIGMOID

Most common type of volvulus (more common in elderly/bed-bound patients); due to torsion around the sigmoid mesocolon.

Plain film
- Coffee bean appearance, lower end points to the pelvis.
- Bowel wall is ahaustral.

Water-soluble enema
- Bird's beak appearance

CAECAL

Tends to occur in younger patients than sigmoid volvulus (30–60 years of age). It is the result of failed peritoneal fixation of the ascending colon. Presents with features of large bowel obstruction.

Plain film
- Marked distension of the caecum.
- Preservation of haustra.
- Long axis of the distended loops arises from the right lower quadrant.
- Gas-filled appendix.

WALDENSTRÖM MACROGLOBULINAEMIA

This condition is a rare, malignant monoclonal gammopathy where there are pathological levels of circulating IgM, elevated serum viscosity and lymphoplasmacytic infiltrate in the bone marrow.

BARIUM FOLLOW-THROUGH
- Micronodularity and fold thickening

CT
- Non-specific lymph node enlargement
- Hepatosplenomegaly

MRI

- Infiltration of the spine is seen in 90% (replacement of the normal fatty bone marrow and bone infarcts).

WHIPPLE DISEASE

Rare, systemic disease due to infection with *Tropheryma whipplei*; it is associated with polyarthritis.

CT

- Low-attenuation retroperitoneal/mesenteric lymph node enlargement
- Small bowel thickening
- Non-dilated small bowel

BARIUM FOLLOW-THROUGH

- Characteristically causes 1–mm sand-like nodules (this is lymphoid hyperplasia) in a non-dilated small bowel.
- Moderate fold thickening of the jejunum and duodenum.

Box 3.28 CAUSES OF LOW-ATTENUATION LYMPH NODES

- Tuberculosis
- Lymphomas
- Necrotic metastases
- Coeliac disease
- Whipple disease

WIDENING OF THE PRE-SACRAL SPACE

A pre-sacral space of <15 mm is normal when measured between the mid-rectum and the sacrum. The most common cause of pre-sacral widening is rectal inflammation or malignancy.

Causes (work from the rectum backwards):

- Bowel (inflammatory bowel disease or tumour)
- Fat (pelvic lipomatosis or fibrosis, previous surgery or radiotherapy or developmental cysts: epidermoid, dermoid or duplication)
- Sacral disease (teratoma, meningocele, chordoma, neurofibroma or osteomyelitis)

ZOLLINGER–ELLISON SYNDROME

In 90% of cases, this is secondary to gastrinoma, a gastrin-secreting islet cell tumour. This leads to increased production of gastric HCl. Patients present with pain, diarrhoea and recurrent ulcers. In total, 25% are associated with multiple endocrine neoplasia type-1. (see Table 3.13).

BARIUM MEAL

- Thickened gastric or duodenal folds.
- Ulcers are most commonly found in the first part of the duodenum (10% have multiple ulcers).
- Dilatation of proximal small bowel due to hypersecretion.

PERITONEUM AND MESENTERY

ASCITES

- Collects in a predictable pattern.
- Morrison's pouch; pouch of Douglas; paravesical; paracolic gutters (right more than left).
- Fluid of density with an HU >30 suggests haemorrhage.

MESENTERIC ADENITIS

Common in patients <25 years of age. It presents with pain, fever and vomiting, usually due to viral enteritis.

US/CT

- Clustered, moderately enlarged nodes in the right lower quadrant
- With or without ileocecal wall thickening

MESENTERIC OEDEMA

Due to e.g. reduced albumin, cirrhosis, heart failure, trauma or ischaemia (latter with thickened bowel wall). A similar appearance is seen post-radiotherapy.

CT

- Diffuse hyperdense mesentery, making distinction of vessels difficult.
- Hyperdense mesenteric fat and mesenteric retraction post-radiotherapy.

MESENTERIC PANNICULITIS

Rare, chronic inflammation of small bowel mesenteric fat. The fibrosing variant is known as fibrosing mesenteritis. Desmoid and carcinoid tumours are important differentials.

CT

- Well-defined, heterogeneous mass at the mesenteric root, which envelops vessels but does not involve bowel.
- Predilection for involvement of jejunal mesentery.
- Look for a low-attenuation halo of spared perivascular fat.

OMENTAL INFARCTION

Most commonly affects the right side of the greater omentum and presents with acute abdominal pain.

CT

- High-attenuation streaks in the omental fat with mass effect
- Normal large and small bowel

PERITONEAL MESOTHELIOMA

Rare—however, it is the most common peritoneal primary. Associated with asbestos (50%) and radiation therapy; prognosis is poor.

CT

- Diffusely thickened/nodular peritoneum, omentum and mesentery
- Foci of calcification
- Pleural thickening
- Often no ascites (therefore can be distinguished from secondary disease)
- Invades adjacent organs

PERITONEAL METASTASIS

Most commonly from the colon, stomach, pancreas or ovary.

CT

- Linear fat stranding adjacent to the site of primary indicates invasion.
- Peritoneal carcinomatosis is associated with ascites and nodules.
- Look for enhancing nodules on the diaphragm and around the liver and spleen—calcified nodules pre-treatment suggest an ovarian or gastric primary.

PERITONITIS

May cause peritoneal/mesenteric thickening. Causes include bacterial, chemical or granulomatous disease, TB (dense ascites) and sclerosing peritonitis (a common complication of peritoneal dialysis).

CT

- Thickened, adherent small bowel loops and bowel dilatation initially.
- Loculated ascites, bowel obstruction and peritoneal/bowel wall calcification typical later.

PSEUDOMYXOMA PERITONEI

Follows rupture of a benign or malignant mucin-producing tumour, most commonly from the appendix or ovary.

CT (FIGURE 3.14)

- Large volume of low-attenuation fluid, may be loculated.
- Peritoneal calcification.
- Scalloping of the liver/splenic contour is a characteristic of mucinous ascites.

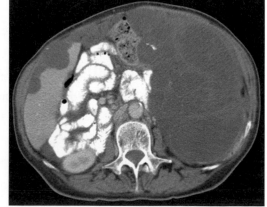

Figure 3.14 Pseudomyxoma peritonei. Axial CT image with intravenous contrast demonstrating loculated low-attenuation fluid with characteristic scalloping of the liver.

RETROPERITONEAL LEIOMYOSARCOMA

These account for about a third of soft tissue sarcomas. They arise from the smooth muscles of the blood vessels (more commonly veins) or bowel and are more common in women. The inferior vena cava (IVC) is most commonly affected.

CT

- May be intra- or extra-luminal (more common), or a combination of either.
- Large, heterogeneous enhancing mass.
- May have a large cystic component—fat and calcification less common.
- Distant metastasis to liver and lung is common with the intravascular type.
- Exclude renal cell carcinoma as the cause of tumour thrombus (appears similar and is much more common).

MRI

- Predominantly high on T2, foci of high T1 due to haemorrhage

RETROPERITONEAL LIPOSARCOMA

This is an uncommon tumour, but it is the most common retroperitoneal sarcoma. It affects adults and is lipomatous with a soft tissue component.

CT

- Fat components easily identified on CT (HU $\leq$–10)—may be slightly higher density than 'normal' fat.
- May be cystic.
- Differentiation from a benign lipoma is not always possible—however, septations >2 mm thick or nodules suggest sarcoma.
- Mass enhances with contrast.

MRI

- High signal on T1 and T2 due to fat content.
- Myxoid type is hyperintense on T2 and shows delayed enhancement post-contrast.

RETROPERITONEAL MALIGNANT FIBROUS HISTIOCYTOMA

Rare, but it is the most common tumour to arise due to previous radiotherapy.
It is an aggressive tumour that is more common in men. About 15% occur in the retroperitoneum.

CT

- Large, heterogenous soft tissue mass.
- Contains areas of necrosis that are low attenuation.
- Calcification in about 25%—this is quite specific to this tumour and rare in other retroperitoneal malignancies.

RETROPERITONEAL VASCULAR MALIGNANCY

Composed of haemangiopericytoma and angiosarcoma. Haemangiopericytoma has a favourable prognosis; angiosarcoma is very aggressive and metastasises early.

CT/MRI

- Amorphous calcification is a rare feature.
- Highly vascular tumours demonstrating brisk enhancement.

LIVER

Box 3.29 COMMON VARIANTS OF HEPATIC ARTERY (HA) ANATOMY

Replaced left (10%)
Left HA comes off left gastric artery

Replaced right (10%)
Right HA comes off superior mesenteric artery

Accessory left (10%)
Extra left HA from left gastric artery

Accessory right (10%)
Extra right HA from superior mesenteric artery

Box 3.30 CROSS-SECTIONAL IMAGING OF THE LIVER

Computed tomography
- Normal liver is 55–60 HU post-contrast, usually 8–10 HU more than the spleen.
- Most liver tumours are arterialised and so show maximal enhancement in the arterial phase (20–40 seconds post-contrast).

Magnetic resonance imaging
- Normal liver returns a signal similar to muscle, except on inversion recovery.
- On T1, spleen is darker than liver; on T2, spleen is brighter than liver.
- Gadolinium is the most commonly used contrast agent.
- Superparamagnetic iron oxide particles shorten T1 and T2 and are taken up by the reticuloendothelial system.
- Hepatocyte-specific agents (e.g. mangafodipir) accumulate in hepatocytes and are then excreted via the bile—normal liver parenchymal enhancement & biliary system.
- See Tables 3.10 and 3.11 new for summary and comparison of the characteristics of focal liver lesions.

ABSCESS—AMOEBIC

Tends to affect younger patients, typically the patient is acutely unwell and may have a history of recent travel.

US

- Large solitary lesion, typically affects the right hepatic lobe
- Hypoechoic with thick nodular walls

ABSCESS—FUNGAL

Occurs in immunosuppressed patients, mostly due to candidiasis.

US

- Most commonly fibrotic changes are seen—hypoechoic liver
- 'Wheel within wheel' appearance is caused early in the disease by a central necrotic hypoechoic nidus of fungal elements, surrounded by an echogenic rim.
- Hyper-reflective areas denote scarring

CT

- Scattered areas of calcification may be seen with fibrosis and scarring
- Multiple small foci of low attenuation post-contrast indicate microabscesses
- Features are often non-specific and biopsy may be required

ABSCESS—PYOGENIC

Most commonly due to ascending cholangitis from benign or obstructive biliary disease or due to haematogenous seeding (e.g. from diverticulitis). *E. coli* is the most common pathogen. Treatment is with percutaneous or surgical drainage.

US

- Poorly defined hypoechoic (hyperechoic in 25%) lesion with internal debris
- Septated with irregular walls
- May contain hyperechoic foci (i.e. gas)

CT (FIGURE 3.15)

- Peripheral rim of enhancement
- Irregular shape
- Attenuation between 0 and 45 HU
- May contain gas locules

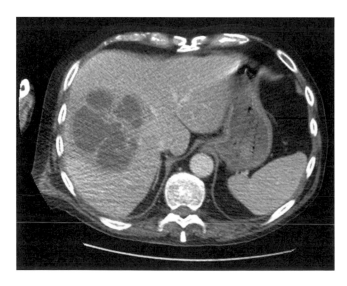

Figure 3.15 Liver abscess. Axial CT image with intravenous contrast demonstrating a low-attenuation liver lesion with peripheral enhancement and enhancing internal septae.

ADENOMA

This is a benign tumour composed of proliferating hepatocytes. It typically affects young women on the oral contraceptive pill or may be linked to glycogen storage disease. There may be rapid growth during pregnancy. There is a small risk of malignant transformation (1%).

US

- Typically 8–10 cm in size, hyperechoic lesion (may mimic haemangioma).
- 80% solitary, right lobe.
- Central areas of low echogenicity caused by haemorrhage or necrosis.
- Check for subcapsular/intraperitoneal haematoma.

CT

- Hypodense.
- Transient arterial enhancement, isodense by portal venous phase.
- There may be mixed enhancement with hypodense patches due to necrosis and degeneration (as they outgrow vascular supply).
- Check for subcapsular or intraperitoneal haematoma.

MRI

- High T1 (most other lesions are low T1) due to glycogen, fat and haemorrhage
- Isointense on in-phase T1, loses signal on out-of-phase images
- Isointense on T2
- Immediate and intense enhancement with rapid washout

NUCLEAR MEDICINE

- Reduced tracer uptake on technetium-99m-labelled sulphur colloid scan (due to non-functioning Kupffer cells)

ANGIOGRAPHY

- Large peripheral arteries feeding into the tumour mass

ADENOMYOMATOSIS

This is an unusual condition, more common in females and associated with gallstones (90%). It often presents with right upper quadrant pain. It is associated with thickening of the smooth muscle of the gallbladder, causing mucosal folding.

US (FIGURE 3.16)

- Bright reflections.
- Comet-tail artefacts from the gallbladder wall—due to the visualisation of cholesterol-filled hyperechoic sinuses (Rokitansky–Aschoff sinuses).

- Characterised by generalised or focal mural thickening with intramural diverticula.
- Main differential for focal thickening is gallbladder cancer.

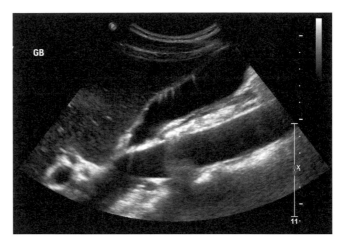

Figure 3.16 Adenomyomatosis. Ultrasound image demonstrating comet tail artefacts from the superior gallbladder wall.

MRI

- The string of beads sign is the hallmark and is highly specific in differentiating it from carcinoma (multiple foci of high signal within the wall of the gallbladder on T2).

AEROBILIA

Mostly iatrogenic, post-sphincterotomy or formation of a Roux loop.

CT

- Most collects in the non-dependent biliary tree.
- Aerobilia in the context of a biliary stent suggests stent patency.

AMIDARONE

Antiarrhythmic agent affecting the liver due to a build-up of iodinated metabolites. More commonly causes pulmonary fibrosis (basal segments).

CT

- Increased liver attenuation of 95–145 HU (normal 30–70 HU)
- Spleen not involved (unlike haemochromatosis) (Table 3.7)

Table 3.7 Causes of altered liver attenuation

Increased	Decreased	Increased or decreased
Amiodarone	Fatty infiltration	Glycogen storage disease
Thorotrastosis	Steroid use	
Cisplatin	Chemotherapy	
Haemochromatosis	Nutritional	
Haemosiderosis	Amyloid	
Iron overload	Hepatic venous congestion	
Wilson disease	Diabetes	

Note: Hyperattenuation is due to high-atomic number element infiltration; hypoattenuation is due to increased low-atomic number elements (e.g. C, H and O).

ANGIOSARCOMA

Aggressive tumour with a poor prognosis. The tumour has a heterogeneous appearance on all imaging modalities.

CT

- Heterogeneous appearance due to multiple haemorrhagic foci within the lesion.
- Enhances heterogeneously and progressively in the venous phase.
- Often multinodular.

BILIARY CYSTADENOMA

This tumour arises from the bile ducts in the right lobe. It is more common in women and may undergo malignant transformation.

US

- Often a multilocular cystic lesion in the right hepatic lobe.
- Contains internal septations.
- Mural papillary projections are characteristic.

CT

- Well-defined cystic lesions with internal septations.
- Septations, cyst walls and solid components may enhance (unlike simple cysts).

BILIARY HAMARTOMAS

This is a benign ductal abnormality; may mimic metastases.

MRI

- Liver normal in size.
- Numerous tiny lesions (<5 mm)—these are predominantly high signal on T2.
- Lesions can contain a small solid component.

BIOPSY

The preferred approach is right lateral for liver biopsy, or anterior sub-costal if there is respiratory compromise (patient can sit up more easily). Traversing normal liver reduces the risk of bleeding.

Consent for:

- Haemorrhage, pneumothorax, biliary peritonitis, bowel/gallbladder perforation, arterioportal shunt (all 1/300, tend to occur in first 24 hours).
- Overall risk of death is 1/10,000 in those with liver disease.

BUDD–CHIARI SYNDROME

It presents with hepatomegaly, ascites and classically paroxysmal nocturnal haemoglobinuria (dark urine in the morning). Caused by membranous obstruction of the suprahepatic IVC (i.e. venous outflow) by a congenital web or hepatic venous thrombosis (due to e.g. thrombophilia or metastases). About two-thirds of cases are idiopathic.

US

- Hepatic veins may not be seen.
- Thrombus within hepatic veins.
- Turbulent or reversed hepatic venous flow.
- Marked peripheral collaterals.
- Hepatosplenomegaly.
- Caudate hypertrophy only occurs with chronic Budd–Chiari syndrome.

CT

- Enlarged liver with ascites when acute
- Hyperenhancing central liver segments on early-phase, post-contrast, peripheral hypoenhancement (this pattern reverses on delayed images—the 'flip-flop' pattern).
- Absent hepatic veins.
- Caudate hypertrophy with chronic Budd–Chiari syndrome (compensatory enlargement, the caudate is spared as it drains directly into the IVC).
- Dysmorphic appearance to liver, mosaic enhancement.
- Gallbladder wall thickening.
- Increased portal vein diameter.

MRI

- Enhancement as per CT, but may also show absence of flow voids on T1 images if thrombus is present.

INTERVENTION

- A 'spider's web' appearance of collaterals is diagnostic.
- Thrombus in hepatic veins.
- Balloon dilatation of the hepatic venous web may be performed for treatment.

CALCULOUS CHOLECYSTITIS

Up to 95% of cholecystitis involves stones.

US

- Gallstones and gallbladder wall >3 mm thick is most sensitive.
- Markedly distended gall bladder (>5 cm), pericholecystic fluid, wall hyperaemia and wall striations are suggestive.

CT

- Intramural or intracystic gas suggests gangrenous cholecystitis or emphysematous cholecystitis.
- Up to 10% of gallbladders perforate with acute cholecystitis.

NUCLEAR MEDICINE

- Hepatic iminodiacetic acid (HIDA) scan: technetium-99m-labelled bilirubin analogue given intravenously; images then gathered over the next 2–4 hours.
- Passage of isotope: liver → bile ducts → gallbladder and duodenum → small bowel.
- Needs gallbladder to be present and cystic duct to be patent.
- Non-visualisation of the gallbladder at 4 hours is diagnostic (i.e. cystic duct is obstructed).

Box 3.31 CAUSES OF GALLBLADDER WALL THICKENING

Intrinsic
- Cholecystitis (acute or chronic)

Extrinsic (three H's and an R)
- **H**epatitis
- **H**ypoalbuminaemia
- **H**eart failure
- **R**enal failure

Focal
- Adenomyomatosis
- Cholesterosis
- Gallbladder carcinoma

Box 3.32 ACALCULOUS CHOLECYSTITIS

Most often seen in the intensive care (ITU) setting. US may show echogenic gallbladder contents and a distended, thick-walled gallbladder. HIDA is most sensitive for diagnosis.

CAROLI DISEASE

Rare, autosomal recessive disease. Patients often present aged 10–30 years with recurrent cholangitis. Predisposes to infection, inflammation, stones and cholangiocarcinoma. Associated with medullary sponge kidney and renal cysts.

US

- Multiple cystic structures converging towards the porta hepatis and communicating with the bile ducts
- No strictures

CT

- Multiple cystic structures with a central enhancing 'dot', representing the portal vein radicles surrounded by dilated ducts—the central dot sign.
- The central dot sign and communication with the bile ducts help distinguish Caroli disease from multiple hepatic cysts.

MRCP

- Ectatic intrahepatic ducts extending to the periphery
- Dilated common bile duct
- No strictures

CHOLANGIOCARCINOMA

Originates in the bile duct epithelium and spreads by direct invasion. In total, 60% are perihilar (i.e. Klatskin tumours). Most present with hilar obstruction and normal extrahepatic ducts. Risk factors include inflammatory bowel disease (10-fold), primary sclerosing cholangitis (15-year latency), choledochal cysts, chronic stones and viral hepatitis. It may appear as a frank mass, intraductal polyp or diffuse duct wall thickening. The tumour commonly invades nerves, infiltrates the liver and metastasises to coeliac lymph nodes and the peritoneum.

Box 3.33 THE BISMUTH CLASSIFICATION OF CHOLANGIOCARCINOMA

I: common bile duct
II: hilar and first-order ducts
IIIA: hilar and extends into the second-order ducts on the right
IIIB: hilar and extends into the second-order ducts on the left
IV: hilar and extends into the second-order ducts bilaterally

---

US

- Right hepatic lobe affected more commonly
- Nodules/focal bile duct wall thickening
- Hyperechoic bile duct walls

CT

- Can be subtle—tumour mass is often isodense.
- Peripheral enhancement.
- Delayed enhancement of the lesion (best seen at 10 minutes).
- Intrahepatic duct dilatation.
- May contain calcification.
- Liver infiltration is common.
- Check for peritoneal disease (10%).

MRCP

- Most sensitive for diagnosis.
- Check for vascular encasement.
- Lesion is high signal on T2, low signal on T1.
- Enhancement characteristics as for CT.
- Does not take up superparamagnetic iron oxide (SPIO).

Box 3.34 FACTORS FAVOURING CHOLANGIOCARCINOMA OVER HEPATOCELLULAR CARCINOMA

- Non-cirrhotic liver.
- No significant central arterial phase enhancement.
- No capsule.
- Dilated bile ducts peripheral to a cholangiocarcinoma in 30%, but only in about 2% of hepatomas.
- Liver capsular retraction.

CHOLANGITIS

This is mostly due to stone-related biliary obstruction.

US

- Dilated intra- and extra-hepatic bile ducts
- Calculi in the gallbladder or ducts

CT

- Useful if an abscess is suspected.

CHOLECYSTODUODENAL FISTULA

Rare—either from cancer or more commonly chronic stone disease. In total, 90% are associated with perforations due to gallstones. Either fistulates to the duodenum or the colon. May lead to gallstone ileus.

PLAIN FILM

- Gallstone ileus: dilated bowel, opaque gallstone in bowel and pneumobilia (rare) (Figure 3.17)

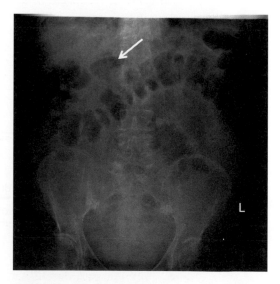

Figure 3.17 Gallstone ileus. Frontal abdominal radiograph demonstrating small bowel dilatation with pneumobilia (white arrow).

CT

- Pneumobilia
- Shrunken gallbladder mimicking a diverticulum of the duodenal bulb

---

Box 3.35 CAUSES OF PNEUMOBILIA

Choledochal fistula
Iatrogenic
Choledochoenterostomies (e.g. Whipple's)
Endoscopic retrograde cholangiopancreatography (ERCP) + sphincterotomy

---

CHOLEDOCHAL CYSTS

These result from congenital focal or diffuse dilatation of the bile ducts. They are the most common congenital lesions of the gallbladder. They are associated with biliary stasis leading to infection, inflammation and stone disease. There is a 20-fold increased risk of cholangiocarcinoma (Table 3.8).

US

- Variable appearances (Table 3.9).
- Most commonly there is simply common bile duct (CBD) dilatation with normal intrahepatic ducts (type I).

Table 3.8 The Todani classification of bile duct cysts

Type	Frequency	Characteristics
I	Up to 90%	Solitary dilatation of the common bile duct, non-dilated intrahepatic ducts
II	2%	True ductal diverticulum arising from the common bile duct
III	2%	Choledochocele—there is dilatation of the last part of the common bile duct within the duodenum
IV	20%	Dominant extrahepatic duct dilatation with multifocal intrahepatic duct dilatation
V	Rare	Caroli disease—multiple, cystic dilatation of the intrahepatic bile ducts

Table 3.9 Characteristics of bile duct cysts on HIDA scan

	Choledochal cyst	Hepatic cyst	Biliary atresia
Photopenia present	Yes	Yes	No; whole liver takes up HIDA
Small bowel visualisation	Paucity of contrast in the small bowel	Small bowel visualised	No contrast in the small bowel

HIDA SCAN

- Demonstrates cystic structure connected to the biliary system.
- Positive result shows a photopenic area that fills within 60 minutes, with a paucity of contrast/lack of visualisation in the small bowel.

CHOLELITHIASIS

In total, 90% of ductal stones come from the gallbladder, with the rest arising from the duct itself. A total of 70% are cholesterol based; they are pigment based if arising in the duct itself. Only about 10% are visible on CT. The biliary system is best imaged following a 4–hour fast (to distend the gallbladder).

Box 3.36 CBD MEASUREMENTS

Post-cholecystectomy, ≤10 mm is acceptable. Otherwise, 1 mm for every 10 years from 5 mm at 50 years of age (i.e. 6 mm at 60 years of age, etc.).

US

- First line, good specificity (>95%).
- Shadow casting calculi in the gallbladder/bile ducts.
- Non-shadowing echogenicity is sludge (could also be blood or pus).
- Mimics include—gas, blood clots, clips, arterial calcification, parasites.
- CBD <4 mm unlikely to contain any stones.
- EUS is most sensitive for detecting CBD stones.

CT

- Stone detected when surrounded by lower density bile.

MRCP

- Bile ducts clearly demonstrated on T2-weighted sequences, best seen in the coronal plane.
- Most sensitive, may be reserved where there is a low likelihood of stone.
- Stones are represented by low-signal filling defects.
- Not reliant on normal liver function.
- Risk of false negative with gas, blood and flow voids.

CIRRHOSIS

Cirrhosis is the final step of liver injury, and is not usually reversible. Hepatocellular necrosis leads to fibrosis and nodule regeneration. The process may occur over weeks or years. Patients have altered immunity and undergo changes in the vascular bed both in the liver and in the lungs. Cirrhotic patients are at increased risk of pulmonary complications including bacterial pneumonia, hydrothorax, pulmonary hypertension and adult respiratory distress syndrome. The top three causes of cirrhosis are hepatitis C, alcohol and idiopathic. Hepatocellular carcinoma (HCC) develops in up to 25% of patients with cirrhosis.

US

- Advised for surveillance every 6 months (rule out hepatocellular carcinoma [HCC]).
- Atrophy of segments VI and VII (i.e. right lobe), hypertrophy of segments I, II and III (left lobe).
- Echotexture has a coarse, 'starry night' appearance.
- Increased arterial flow, surface nodularity in advanced cirrhosis.
- Regenerative nodules are hypoechoic.
- Ascites.

CT

- CT and MRI are insensitive to early cirrhotic change.
- Reduced attenuation due to fatty infiltration.
- Irregular heterogeneous liver with low attenuation and ascites.
- Retracted capsule with low attenuation beneath may represent focal fibrosis—rare, diagnosed by biopsy.

MRI

- Regenerative nodules may be high signal on T1 (due to iron accumulation, 'siderotic nodule') and low signal on T2—opposite pattern to a metastasis.
- HCCs have enhancing pseudocapsules, whereas dysplastic nodules do not.

Box 3.37 CYSTIC FIBROSIS LIVER MANIFESTATIONS

- Cirrhosis, fibrosis and portal hypertension.
- Steatosis.
- Sclerosing cholangitis.
- Cholelithiasis.
- Micro-gallbladder is commonly seen.

EPITHELIOID HAEMANGIOENDOTHELIOMA

This is more common in women. There are multiple peripheral nodules that may coalesce and cause capsular retraction. Spared segments hypertrophy.

US

- Solid, hypoechoic lesions

CT

- Multiple slow-growing, peripheral, low-density foci that may coalesce.
- Punctuate calcification.
- Prominent rim enhancement with contrast ('halo sign').
- There may be capsular retraction adjacent to a nodule.

MRI

- Lesions are non-specific, low signal on T1, high on T2.

FATTY INFILTRATION

Box 3.38 IMAGING PITFALLS WITH DIFFUSE FATTY INFILTRATION
Due to accumulation of fats in hepatocytes.
Imaging with CT:
• Liver density of <40 HU is specific, but not sensitive.
• Note—the spleen enhances earlier than the liver, so comparing densities in the arterial or early portal venous phases is unhelpful.
Source: Hamer, O.W. et al. Fatty liver: Imaging patterns and pitfalls. *Radiographics* 26:1637–1653.

Increased triglyceride loading of hepatocytes due to excess alcohol, obesity, diabetes, CF, malnutrition, total parenteral nutrition, drugs (steroids, methotrexate, chemotherapy and amiodarone), hepatitis or pregnancy. The stages are:

1. Steatosis (common, affects 15% of the population)
2. Non-alcoholic steatohepatitis (NASH) (6%–8% progress to this)
3. Cirrhosis (15% progress to cirrhosis)

US

- Diffusely hyper-reflective liver—adjacent renal cortex is hypo-reflective compared to the adjacent liver (the reflectivity is normally similar).
- Loss of definition of the diaphragm.
- Poor visualisation of the intrahepatic architecture.

CT

- Liver is diffusely hypodense—eventually, hepatic vessels look as if they contain contrast when they do not.
- Density of <40 HU is diagnostic.
- Density >10 HU less than that of the spleen on an unenhanced scan.

MRI

- In- and out-of-phase imaging is best for diagnosis: there is loss of signal on out-of-phase imaging compared to in-phase imaging.
- Increased signal on T1 and mildly so on T2.
- Low signal on STIR.

Box 3.39 IN- AND OUT-OF-PHASE IMAGING
Fat and water in the same voxel cancel out when out of phase (check the vertebral body—this should also appear low signal due to fatty bone marrow).

FIBROLAMELLAR CARCINOMA (FLC)

This is an uncommon variant of HCC affecting young patients with no risk factors. The tumour is typically large at diagnosis. The overall prognosis is better than HCC, with a 5–year mortality rate of 30%–40% (90% with HCC). Local recurrence and nodal metastases are common.

US

- Solid, encapsulated mass of 5–20 cm at presentation
- Calcification
- Hyperechoic scar (60%)

CT

- Lobulated margin.
- Hypodense, particularly the central scar.
- Punctate calcification in 50%.
- Moderate, peripheral arterial enhancement post-contrast.
- Low attenuation on the portal phase (i.e. rapid washout).
- Scar does not enhance, but often contains calcification.

MRI

- Mass low signal on T1, high on T2

Box 3.40 FIBROLAMELLAR CARCINOMA VERSUS HEPATOCELLULAR CARCINOMA

- Not associated with elevated alpha-fetoprotein (AFP).
- Not associated with cirrhosis.
- Often calcified.
- Better prognosis than hepatocellular carcinoma.
- Does not washout as much as hepatocellular carcinoma—isointense in venous phase.

Box 3.41 FIBROLAMELLAR CARCINOMA VERSUS FOCAL NODULAR HYPERPLASIA (FNH)

- Calcification in fibrolamellar carcinoma.
- Scar is low T2, whereas in FNH it is high T2.
- Central scar does not enhance with fibrolamellar carcinoma (it does with FNH).

FOCAL FATTY INFILTRATION

This is associated with obesity, diabetes and alcohol excess.

CT

- 'Geographic' distribution of low density, typically in the gallbladder fossa, adjacent to the falciform ligament or at the porta hepatis.
- No enhancement or mass effect.

MRI

- Geographic area of increased T1 signal, isointense/low T2 signal.
- Signal loss on out-of-phase images.
- Adenomas and HCCs also lose signal on out-of-phase images—however, these display mass effect/displace vessels.

FOCAL NODULAR HYPERPLASIA (FNH)

This is a benign, hamartomatous malformation that is most common in young women. It is the second most common benign tumour after haemangioma. The tumour is made up of hyperplastic liver tissue arranged in an abnormal fashion. They are asymptomatic and rarely bleed.

US

- Well-defined lesion, usually peripheral right lobe
- Usually <5 cm
- Mostly solitary (about 20% are multiple)
- Large central vessel that may be detectable on Doppler
- Basket/spoke wheel pattern on contrast US

MRI (FIGURE 3.18)

- Calcification, necrosis and haemorrhage are rare.
- Isointense and resembles normal liver.
- Marked enhancement post-contrast on the arterial phase with radiating septa.
- Arterial enhancement of the lesion, delayed enhancement of the scar.
- FNH retains gadobenate and appears isointense, building to hyperintense 1–3 hours later.
- 50% have a central scar.
- Central scar is bright on T2 (central scar of FLC shows low T2 signal), low on T1.

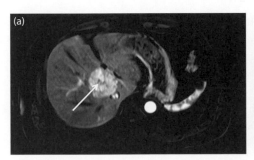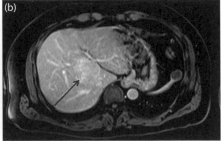

Figure 3.18 Focal nodular hyperplasia. Post-contrast axial images from an MRI of the liver. (a) Arterial phase imaging shows an avidly enhancing lesion with a hypointense central scar (white arrow). (b) Delayed phase imaging shows the lesion to become isointense to the background lines with enhancement of the central scar (red arrow).

CT

- Isodense/slightly hypoattenuating lesion on unenhanced CT.
- Hypodense scar may enhance.
- Intense transient arterial enhancement, isodense to liver on the venous phase.

NUCLEAR MEDICINE

- 70% show normal or increased uptake on technetium-99m-labelled sulphur colloid scan—specific to FNH (colloid is a Kupffer cell agent, Kupffer cells are present in normal liver and FNH—not present in e.g. FLC).
- Technetium-99m HIDA scan shows immediate uptake and delayed clearance in 90%.

Box 3.42 LIVER TUMOURS WITH A CENTRAL SCAR

- Adenoma
- Fibrolamellar carcinoma
- Giant cavernous haemangioma
- FNH

Box 3.43 FNH VERSUS ADENOMA

- Central stellate scar.
- Uptake of hepatobiliary contrast agents on magnetic resonance imaging.
- FNH not associated with the oral contraceptive pill.
- Adenoma has propensity for spontaneous haemorrhage.
- Size.
- T1 high in adenoma.

GALLBLADDER CANCER

Rare—prognosis is poor. It presents with biliary obstruction, and mostly occurs in the context of stones. Melanoma, breast cancer and lymphoma may metastasise to the gallbladder.

US

- Focal area of wall thickening
- Vascular mass on Doppler US
- Gallstones in up to 90%

CT

- Gallbladder mass that commonly spreads by direct extension into the liver.
- Enhances with contrast.
- Nodes at the porta hepatis.
- Peritoneal disease is common.

GALLBLADDER POLYPS

These are common, mostly benign and cholesterol based. The risk of malignancy is increased significantly with polyps >10 mm, and these are removed. Lesions >6 mm are followed up with US.

US

- Non-mobile polypoid lesion in the lumen of the gallbladder.
- No posterior acoustic shadow.
- May be mobile if the stalk is long.

HAEMANGIOMA

This is the most common benign liver tumour and affects 2%–5% of the population. It is more common in women and is composed of blood-filled spaces contained by fibrous walls lined by epithelial cells. They are often asymptomatic, but may present with hepatomegaly or, rarely, spontaneous haemorrhage. There are two types:

- Simple (most common, multiple in 10%, may enlarge during pregnancy)
- Cavernous/giant (rare, >5 cm, may cause symptoms due to haemorrhage or necrosis)

US

- Hyperechoic, well defined and lobulated
- Large haemangioma may appear heterogeneous
- Can be hypoechoic, especially in paediatric patients = cavernous haemangioma
- No flow within, may have adjacent flow (cavernous haemangioma may show internal flow)

CT

- Well-defined, hypodense mass pre-contrast
- Early peripheral nodular enhancement with central fill in on delayed scan

MRI (FIGURE 3.19)

- Hypointense on T1
- Very bright on T2, 'light bulb sign'
- Early peripheral nodular enhancement and central fill-in as for CT

NUCLEAR MEDICINE

- Low uptake on single photon emission computed tomography (SPECT) with technetium-labelled erythrocytes—the lesions fill in and demonstrate increased activity on delayed scan.

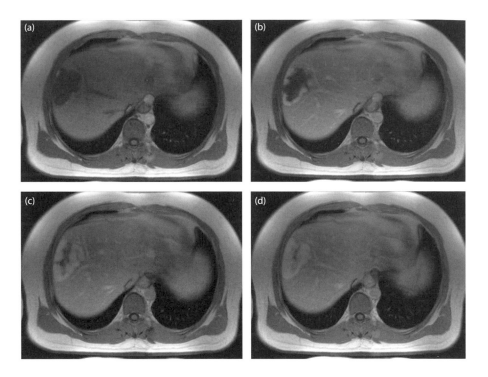

Figure 3.19 Hepatic haemangioma. Dynamic post-contrast axial images from a magnetic resonance image of the liver. There is a lesion in the right hepatic lobe which shows early peripheral enhancement (a, b) and progressive centripetal fill-in (c, d).

HAEMOCHROMATOSIS

This is an inherited or acquired multi-system disease due to iron deposition (including out of the reticuloendothelial system). The primary form is inherited by autosomal recessive inheritance. There is an increased risk of malignancy in the liver, especially HCC. Iron is also deposited to the skin (90%), myocardium (15%), endocrine glands and joints (20%). 30% of patients are diabetic due to pancreatic damage.

CT
- Hepatosplenomegaly
- Liver attenuation 75–135 HU non-contrast

MRI (FIGURE 3.20)
- Iron causes signal loss— best seen on T2* gradient echo (also seen on T1).

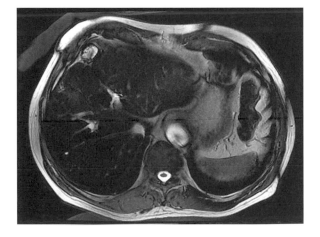

Figure 3.20 Haemochromatosis. Axial T2-weighted images of the abdomen demonstrating marked signal loss within the liver.

- Significant signal loss on T2 is characteristic.
- Signal loss in liver and pancreas—the spleen is spared.

HAEMOSIDEROSIS

This is due to haemosiderin deposition (mostly in the reticuloendothelial system), associated with repeated blood transfusions. There is iron deposition without organ dysfunction mostly in the liver, spleen and bone marrow.

CT

- Liver density is >75 HU, greater than expected (usually 55–60 HU).

MRI

- Low signal T1, T2 and T2* in the liver and spleen—the pancreas is spared.
- Best demonstrated by signal loss on T2* gradient echo sequences (GRE)—the more iron there is, the more signal is lost.
- The spleen is usually less infiltrated than the liver (therefore brighter on MRI).

HEPATIC ARTERY ANEURYSM

This is the second most common splanchnic aneurysm due to atherosclerosis, trauma or infection. In total, 60% are symptomatic with right upper quadrant pain, GI haemorrhage and obstructive jaundice being most common.

CT

- May have curvilinear calcifications
- Usually extrahepatic (20% intrahepatic)
- Intense enhancement if not thrombosed

HEPATIC INFARCTION

Uncommon due to the dual blood supply of the liver. Causes include transjugular intrahepatic portosystemic stunt (TIPS), cholecystectomy, chemoembolisation, liver transplant, arterial emboli and hypercoagulable states (e.g. sepsis). Abscess, scarring and failure of transplanted livers are complications.

CT

- Solitary/multiple peripheral wedge-shaped areas of low attenuation and poor enhancement.
- Review hepatic artery and portal vein for evidence of thrombosis.

HEPATIC VENOUS CONGESTION

Passive hepatic congestion refers to the effects of impaired hepatic venous drainage due to cardiac disease. Cardiac failure and tricuspid valve disease are common causes. It may be a sign of right heart strain in the setting of pulmonary emboli.

US

- Hepatomegaly with distended hepatic veins and IVC when acute.
- 'To-and-fro' blood flow in hepatic veins on Doppler (note—this is when hepatic venous flow occurs in both anterograde and retrograde directions due to raised right-sided cardiac pressure; normal hepatic venous (HV) flow should just be anterograde [i.e. flowing towards the heart]).
- Chronic congestion may cause cirrhosis.

CT

- Enlarged liver with distended hepatic veins and IVC
- Early filling of hepatic veins on arterial phase (due to reflux of contrast)
- Patchy parenchymal heterogeneous enhancement on venous phase
- Peri-portal low attenuation (oedema)
- Ascites
- Pleural effusions/cardiomegaly
- Cirrhosis with or without its complications with chronic disease

HEPATOBLASTOMA

More common in children aged <3 years, but can occur at any age. It is the third most common intra-abdominal tumour in children. AFP is grossly elevated.

CT

- Large, heterogeneous mass, confluent nodules
- Arterial enhancement with areas of central necrosis

HEPATOCELLULAR CARCINOMA (HCC)

This is the most common liver primary occurring mostly in patients with chronic liver disease and cirrhosis. AFP is the tumour marker, and gross elevation is diagnostic. The tumour derives its blood supply from the hepatic artery and often invades the portal vein. The most frequent site of metastasis is the lungs. Surgical resection and liver transplant are the only options for cure.

US

- Hyper- or hypo-echoic liver lesions—solitary, multifocal or diffuse.
- May show arterial vascularity.
- Heterogeneous reflectivity due to areas of necrosis.
- Smaller lesions are typically of homogeneous low reflectivity.
- Check the patency of the portal vein.

CT (FIGURE 3.21)

- Ill-defined and low-density (can be isodense) lesions.
- 10% have calcifications.
- May contain fat.
- Invasion of the portal vein is typical, look for an enlarged portal vein.
- Encapsulated low-density mass pre-contrast.
- Rapid arterial enhancement with washout in the venous phase.

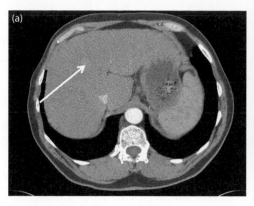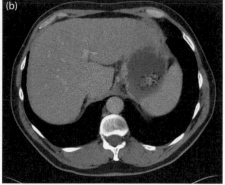

Figure 3.21 Hepatocellular carcinoma, axial CT images of the liver. (a) The arterial phase scan shows a small enhancing lesion in the right lobe. (b) The venous phase scan shows the lesion to washout.

MRI

- Marked enhancement in the arterial phase (20 seconds); there may be peripheral enhancement in the venous phase (60 seconds) due to pseudocapsule.
- Lesion is high signal on a T2* post-superparamagnetic iron oxide.

Box 3.44 SUPERPARAMAGNETIC IRON OXIDE (SPIO)

SPIO and gadolinium are useful for the detection of hepatocellular carcinoma in cirrhotic patients in whom the detection is difficult with gadolinium alone.

- SPIO is taken up by hepatocytes and causes marked T2 shortening (i.e. signal loss).
- The lesion composed of abnormal cells does not take up SPIO and therefore appears high signal.

INTERVENTION

- Thermal ablation/transarterial chemoembolisation (TACE) should only be performed in Child–Pugh score A or B patients.
- Thermal ablation is used for small tumours that are not amenable to surgery to give local control and increase life expectancy.
- Thermal ablation may also be used to control tumours in patients waiting for a transplant.
- TACE may be used for large, unresectable tumours.
- Can be combined—TACE to reduce tumour volume, followed by ablation.
- TACE after ablation may also decrease recurrence.

Box 3.45 CHILD–PUGH SCORE

System for grading liver function in chronic liver disease based on points awarded for international normalized ratio (INR), bilirubin, albumin, hepatic encephalopathy and ascites to determine grade A, B or C (severe).

HYDATID CYST

The liver is most commonly affected by this zoonosis. The cause is the *Echinococcus granulosus* or *Echinococcus multilocularis* tapeworm. The lungs are also commonly affected. In total, 50% have a blood eosinophilia. The Casoni skin test is useful for diagnosis.

US

- Variable appearance from a simple unilocular cyst to a complex heterogeneous cystic mass.
- Daughter cysts are a characteristic but rare finding—large central cyst with multiple small daughter cystic spaces peripherally.
- Detachment of the endocyst gives rise to 'floating membranes' within the cyst cavity.
- The 'water lily sign' is characteristic—a cyst with an undulating, floating membrane with a detached endocyst.
- 20%–30% of cysts calcify—usually curvilinear or ring-like.
- There is a risk of anaphylaxis with cyst aspiration due to intravascular transfer of cyst contents.

CT

- High-attenuation cyst wall (even without calcification).
- Wall and septae enhance with contrast (unlike a simple liver cyst).
- Predilection for the lower lobes of the lungs, with disease more common on the right (multiple in 20%, bilateral in 20%).

Box 3.46 CAUSES OF CALCIFIED LIVER LESIONS

Primary liver tumours
- Hepatocellular carcinoma
- Hepatoblastoma
- Fibrolamellar carcinoma
- Mucinous cystadenocarcinoma

Metastases

Inflammation and infection
- Granulomatous infection
- Parasitic (including hydatid)
- Abscess
- Sarcoid

Vascular
- Giant haemangioma
- Haematoma

KAPOSI SARCOMA

This is an AIDS-defining illness that primarily affects the skin. It is the most common AIDS-related neoplasm and often presents with multiple raised, purplish skin lesions. Lymph node enlargement is the second most common feature.

CT

- Enhancing abdominal lymph nodes
- Multiple 5–12–mm, low-attenuation nodules in the liver
- Skin lesions help to distinguish from fungal microabscesses and multiple haemangioma

LIVER TRANSPLANT

One arterial anastomosis, two venous (portal vein and IVC) and a biliary anastomosis. Hepatic artery thrombosis is the most common and serious early vascular complication post-transplant. In total, 30% of cases experience biliary complications (e.g. ischaemic stricture).

US

- Hepatic artery stenosis—tardus parvus waveform (low restistive index, prolonged systolic acceleration time).
- A small amount of perihepatic intraperitoneal fluid, periportal oedema and a right pleural effusion are expected for several weeks post-transplant.

Box 3.47 LIVER RESECTION
• Left hepatectomy—II and III resected.
• Right hepatectomy—V, VI, VII and VIII resected.
• IV is resected in an extended left or right hepatectomy.
• I is only resected in transplantation.

METASTASES

The liver is mostly involved by the haematogenous route via the hepatic artery. GI malignancy affects the liver via the portal vein. The top three tumours that metastasise to the liver are colorectal, gastric and pancreatic.

US

- Homogeneous, hyper- or hypo-echoic lesions.
- May be cystic (beware ovarian metastases that mimic simple cysts).
- Calcification, especially with mucinous tumours.
- Hyperechoic metastases most commonly from colonic adenocarcinoma, also renal cell carcinoma (RCC), choriocarcinoma and neuroendocrine tumours.

CT

- May show complete peripheral enhancement rather than solid (only haemangiomas show nodular).
- 2%–3% of liver metastases calcify, most commonly due to mucinous tumours (e.g. colon, gastric, ovarian, treated lymphoma or neuroblastoma in children).
- Most metastases are relatively hypovascular.
- Carcinoid, melanoma, thyroid, renal, pancreatic islet cell tumours and pheochromocytoma metastases are hypervascular.
- Peripheral washout is virtually diagnostic of malignancy.

MRI

- Most metastases have a non-specific appearance on MRI: low T1 signal, high T2 signal.
- Post-contrast, there is early peripheral enhancement with prolonged central enhancement and early peripheral washout.
- Diffusion-weighted imaging is especially useful for detecting small lesions, look for high diffusion-weighted imaging signal with corresponding low signal on the apparent diffusion coefficient map.

INTERVENTION

- Thermal ablation is considered for tumours <5 cm that are unsuitable for surgery or control of small-volume disease post-resection.
- Approaches include radiofrequency ablation, microwave, cryoablation and irreversible electroporation.

Box 3.48 BENIGN MIMICS OF LIVER METASTASES

- Focal fatty infiltration
- Regenerating nodules
- Focal fibrosis
- Abscess
- Focal nodular hyperplasia
- Adenoma

MIRIZZI SYNDROME

This is a rare syndrome due to obstruction of the common bile duct owing to extrinsic compression from a large calculus in the cystic duct. Fistulation may occur.

US

- Dilatation of the common bile duct to the level of a stone that lies outside of the CBD (i.e. in the cystic duct).

NODULAR REGENERATIVE HYPERPLASIA (NRH)

In the context of cirrhosis, some nodules of regenerating parenchyma may dominate—this may be confused with HCC. NRH represents reparative attempts by hepatocytes in response to liver injury.

US

- Hypoechoic nodules, typically <1 cm

CT

- Typically under 1 cm.
- Isodense to liver parenchyma unless they contain iron deposits (siderotic nodules), in which case they are hyperdense.
- Dysplastic nodules typically are >1 cm, seen in up to 25% of cirrhotic livers.

Table 3.10 Typical enhancement characteristics of focal liver lesions

Arterial enhancement	Delayed enhancement
Adenoma	Haemangioma
Hepatocellular carcinoma	Cholangiocarcinoma
FNH	Solitary fibrous tumour
	Treated metastases

Box 3.49 MAGNETIC RESONANCE IMAGING SIGNAL CHARACTERISTICS

- T1—liver > spleen > muscle
- T2—spleen > liver
- Lesions with high signal on T1: fat-containing (including adenoma), proteinaceous, blood products, melanoma, contrast

---

PERCUTANEOUS TRANSHEPATIC CHOLANGIOGRAPHY/ PERCUTANEOUS TRANSHEPATIC BILIARY DRAINAGE

Rarely done for diagnostic reasons, mostly used for relief of biliary obstruction/palliation where surgery is not possible. Metal stents preferred if surgery is not planned, otherwise plastic.

- Complications include sepsis, haemorrhage and death (1%–2%).
- Sepsis/haemorrhage in 2% post-procedure, death in 1.7%.
- US-guided puncture of right hepatic ducts via right flank, left-sided ducts via epigastrium

POLYCYSTIC LIVER DISEASE

This is a benign, hereditary disease that may or may not be associated with autosomal dominant polycystic kidney disease (ADPKD). There is no malignant potential. Complications include haemorrhage, portal hypertension and infection. Aspiration provides short-term relief of symptoms.

PORCELAIN GALLBLADDER

Due to chronic cholecystitis, there is dense wall calcification. Associated with malignancy in up to 30%, therefore a prophylactic cholecystectomy should be offered.

US

- Dense acoustic shadowing from the calcified wall—easily mistaken for gas

CT (FIGURE 3.22)

- Circumferential, dense gallbladder wall calcification

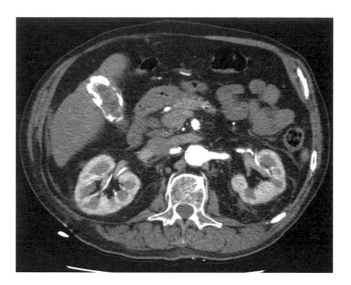

Figure 3.22 Porcelain gallbladder. Axial computed tomography images of the abdomen with intravenous contrast demonstrating a circumferential dense mural calcification of the gallbladder.

PORTAL HYPERTENSION

Defined as an increase in portal venous pressure >10 mmHg. Causes include thrombus, cirrhosis, veno-occlusive disease and heart failure. The normal portal vein measures up to 13 mm in diameter with a hepatopetal flow rate of 12–30 cm/second, varying with respiration.

US

- Doppler to establish presence and direction of flow (flow <10 cm/second is abnormal).
- Portal vein diameter ≥15 mm is suggestive.
- Severe portal hypertension may cause flow reversal (hepatofugal).
- Check for portosystemic collaterals, splenomegaly and ascites.

CT

- Portosystemic collaterals (splenogastric, gastro-oesophageal, splenorenal, paraumbilical)
- Ascites
- Bowel/gallbladder oedema
- Splenomegaly

PORTAL VEIN THROMBOSIS

Causes are either intrahepatic (e.g. cirrhosis, tumour invasion or hypercoagulability) or extrahepatic (e.g. post-surgical, tumour invasion, sepsis or clot propagation). CT/MRI are useful if US is non-diagnostic.

US

- Echogenic material in the portal vein—if the material has vascularity, then it is likely to be tumour.
- Portal vein diameter >15 mm.
- No flow in the portal vein.
- Ascites.
- Splenomegaly.

PORTAL VENOUS GAS

This is always abnormal, due to necrotic gut from e.g. gastric emphysema, volvulus, infection, Crohn disease, post-trauma, etc. Associated with necrotising enterocolitis in neonates.

CT

- Gas is seen extending peripherally in the liver (more peripheral than pneumobilia).

PRIMARY BILIARY CIRRHOSIS (PBC)

Primary biliary cirrhosis is the inflammatory destruction of peripheral bile ducts leading to cirrhosis. In total, 90% of patients are female. It is associated with autoimmune disorders including rheumatoid arthritis, Sjogren syndrome, scleroderma and Hashimoto thyroiditis. The disease is limited to the intrahepatic bile ducts.

US

- Cirrhosis—check for areas of atrophy, compensatory hypertrophy (segment I) and regenerative nodules.
- Peripheral duct abnormalities in advanced disease.

CT

- Dilated intrahepatic ducts that do not communicate with the main ducts.
- Hyperattenuating, hypertrophied caudate lobe.
- Surrounded by hypoattenuating, rind-like right lobe (pseudotumour).
- Shrunken left lobe.

PRIMARY SCLEROSING CHOLANGITIS (PSC)

More common in males aged 20–40 years, it is an idiopathic, progressive, fibrosing inflammatory disorder of the biliary tree. Associated with ulcerative colitis (UC), Riedel thyroiditis, Sjogren syndrome, cystic fibrosis (CF), retroperitoneal fibrosis, etc. Pathologically, there are multifocal areas of periductal fibrosis that narrow ducts with intervening normal ducts. The stenoses cause cholestasis, sepsis and biliary cirrhosis (hepatic failure). There is an increased risk of cholangiocarcinoma.

US

- Areas of intrahepatic duct dilatation with strictures.
- Both intrahepatic and extrahepatic ducts are usually involved.
- Increased echogenicity of the portal triads.
- 10% have bile duct stones.

MRCP (FIGURE 3.23)

- Irregular strictures of the intrahepatic/extrahepatic ducts.
- Classic 'string of beads' appearances with alternating segments of dilatation and stenosis.
- Pruned tree appearance due to obliterated peripheral ducts.
- Up to 25% have ductal diverticula.

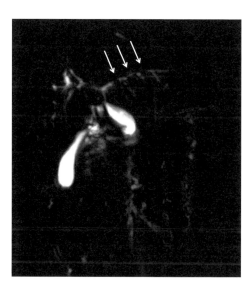

Figure 3.23 Primary sclerosing cholangitis. Maximum intensity projection (MIP) image from an MRCP demonstrating multiple strictures of the intrahepatic ducts (white arrows).

SCHISTOSOMIASIS

The radiological features rarely develop until the late stages of the disease and are signs of cirrhosis and fibrosis. There is an increased risk of HCC.

US

- Grossly cirrhotic liver
- Markedly hyperechoic septa separating areas of relatively normal liver, the 'turtle back' appearance

SHUNTS

The shunt is either between the artery and portal vein or between the artery and hepatic vein. May be due to trauma (including biopsy), cirrhosis, portal hypertension, tumour or hereditary haemorrhagic telangiectasia (Osler–Weber–Rendu disease).

US

- Increased colour flow

CT

- Blush of contrast.
- Large shunts can cause heart failure.

THOROTRASTOSIS

Thorotrast is an α-emitting radioactive isotope used as a contrast agent until the mid-1950s. It remains in the reticuloendothelial system indefinitely and is associated with delayed malignancies—angiosarcoma, cholangiocarcinoma and HCC.

PLAIN FILM

- Opaque liver and spleen with a stippled appearance

TRANS-JUGULAR INTRA-HEPATIC PORTO-SYSTEMIC SHUNT (TIPS)

Performed for bleeding oesophageal or gastric varices due to portal hypertension when endoscopic therapy has failed. The aim is to stop bleeding and prevent re-bleeding. A pathway is created between the portal vein and hepatic veins, which is kept patent with a stent, typically with jugular access. Complications include arteriovenous (AV) fistula and stent stenosis/occlusion.

TRAUMA

Second most commonly injured solid organ after the spleen, but two-fold greater morbidity of the spleen. A laceration involving a major vessel is life threatening.

US

- Useful for follow-up only, to monitor for complications (e.g. abscess)

CT

- Linear, low-density defect—right lobe, posterior segments most commonly (V–VIII).
- Haemoperitoneum (due to capsular rupture).
- Laceration involving the hilum/evident perfusion deficit mandates arterial phase imaging.

INTERVENTION

- Angiograms performed in the setting of active bleeding with intent to embolise

---

Box 3.50 AMERICAN ASSOCIATION FOR THE SURGERY OF TRAUMA (AAST) GRADING OF LIVER LACERATION

I.	Haematoma <10%, laceration <1 cm deep
II.	Haematoma <50%, laceration <3 cm deep/10 cm long
III.	Haematoma >50%, laceration >3 cm deep and >10 cm long
IV.	Active bleeding, laceration involving ≤ segments
V.	Laceration of greater than three segments, juxtahepatic venous injuries—IVC, major hepatic, vein, etc.
VI.	Avulsion

VIRAL HEPATITIS

Caused by a hepatitis virus or Epstein–Barr virus. Associated with raised transaminases and positive serum antibodies.

US

- Hepatosplenomegaly
- Diffuse decrease in liver echogenicity
- Increased brightness of the portal triads resulting in 'starry sky' appearance
- Oedema of the gallbladder fossa and gallbladder wall thickening

CT

- Hepatosplenomegaly.
- Gallbladder wall thickening.
- Periportal oedema.
- Regenerative nodules and lymph node enlargement (porta hepatis, gastrohepatic ligament and retroperitoneum) are features of chronic hepatitis.

WILSON DISEASE

This is a rare, autosomal recessive disorder of copper metabolism. Copper accumulates in the liver initially; once the liver is saturated, copper deposition occurs in the basal ganglia, renal tubules, cornea (Kayser–Fleischer rings), bones, joints and parathyroid glands.

US

- Imaging features are non-specific.
- Fatty infiltration.
- Acute or chronic hepatitis.
- Cirrhosis or liver necrosis.

MRI

- Cirrhosis.
- Findings are non-specific.

XANTHOGRANULOMATOUS CHOLECYSTITIS (XGC)

This is an uncommon inflammatory disorder of the gallbladder characterised by multiple intramural nodules and proliferative fibrosis. Similar imaging appearance to gallbladder carcinoma.

CT

- Pericholecystic infiltration to the liver.
- Biliary obstruction.
- Regional lymphadenopathy.
- Multiple intramural, low-density nodules (xanthogranulomas) suggests XGC over gallbladder malignancy.

Table 3.11 Imaging characteristics and differentiators of focal liver lesions

Lesion	Definable characteristics	US	CT	MRI
Focal nodular hyperplasia	Arterial enhancement but slow washout Usually progressively enhancing central scar Scar high T2 Usually takes up SPIO—implying it is benign and contains Kupffer cells No cirrhosis No pseudocapsule	Well-defined lesion Large central vessel that may be detectable on Doppler	**Unenhanced** Isodense Well-circumscribed, slightly hypoattenuating mass **Contrast – Arterial** Intense transient arterial enhancement **Contrast – Portal phase** Isodense **Contrast – Delayed** Central scar may demonstrate enhancement	**T2 fat saturated** Isointense High signal of the central scar due to vascular channels and oedema Central scar bright on T2, but fibrolamellar carcinoma is dark **T1 fat saturated** Isointense Low signal scar **Aortic–gadolinium–arterial** Enhancement of the lesion **1 hour post-gadolinium** Isointense apart from scar, which enhances Hepatobiliary contrast agents (MultiHance or Gd-BOPTA) not taken up by adenoma Increased diagnostic significance with gadobenate FNH will retain gadobenate and appear isointense building to hyperintense in the liver on hepatobiliary (HPB) phase images (1–3 hours post-gadolinium)

continued

Table 3.11 (*Continued*) Imaging characteristics and differentiators of focal liver lesions

Lesion	Definable characteristics	US	CT	MRI
Hepatic adenoma	Peripheral arterial enhancement, variable washout	Large hyperechoic lesion	Hypodense	Most lesions are low T1 including FNH
	Has pseudocapsule	Central areas of low density caused by haemorrhage or necrosis	**Contrast – Arterial phase** Transient arterial enhancement	Adenoma are high T1
	No cirrhosis			Due to the presence of glycogen and fat
	Minimal SPIO uptake		Isodense portal phase	Isointense on in-phase T1
	Non-enhancing scar			Isointense on T2
	Usually large with areas of haemorrhage			Loses signal on out-of-phase images
	May contain fat–high T1			Immediate and intense enhancement with gadolinium
				Equilibrate in the portal phase
Fibrolamellar carcinoma	Calcification	Solid	Lobulated margin	T1–low signal
	Central scar that does not enhance and is low T2	Hyperechoic scar	Hypodense, particularly the central scar	T2–high signal
			Contrast – Arterial phase Enhances moderately and peripherally	This differentiates it from focal nodular hyperplasia as FNH does not contain calcification
			Contrast – Venous phase Isointense in the venous phase	Central scar is typically low signal on T1 and T2–this differentiates it from FNH, for which the scar is high
			Scar often contains calcification	T2 + scar enhances with FNH

continued

Table 3.11 (*Continued*) Imaging characteristics and differentiators of focal liver lesions

Lesion	Definable characteristics	US	CT	MRI
HCC	Arterial enhancement with washout in venous phase and pseudocapsule	May be hyper- or hypo-echoic	**Unenhanced**	**Dynamic T1 MRI**
	HCCs wash out more avidly than the other lesions	May occlude the portal vein	Encapsulated	Marked enhancement on the arterial phase—the arterial phase is at 20 seconds
	Usually does not take up SPIO	May show arterial vascularity	Hypodense mass	Less marked on the venous phase—the venous phase is at 60 seconds
	Associated with cirrhosis	Heterogeneous reflectivity due to areas of necrosis	**Contrast – Arterial**	The peripheral enhancement in the venous phase is due to the pseudocapsule
	Often shows invasion of portal veins	Smaller lesions are typically of homogeneous low reflectivity	Rapid enhancement during arterial phase	**T2* post-SPIO**
			Hyperenhancing in the acute phase	Dark, iron-laden liver with the bright lesion, as this does not take up SPIO
			Contrast – Portal phase	T2 hyperintensity
			Early washout of contrast on delayed images	
			Washout in the venous phase	

continued

Table 3.11 (*Continued*) Imaging characteristics and differentiators of focal liver lesions

Lesion	Definable characteristics	US	CT	MRI
Metastases	Peripheral washout sign is diagnostic of mets	Homogeneous Hyper- or hypo-echoic May be cystic	May show complete peripheral enhancement rather than nodular Only haemangiomas show nodular Washout on delayed phase	T1–low T2–high T2 fat sat–high **T1 arterial phase** Early peripheral enhancement **T1 equilibrium phase** Prolonged central enhancement with low signal peripherally Peripheral washout sign
Dysplastic nodules	Cirrhosis No raised AFP Often take up SPIO Bright enhancement Usually no pseudocapsule Simple regenerative nodules do not usually enhance	The nodules are generally hypoechoic	—	T1 high signal intensity
Regenerative nodules	High T1 <1 cm Cirrhosis Isodense on unenhanced CT	—	Isodense on unenhanced <1 cm	High T1

continued

Table 3.11 (*Continued*) Imaging characteristics and differentiators of focal liver lesions

Lesion	Definable characteristics	US	CT	MRI
Haemangioma	Early peripheral enhancement with gradual filling in on delayed imaging High signal on heavily T2 sequences Does not take up SPIO However, atypical haemangiomas do occur, which can be difficult to diagnose	Hyperechoic lesions	Hypodense Early periperal nodular enhancement Centripetal fill in on delayed phase	T1–hypointense T2 fat sat–hyperintense Lobulated, well-defined margin T1 post-gad arterial phase Early peripheral nodular discontinuous enhancement T1 post-gad portal venous and delayed phases Progressive enhancement Enhancement is equal to the vessels
Cholangiocarcinoma	Does not take up SPIO	Nodules/focal bile duct wall thickening Hyperechoic bile duct walls	Tumour mass is often isodense Peripheral enhancement Demonstrates delayed enhancement—best seen on late venous enhancement (10 minutes) Intrahepatic duct dilatation May contain calcification	Peripheral enhancement in cholangiocarcinoma, but less than in the vessels Capsular retraction T1–hypointense T2–hyperintense

Note: CT: computed tomography; HCC: hepatocellular carcinoma; MRI: magnetic resonance imaging; SPIO: superparamagnetic iron oxide; US: ultrasound.

PANCREAS

AMPULLARY TUMOURS

These tend to be small and are often not seen with imaging. They are strongly associated with FAP.

CT

- Low-density mass centred on the ampulla
- Double duct sign (dilated common bile duct and pancreatic duct) with no detectable pancreatic head mass

MRCP

- Abrupt cut-off of the distal common bile duct

ANNULAR PANCREAS

Due to a failure of rotation during development, leading to pancreatic tissue partially or completely encircling the duodenum. It is associated with Down syndrome.

CT

- Pancreatic tissue encircling D2
- Proximal duodenal dilatation
- Pancreatic inflammation

BIOPSY

Either guided by US, EUS or CT. The bowel can be crossed safely with a 20– or 22–G needle (not spleen). About 3% get pancreatitis; haemorrhage occurs rarely.

CYSTIC FIBROSIS (CF)

In total, 85% of patients with CF have a severe exocrine deficiency due to pancreatic atrophy following chronic ductal obstruction.

CT

- Atrophic, fatty, calcified pancreas is typical.
- Pancreatic cysts from ductal obstruction.

Table 3.12 Pancreatic mucinous cystadenoma versus serous cystadenoma

	Serous microcystic adenoma (benign) (Figure 3.24)	Mucinous cystic neoplasm (malignant potential)
Frequency	Less common	More common
Number of cysts	>6	<6
Size of individual cysts	<2 cm	>2 cm (average 5 cm)
	Swiss cheese pattern due to innumerable cysts	
Calcification	40%, amorphous, starburst	20%, rim calcification
	Central calcification is the rule	
Enhancement	Hypervascular	Hypovascular
Cyst contents	Glycogen	Mucin
Other features	Central scar 15%	Peripheral enhancement spread: local, lymph nodes, liver
Demographics	Older patients (>60 years of age)	Younger patients (40–60 years of age)
Location	70% head of pancreas	95% in body or tail
Associations	Von Hippel–Lindau disease	

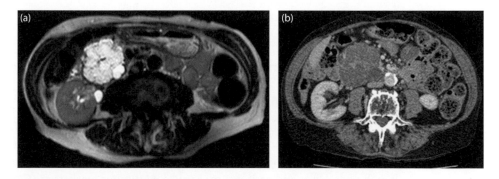

Figure 3.24 Serous cystadenoma. (a) Axial T2 weighted MRI of the abdomen demonstrating a multicystic lesion. (b) Axial CT image of the abdomen with intravenous contrast demonstrating a multicystic lesion within the region of the pancreatic head with visible septae.

DIVISUM

Due to a failure in fusion of the dorsal and ventral ducts. The major papilla drains the ventral duct (head) and a minor papilla drains the dorsal duct (body and tail). It may cause a functional stenosis and pancreatitis and is associated with an increased risk of pancreatic cancer.

CT

● Lobulation/enlargement of the pancreatic head
● Separation of the ventral and dorsal portion of the pancreas by a cleft of fat
● Actual visualisation of the divided ducts

MRCP

- Long, narrow dorsal duct that is dominant (drains most of the pancreas) and empties via the minor papilla—this duct may be dilated due to stenosis at the minor papilla.
- Short ventral duct empties to the major papilla.
- 'Crossing duct sign'—best seen on coronal MIPs.

Table 3.13 Multiple endocrine neoplasia (MEN) syndrome associations

MEN 1	**'PAN PAR PIT'**
	Pancreatic tumours
	Parathyroid adenoma
	Pituitary adenoma
MEN 2A	**'PARAMEDPHE'**
	Parathyroid adenoma
	Medullary thyroid carcinoma
	Pheochromocytoma
MEN 2B	**'MPMPMC'**
	Medullary thyroid carcinoma
	Pheochromocytoma
	Mucosal neuromas of the gastrointestinal tract
	Prognathism
	Marfanoid
	Cutaneous neuromas

DUCTAL ADENOCARCINOMA

This is the most common pancreatic malignancy, accounting for 90% of pancreatic cancers. Risk factors include chronic pancreatitis and smoking. These are aggressive tumours that invade adjacent vessels, nerves and lymphatics. Tumours metastasise to lymph nodes, liver and peritoneum. Associated tumour markers are Ca19-9, Ca242 and carcinoembryonic antigen (CEA). About 10% can be resected at diagnosis (Whipple procedure); 5-year survival is up to 3%. See Table 3.14.

Box 3.51 STAGING PANCREATIC CANCER

T1—pancreas only, <2 cm size
T2—pancreas only, >2 cm size
T3—beyond pancreas but not involving superior mesenteric artery or coeliac
T4—involves superior mesenteric artery/coeliac

Source: American Cancer Society. 2013. American Joint Committee on Cancer (AJCC) TNM staging system. Available at: http://www.cancer.org/cancer/pancreaticcancer/detailedguide/pancreatic-cancer-staging

---

Table 3.14 Factors determining suitability for surgical management of pancreatic malignancy

Resectable	Not resectable
The tumour extends to less than 25% of the circumference of the superior mesenteric vein	Extends beyond the pancreatic margin
	Invasion of adjacent organs
The tumour extends to 25% and 50% of the circumference of the superior mesenteric artery	Tumour is in contact with more than half of the superior mesenteric artery
Invasion of the duodenum (would be resected with Whipple procedure)	Enlarged regional lymph nodes outside resection boundaries

US

- Hypoechoic mass.
- Pancreatic head tumours cause biliary obstruction early on.
- EUS also useful for diagnosis and T-staging.

CT

- Arterial (assess pancreas) and portal venous phases (assess liver).
- Look for a hypovascular, hypoattenuating mass post-contrast.
- The portovenous confluence is often invaded—look for venous collaterals.
- Check for local lymph node enlargement then coeliac, common hepatic, mesenteric and para-aortic. Note that nodes may be involved without being enlarged.
- Peritoneal nodules may be too small to be detected—ascites implies peritoneal disease.

MRI

- Pancreatic tumours are typically seen as low-signal abnormalities on T1-weighted fat saturated MRI.

NUCLEAR MEDICINE

- PET is useful for assessing local disease recurrence.

ECTOPIC PANCREAS (PANCREATIC REST)

Ectopic pancreatic tissue typically occurs in the greater curvature, pylorus, duodenal bulb or proximal jejunum.

BARIUM STUDY

- Submucosal nodule (up to 5 cm diameter) with rudimentary central duct—this appears as a filling defect with tiny central barium collection.

CT

- Often too small to be diagnosed on CT.
- Look for a rounded mass protruding into the gut lumen.

INTRADUCTAL PAPILLARY MUCINOUS NEOPLASM (IPMN)

Mucin-producing tumour that arises from the epithelium of the main pancreatic duct or a branch. It can be a cause of recurrent pancreatitis and so pancreatic atrophy is often present. Cystic pancreatic lesions may be benign, see Table 3.12.

MRCP

- Cystic lesions communicating directly with the main pancreatic duct suggests branch duct IPMN.
- Markedly dilated main duct with or without luminal soft tissue lesion (low signal on T2) with main duct IPMN.
- The mucinous secretions are high signal on T2 (aggregations of mucin can mimic the tumour itself and are low signal on T2).

ISLET CELL TUMOURS

These are rare, endocrine, pancreatic tumours (1%–2% of pancreatic malignancies). EUS is most sensitive for diagnosis. Insulinomas are the most common islet cell tumour (other types include gastrinoma, non-functioning tumour, glucagonoma, VIPoma and somatostatinoma).

CT (FIGURE 3.25)

- Characteristic intense arterial enhancement
- Insulinoma tend to be <2 cm
- Vascular invasion
- Pancreatic calcification is common
- Hypervascular metastases (often extensive liver disease)

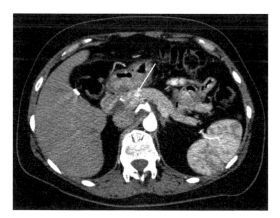

Figure 3.25 Insulinoma. Axial CT image of the abdomen in the arterial phase demonstrating a small arterially enhancing lesion in the neck of the pancreas (white arrow).

PANCREATICOBLASTOMA

Rare tumour, but the most common pancreatic malignancy in children (most <10 years of age). It is an exocrine tumour.

US

- Well-defined mass, heterogeneous internal echogenicity

CT

- Heterogeneous mass often with a prominent cystic component.
- Mass necrosis and punctate calcification.
- The majority are found in the pancreatic head.
- Hypoenhancing compared to adjacent normal gland.

SOLID AND PAPILLARY EPITHELIAL NEOPLASM

This is a rare, low-grade exocrine tumour occurring mainly in young females.

CT

- Well-circumscribed mass of mixed attenuation anywhere in the pancreas
- Spectrum of CT findings, from almost completely cystic to solid

METASTASES

The primary lesions most commonly associated with pancreatic metastases are kidney, breast, lung, colon (usually right-sided) and melanoma.

CT

- Look for a pancreatic nodule typically enhancing in the arterial phase.

PANCREATITIS—ACUTE

There is no obvious cause in up to 30%. For the remainder, alcohol and stones are most common. Fluid collections that do not resolve within 4-weeks are pseudocysts. These complicate about 10% of cases, though half of these resolve without treatment. Overall mortality is about 5%, but is up to 30% with severe pancreatitis. Necrosis is the hallmark of severe inflammation and is complicated by infection in up to 70%.

US

- May be normal.
- Generalised/focal gland enlargement with ill-defined margins.
- Reduced reflectivity of the pancreas.
- With or without peripancreatic fluid.
- Check for gallstones.

CT (FIGURE 3.26)

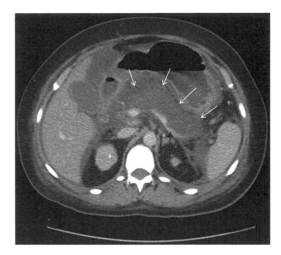

Figure 3.26 Acute pancreatitis with pancreatic necrosis and splenic vein thrombus. Axial computed tomography image of the abdomen following intravenous contrast demonstrating the pancreas to be poorly enhancing (white arrows) with a small filling defect in the splenic vein (red arrow).

- May be normal.
- Pancreas enlarged, peripancreatic fat stranding.
- Normal enhancement pattern initially.
- Check for pathology at the left lung base (e.g. atelectasis, pleural effusion, consolidation).
- Areas of reduced enhancement/non-enhancement in the pancreas suggest necrosis.
- Hyperdense areas (50–70 HU) within the gland suggest haemorrhagic inflammation.
- Look for an abscess (i.e. rim-enhancing fluid collection with or without gas bubbles)—forms about 3-weeks after the attack in about 5%.
- Pseudocysts are often within/adjacent to the pancreas and managed with large-bore drain (e.g. 24 F) or cyst-gastrostomy.
- Large pseudocysts may cause biliary obstruction.
- Check for vascular complications: splenic artery aneurysm or splenic/portal venous thrombosis (Note: Splenic vein thrombosis causes gastric fundal varices and splenomegaly).
- Other complications include bowel oedema, necrosis and perforation (Table 3.15).

Table 3.15 Computed tomography severity index of acute pancreatitis (>7 is associated with 20% mortality)

Pancreas			Necrosis	
Normal	0		None	0
Focal/diffuse enlargement	1	+	<30%	2
Peripancreatic inflammation	2		30%–50%	4
Single fluid collection	3	+	>50%	6
≥2 collections/abscess	4			

Source: Balthazar, E.J., Freeny, P.C., Vansonnenberg, E. 1994. Imaging and intervention in acute pancreatitis. *Radiology* 193:297–306.

PANCREATITIS—AUTOIMMUNE

Associated with IgG4. More common in Japan, although still rare overall. May be managed with steroids.

CT

- Diffuse enlargement of the pancreas ('sausage' or 'banana' pancreas).
- Peripancreatic halo of low density.
- Focal forms may demonstrate an enhancing mass (often misinterpreted as malignancy).
- Not associated with pseudocysts.

PANCREATITIS—CHRONIC

Typically appears after multiple previous attacks of acute pancreatitis. It represents irreversible damage associated with pain and loss of exocrine/endocrine function.

CT

- Calcification.
- Atrophic gland (but can enlarge too).
- Dilated pancreatic duct (>3 mm).
- With or without CBD dilatation.
- Intraductal calcification is a highly reliable sign of chronic pancreatitis (differentiates from carcinoma).

MRCP

- Dilated, irregular pancreatic duct with multifocal stenoses
- Thickening of the duct wall with some side duct dilatation

PANCREATITIS—HEREDITARY

Hereditary pancreatitis is associated with repeated attacks in childhood. It is autosomal dominant and often complicated by pseudocysts. Up to 40% develop pancreatic malignancy.

CT

- Large, spherical pancreatic calcification
- Pseudocysts in 50%

PANCREATIC TRANSPLANT

The anastomosis is either enteric (exocrine enzymes empty to the bowel) or cystic (enzymes empty to the bladder). Cystic connection is associated with lower rejection rates. Most are performed as simultaneous pancreas/kidney transplants. Up to 35% have mild pancreatitis in the first 4-weeks after transplant. Graft failure is mostly due to rejection (25%) or graft vein thrombosis.

US

- Check for a perigraft collection.
- Doppler used to assess vascularity—look for diastolic flow reversal suggesting venous thrombosis (usually within 6-weeks of transplantation).
- Graft rejection is suggested by organ heterogeneity, pancreatic duct dilatation or a poorly defined gland.

CT

- May be used to assess arterial/venous patency where there is suspicion of thrombosis.

MRI

- Useful for assessing graft vessels without intravenous contrast.

Box 3.52 READ MORE ABOUT PANCREATIC TRANSPLANT IMAGING
Vandermeer, F., Manning, M., Frazier, A., Wong-You-Cheong, J. 2012. Imaging of whole-organ pancreas transplants. *Radiographics* 32:411–435.

TRAUMA

Injured in about 10% of blunt abdominal traumas due to crushing of the upper abdomen against the vertebral column ('handlebar injury' in children). It tends to coexist with a liver/duodenal laceration.

CT

- Peripancreatic stranding.
- Linear defect through the gland; ill defined and low density suggests a contusion.

MRCP

- Useful for assessing the integrity of the duct—if it is compromised/transected, then surgical resection is necessary.

SPLEEN

ABSCESS

Uncommon, more prevalent in patients with e.g. sickle cell disease, diabetes, contiguous infection (pyelonephritis or pancreatitis) or immunocompromise. In 75%, splenic abscesses are due to haematogenous spread. Fungal infection is common and causes multifocal small abscesses.

US

- Bright central echogenic focus with surrounding hypoechoic band and 'bull's eye' appearance

CT

- Multiple low-density lesions in the liver/spleen (<1 cm) with central area of high density (could also be lymphoma or metastases)
- Or, thick-walled, irregular, low-density lesion that shows rim enhancement

ACCESSORY SPLEEN (SPLENUNCULUS)

Very common incidental finding affecting up to 30% of the population. It is a congenital anomaly. Splenunculi may hypertrophy if the main organ is removed. Splenosis is ectopic splenic tissue that may develop after splenectomy or splenic rupture (may mimic malignant peritoneal nodules).

CT

- Small (10 mm), well defined
- Identical attenuation and enhancement characteristics to the spleen
- Usually located near the splenic hilum

NUCLEAR MEDICINE

- Technetium-99m heat-denatured erythrocyte scan shows uptake in ectopic splenic tissue.

ANGIOSARCOMA

Very rare, aggressive primary splenic tumour associated with liver metastases at presentation.

MRI

- Diffuse/focal low signal on T1 and T2 due to haemorrhage, which results in iron deposition.
- Spontaneous splenic rupture.
- Calcification (may appear high signal on T1).

CYSTS

Splenic cysts may be primary (e.g. hydatid, epidermoid or lymphangioma) or secondary (e.g. post-trauma, infarction or adjacent pancreatitis). They represent the end stage of a disease process.

US

- Well-defined, rounded.
- Curvilinear rim calcification.
- Low-level internal echoes.
- Lymphangiomas tend to be subcapsular.

CT (FIGURE 3.27)

- Low-density lesion (20 HU) showing no enhancement
- Rim calcification

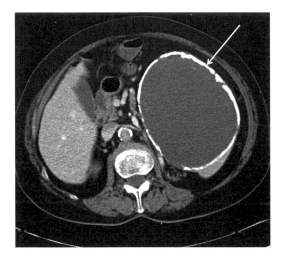

Figure 3.27 Post-traumatic splenic cyst. Axial computed tomography image of the abdomen following intravenous contrast demonstrating a large splenic cystic lesion with rim calcification (white arrow).

HAEMANGIOMAS

These are the most common benign neoplasms of the spleen. Large lesions may rupture. Associated with Kasabach–Merritt syndrome. Imaging characteristics are identical to hepatic haemangioma.

CT

- Early peripheral nodular enhancement with central filling in on delayed scans

MRI

- Lesions are low signal on T1 and high signal on T2.
- Lobulated margin.
- Enhancement characteristics as for CT.

INFARCT

Mostly due to embolic phenomenon. Associated with fever and raised inflammatory markers.

CT

● Peripheral/wedge-shaped/rounded areas of hypoenhancement extending to the splenic capsule

---

Box 3.53 NODULES IN THE SPLEEN

Metastases (e.g. melanoma [most common], lung, breast)
Lymphoma
Abscesses (candidiasis most common in the immunocompromised)
Granulomatous disease (e.g. tuberculosis, sarcoidosis, fungal)

LYMPHOMA

This is the most common splenic malignancy. May be focal or diffuse.

CT/US

● The spleen may be normal, but enlarged.
● May show focal hypodense/hypoechoic lesions (single or multiple) or a solitary mass—or may just be diffusely abnormal.
● Cystic components due to necrosis.
● Calcification, particularly post-treatment.
● Bulky lymph node enlargement.

POLYSPLENIA

This is a rare disorder associated with situs ambiguous. It is characterised by multiple small spleens, usually seen in the right abdomen. It is associated with malrotation in 80% (Table 3.16).

Table 3.16 Polysplenia versus asplenia

Polysplenia	Asplenia
50%–60% mortality in the first year	80% mortality in the first year
Females > males	Males > females
Left isomerism	Right isomerism
Semi annular pancreas	Annular pancreas
Partial anomalous pulmonary venous return	Total anomalous pulmonary venous return
Malrotation 80%	

SARCOIDOSIS

This is a multisystem granulomatous disease. Splenomegaly is the most common abnormality affecting the spleen.

MRI

- Hepatosplenomegaly
- Hepatic and splenic nodules up to 3 cm—low signal on all sequences (hypoattenuating on CT) (Figure 3.28)
- Lymphadenopathy
- Pancreatic mass

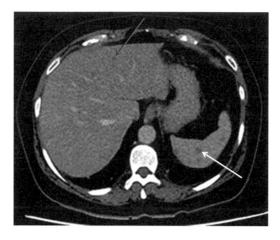

Figure 3.28 Sarcoidosis. Axial computed tomography image of the abdomen following intravenous contrast demonstrating small low-attenuation lesions in the liver (red arrow) and spleen (white arrow).

Box 3.54 LOW-ATTENUATION SPLENIC LESIONS
• Lymphoma
• Metastases
• Haemangioma
• Abscess
• Sarcoidosis

SPLENIC ARTERY ANEURYSM

This is the most common aneurysm of the gut. Due to atherosclerosis, trauma (pseudoaneurysm), pancreatitis (pseudoaneurysm), portal hypertension, infection and pregnancy.

CT

- Calcification is common.
- Diameter >1.5 cm is at risk of rupture.

TRAUMA

The spleen is the most commonly injured solid organ in abdominal trauma. Rib fractures and left renal injury often coexist.

CT

- Low-density, linear, parenchymal lacerations.
- Areas of mottled parenchymal enhancement represent contusions.

ABDOMINAL AIDS (TABLE 3.17)

Table 3.17 Opportunistic infections associated with CD4 count

Infection	CD4 count (μL)
Mycobacterium tuberculosis	300–400
Mycobacterium avium-intracellulare	50–100
Candida	<200
Cryptosporidium	<200
Herpes simplex virus, cytomegalovirus	<100

AIDS-RELATED CHOLANGIOPATHY

Cryptosporidium and CMV are the causes of cholangiopathy (more commonly CMV). It results in intrahepatic and extrahepatic duct dilatation due to periductal fibrosis. The presence of papillary stenosis is useful in distinguishing these conditions from primary sclerosing cholangitis.

MRCP

- Irregular strictures of intra- and extra-hepatic ducts with associated duct dilatation
- Papillary stenosis and intraluminal filling defects due to granulomas
- Duct wall thickening
- Acalculous cholecystitis with or without fluid collections

CANDIDIASIS

Candidiasis occurs at a CD4 count of <100 cells/μL. The oesophagus is most commonly affected. Disseminated candidiasis is less common due to the relative preservation of neutrophil function.

BARIUM SWALLOW

- Longitudinal, linear plaques (these are thickened folds)

CT

- Haematogenous spread can lead to microabscesses within liver, spleen and kidneys.

CYTOMEGALOVIRUS

This is the most common opportunistic infection following HIV/AIDS. It frequently results from reactivation of a latent infection when the CD4 count falls below 100 cells/μL. The caecum is most commonly affected (then small bowel, oesophagus and stomach). It may also cause a biliary periductal fibrosis.

CT

- Pan-colitis, ascites and aphthous ulceration on a background of normal mucosa.
- Large ulcers.
- Caecum typically affected.
- Toxic megacolon and perforation may result in untreated cases.
- Lymph nodes are not enlarged.

GIARDIASIS

This is a protozoal infection that causes diarrhoea and malabsorption.

BARIUM FOLLOW-THROUGH

- Nodularity
- Marked jejunal spasm and jejunal thickening
- Normal ileum

HISTOPLASMOSIS

In regions where the disease is endemic, disseminated disease may occur with CD4 counts of less than 100 cells/μL. Radiologically, this disease is the mimic of mycobacterium tuberculosis (MTB). The bowel can be involved in 75% of infections.

CT

- Thickening of the ascending colon and terminal ileum.
- Annular strictures in chronic disease.
- Low-attenuation retroperitoneal and mesenteric nodes are common.

IMMUNE RECONSTITUTION INFLAMMATORY SYNDROME

In the context of treatment and rising CD4 counts, patients may suffer the effects of disease that were previously masked by impaired immunity. Pyrexia and lymph node enlargement are the cardinal symptoms.

CT

- For example, with extrapulmonary MTB, there can be a large increase in the size of lymph nodes.

KAPOSI SARCOMA

This is the most common neoplasm in AIDS. The stomach, duodenum and proximal small bowel are most commonly involved, but any part of the GI tract may be affected.

CT

- Gastric involvement is expected.
- Enhancing lymph node masses.

MYCOBACTERIUM TUBERCULOSIS/MYCOBACTERIUM AVIUM INTRACELLULARE (MTB/MAI)

Considerable overlap occurs in the CT features of MTB and MAI; however, MAI usually occurs at a greater degree of immunosuppression when the CD4 count falls below 50–100 cells/μL.

CT

- Cardinal imaging features are lymph node enlargement, hepatosplenomegaly and focal lesions in the liver (MTB more), spleen (MTB more) or kidneys.
- Fibrotic fixed peritonitis less common—look for large omental masses, matted and tethered bowel loops and mesentery and loculated ascites.
- Proximal small bowel thickening is a feature of MAI and can resemble Whipple disease.

LYMPHOMA

This is the second most common neoplasm in AIDS. Non-Hodgkin lymphoma occurs as a result of B-cell proliferation induced by Epstein–Barr virus.

CT

- GI tract infiltration is often seen.
- Liver, spleen and renal lesions are common with abdominal Kaposi sarcoma.
- Bulky lymph node enlargement.

CHAPTER 4

Genitourinary, Adrenal, Obstetrics and Gynaecology and Breast

URINARY TRACT

ABSCESS

Renal abscess usually occurs as a complication of pyelonephritis.

ULTRASOUND (US)
- Cortical/corticomedullary, well-defined, hypoechoic area.
- Also look for a perinephric collection.

COMPUTED TOMOGRAPHY (CT)
- Low-attenuation mass with an irregular enhancing thick wall.
- Gas within the mass supports the diagnosis.
- Perinephric fat stranding/fluid collection likely.
- Extrarenal abscess may involve the psoas and extend to the groin.

ACQUIRED UREMIC CYSTIC DISEASE

Multiple bilateral renal cysts developing in patients with end-stage renal failure (ESRF) on dialysis; 90% have it after 5–10 years on dialysis. Greater risk of adenoma, renal cell carcinoma (RCC) and haemorrhage.

US
- Suspect when there are greater than three cysts in a patient with ESRF on dialysis.
- Suspect RCC if there are nodules on cyst.

CT

- Areas of cyst enhancement suggest RCC—tumours usually small.
- Cyst walls may calcify.

ACUTE PYELONEPHRITIS

Usually due to *Escherichia coli* ascending the urinary tract. Most common in women aged <40 years and men aged >65 years. Imaging only if no response to treatment or severely unwell in order to assess for abscess.

CT

- Best clue is wedge-shaped areas of hypoattenuation that extend to the renal capsule (i.e. oedema) on the excretory phase post-contrast, 'striated nephrogram' (Figure 4.1).

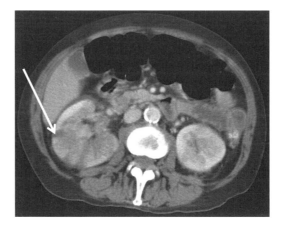

Figure 4.1 Post-contrast axial computed tomography scan of a patient presenting with sepsis and right loin pain. The right kidney is enlarged and contains streaks of low density (white arrow) extending to the renal cortex, the so-called 'striated nephrogram'. This appearance is characteristic of acute pyelonephritis.

US

- Non-specific, most commonly diffusely hypoechoic appearance with loss of corticomedullary differentiation.
- Kidney may be enlarged.

ANGIOMYOLIPOMA (AML)

Most common benign renal tumour, mostly incidental, unilateral and solitary. Composed of vessels, muscle and fat. In total, 20% are found in patients with tuberous sclerosis (TS), and 80% of patients with TS have them (then they are usually multiple and bilateral). Also more common in those with neurofibromatosis and Von Hippel–Lindau disease. Prone to haemorrhage >4 cm in size—treatment is with embolisation or partial nephrectomy. Not thought to be associated with malignancy.

US

- Hyperechoic, solid mass—often brighter than renal sinus fat.
- May appear exophytic.
- Lesions <3 cm need CT or magnetic resonance imaging (MRI) to characterise fully.

CT (FIGURE 4.2a)

- Preferred for diagnosis; diagnostic if fat containing.
- May enhance avidly and be lipid poor, in which case cannot be distinguished from RCC.
- The presence of central necrosis or calcification suggests RCC.

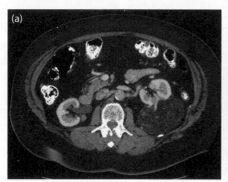 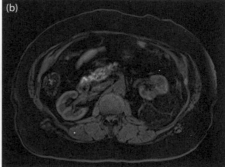

Figure 4.2 (a) Post-contrast axial computed tomography scan showing a large, fat-density lesion arising from the left kidney in keeping with an angiomyolipoma. (b) Corresponding post-contrast T1 fat saturated magnetic resonance image shows some internal vascularity and peripheral enhancement of the lesion, with mainly low signal with fat saturation.

MRI (FIGURE 4.2b)

- Signal loss on out-of-phase gradient echo/fat suppression due to the presence of fat.

AUTOSOMAL DOMINANT POLYCYSTIC KIDNEY DISEASE (ADPKD)

Progressive replacement of the renal parenchyma by cysts, the renal volume is massively increased. Cystic haemorrhage is common. Most present clinically in patients aged 30–50 years. In total, 75% have concurrent hepatic cysts, 10% are pancreatic and 10% have intracerebral berry aneurysms, valvular pathology and arterial dissections. Cyst haemorrhage, infection and renal failure are common—malignancy is rare.

CT (FIGURE 4.3)

- Massively enlarged kidneys with parenchyma replaced by cysts.
- Cysts may be of water density or commonly hyperdense from haemorrhage.

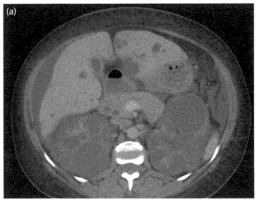
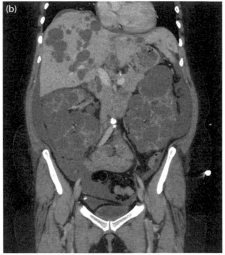

Figure 4.3 Post-contrast axial (a) and coronal (b) computed tomography scans showing grossly enlarged kidneys that are completely replaced by multiple cysts. Note also multiple liver cysts and a small volume of ascites. The appearance is typical of polycystic kidney disease.

AUTOSOMAL RECESSIVE POLYCYSTIC KIDNEY DISEASE (ARPKD)

More severe than ADPKD. Causes oligohydramnios and presents in the neonatal period. Associated with hepatic fibrosis and other abnormalities.

US

- Symmetrically grossly enlarged kidneys, poor corticomedullary differentiation, small cysts (not universally) and dilated tubules

BLADDER EXSTROPHY

Deficient midline abdominal wall with bladder open and everted. Associated with deficient genitalia and bony pelvis.

OBSTETRIC US

- Absent bladder

PLAIN FILM

- Postnatal films show characteristic marked diastasis of the symphysis pubis.

BLADDER MALIGNANCY

In total, 90% of transitional cell carcinomas (TCCs) affect the bladder. Up to 95% of bladder malignancies are TCCs, with the rest being either squamous cell carcinoma (SCC; more with infection or stones) or adenocarcinoma (e.g. urachal anomalies). Rarely secondary malignancy.

US

- Focal bladder wall thickening in a well-distended bladder

CT

- Focal thickening of the bladder wall that enhances more than adjacent normal bladder.
- Enlarged pelvic or common iliac lymph nodes.
- CT intravenous urogram (IVU) used to screen the upper tracts and for long-term follow-up in high-risk patients (e.g. aggressive tumours or muscle-invasive TCCs).

BLADDER RUPTURE—EXTRA-PERITONEAL

The bladder is punctured by bone fragments, typically from an adjacent pelvic fracture. Managed conservatively.

CT CYSTOGRAM

- The bladder is catheterised and drained prior to distension (i.e. 250–300 mL) with dilute (e.g. 5%–10% Omnipaque 350) contrast.
- Look for leak of contrast from the lateral bladder base; leak may extend into the abdominal wall, thigh or scrotum.

URETHROGRAM

- Check for urethral injury (common with extra-peritoneal rupture), usually posterior urethra.

BLADDER RUPTURE—INTRA-PERITONEAL

Results from force to the lower abdomen over a distended bladder (e.g. car seat belt). Biochemical picture suggests acute renal failure due to reabsorption of excretory products. Managed surgically.

CT CYSTOGRAM

- Free fluid in the abdomen that opacifies with bladder filling.
- The site of rupture is at the dome of the bladder (lies within the peritoneum).

BLADDER WALL THICKENING

May be focal (e.g. malignancy) or diffuse (outflow obstruction, neurogenic bladder or chronic infection).

US

- Bladder wall measures >5 mm when distended.
- Trabeculation and diverticula suggest chronic outflow obstruction.
- Debris or stones in the bladder seen with neurogenic bladder.
- Small, thick-walled fibrotic bladder suggests tuberculosis (TB) or schistosomiasis.

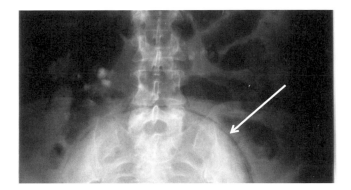

Figure 4.4 Coned in view of a plain abdominal radiograph of the lower abdomen showing gas within the wall of the urinary bladder (white arrow). The diagnosis is emphysematous cystitis.

CT

- Emphysematous cystitis (gas in the bladder wall) (Figure 4.4)
- Calcification in the bladder wall seen with TB, schistosomiasis and malignancy

CHRONIC PYELONEPHRITIS/REFLUX NEPHROPATHY

Due to chronic reflux in children, a gradual process of calyceal blunting and cortical scarring (same as reflux nephropathy). In adults, this is usually due to stones.

US/CT

- Deep cortical scar overlying a blunted ('ectatic') calyx

CYSTS

Very common, affects about 50% of those aged >50 years. Large cysts may cause pain, urinary obstruction, haematuria or hypertension. Often multiple and bilateral. Most cysts are benign. Risk of malignancy can be assessed with the Bosniak classification. Bosniak 2f cysts are followed up; the risk of malignancy is approximately 5%.

US

- Round or oval, anechoic contents and imperceptible wall
- Posterior acoustic enhancement

CT

- Non-enhancing, well defined
- May be of water density or commonly higher due to proteinaceous contents

Box 4.1 BOSNIAK CLASSIFICATION OF RENAL CYSTS
1.   Characteristic simple cyst. No follow-up.
2.   Septated (≤2 mm thick), thin wall/septal calcification, high-density cyst (60–100 HU). No follow-up.
3.   2f. Thickened cyst walls or septate, no contrast enhancement. Thickened/nodular calcification of walls or septae. Most likely benign. Follow-up at 3, 6 and 9 months.

4. Indeterminate, most surgically excised. Thick, irregular calcification, thick septae with or without enhancement, irregular margins, multilocular mass.
5. Frankly malignant, necrotic neoplasm arising from cyst wall. Irregular nodules, nodular septation, thick/shaggy walls/septae, solid areas with enhancement.

Read more:
Whelan, T. 2010. Guidelines on the management of renal cyst disease. *Canadian Urology Association Journal* 4:98–99.

CONGENITAL MEGAURETER

May present prenatally or later in life. Ureter with diameter ≥7 mm is diagnostic. May be due to obstruction or reflux.

US

- Mostly unilateral (more on the left) hydroureter with or without hydronephrosis.
- Look for a transition point in the distal ureter.

NUCLEAR MEDICINE

- Micturating cystourethrogram to assess for reflux
- Mercaptoacetyltriglycine (MAG3) to diagnose obstruction and for follow-up

---

Box 4.2 AAST ORGAN INJURY SCALE—RENAL TRAUMA (FIGURE 4.5)

I. Haematoma/contusion only
II. Haematoma and <1 cm laceration, no urine leak
III. >1 cm laceration, no urine leak*
IV. Cortex laceration and urine leak, vascular injury*
V. Shattered kidney, avulsed pedicle, main artery thrombosis*

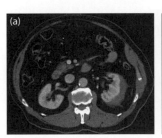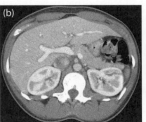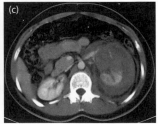

Figure 4.5 Renal trauma—note grades III and above are managed surgically.
(a) Haematoma and contusion only (grade I). (b) >1 cm of laceration without urine leak (grade III). (c) Laceration of the renal cortex with vascular injury (grade IV).

*Managed surgically
Source: Ramchandani, P., Buckler, P.M. 2009. Imaging of genitourinary trauma. *AJR. American Journal of Roentgenology* 192:1514–1523.

CROSSED FUSED ECTOPIA

Both kidneys on the same side of the abdomen (more on right) and fused together. May present as an abdominal mass. Ureters insert normally to the bladder.

EMPHYSEMATOUS PYELONEPHRITIS

Gas within the renal parenchyma due to multiple small abscesses, mostly in patients with diabetes, obstruction or immunodeficiency. It is a life-threatening, fulminant infection. Emphysematous pyelitis is gas only in the collecting system. Pyonephrosis indicates an infected, obstructed system.

CT

- Bubbles of gas seen within the renal parenchyma and/or collecting system
- May extend to the perinephric space and retroperitoneum

FIBROMUSCULAR DYSPLASIA

Non-atherosclerotic disease affecting the arterial wall, most commonly involving mid-distal renal arteries. Associated with collagen vascular diseases. Tends to affect young women. Presents with refractory hypertension.

INTERVENTION

- Classic appearance is the 'string of beads' sign (this is pathognomic), made up of multiple stenoses and dilated segments.
- Responds well to angioplasty.

HIV

Kidney may be affected directly by the virus. Also with HIV, the kidney is more prone to secondary infections, malignancy (lymphoma and Kaposi sarcoma) and side effects of antiretroviral treatment.

US

- Echogenic, enlarged kidneys in the context of HIV infection

CT

- 'Striated nephrogram' appearance

HORSESHOE KIDNEY

Most common abnormality of renal fusion. Associated with syndromes and anomalies elsewhere. Morbidity from traumatic injury, recurrent infections, stones and pelvi-ureteric junction (PUJ) obstruction. Higher risk of malignancy.

US

- Fibrous or parenchymal band fusing the lower poles across the midline

- Low position (inferior mesenteric artery prevents migration superiorly)
- Lower renal poles point medially, pelvices anteriorly

CT

- Multiple, ectopic renal arteries e.g. arising from common iliac/internal iliac etc.

LEUCOPLAKIA

Linked to chronic infection/stones. There is squamous metaplasia with keratinisation and desquamation. Plaque flakes may then be passed in the urine.

CT

- May cause strictures in the urinary tract (seen on CT IVU).

LYMPHOMA

In total, 90% of cases are secondary, mostly by haematogenous metastases (mostly non-Hodgkin lymphoma). Mostly asymptomatic, 60% complete remission after treatment. Look for lymphoma elsewhere—liver, lung, central nervous system, bones, etc.

US

- Diffuse renal enlargement with early disease, more discrete mass with late disease
- Less likely to cause venous thrombosis compared to RCC
- Expect lymph node enlargement and splenomegaly

CT

- Diffuse renal enlargement or poorly enhancing renal lesion with lymph node enlargement
- Splenomegaly

MALAKOPLAKIA

Rare granulomatous reaction to chronic infection, usually with *E. coli*. More common in females.

US/CT

- Diffuse bladder wall thickening

MEDULLARY SPONGE KIDNEY

Dysplastic dilatation of the papillary collecting tubules leading to papillary urinary stasis, stones and infection. Usually bilateral and symmetrical and does not progress to renal failure—asymptomatic. In total, >80% get medullary nephrocalcinosis.

CT

- Bilateral medullary calcification
- 'Paintbrush' appearance with contrast—contrast in dilated tubules

METASTASES

Most renal tumours are metastases, mostly from lung, breast or gastrointestinal malignancy. Mostly asymptomatic, they present late and prognosis is poor.

US

- Small, round, typically bilateral with varying reflectivity (i.e. anything)
- Normal colour flow patterns
- Rarely breach of renal capsule

CT

- Multiple foci enhancing poorly compared to adjacent renal parenchyma.
- Expect widespread disease elsewhere on the scan.
- Note—melanoma metastases are hypervascular and mimic RCC.

MULTICYSTIC DYSPLASTIC KIDNEY

Congenital cystic renal destruction thought to be due to ureteral obstruction *in utero*. Contralateral abnormalities are common (e.g. PUJ obstruction).

US

- Multiple cysts separated by echogenic fibrous tissue, minimal vascularity, may mimic hydronephrosis

NUCLEAR MEDICINE

- No excretion on MAG3

MULTILOCULAR CYSTIC NEPHROMA

Tends to affect boys in childhood and women in adulthood. This is a collection of cysts separated by thin septae and enveloped in a thick capsule. Bosniak 3–4, but benign. Excised as cannot be distinguished from RCC on imaging.

US

- Well-defined, multi-loculated cystic mass
- Hyper-reflective capsule

CT

- Solitary, well-defined cystic mass with enhancing capsule and internal septations
- May herniate into the renal pelvis

NEPHROCALCINOSIS

Calcium deposition in the renal parenchyma, usually bilateral and from systemic disease. Either found in the renal medulla (common) or cortex (rarely).

MEDULLARY

Arises from increased levels of calcium in the circulation, mostly due to primary hyperparathyroidism, medullary sponge kidney, increased vitamin D, renal tubular acidosis (most common cause in children) or milk-alkali syndrome.

US (Figure 4.6)
- Renal pyramids may appear echogenic (i.e. calcified).

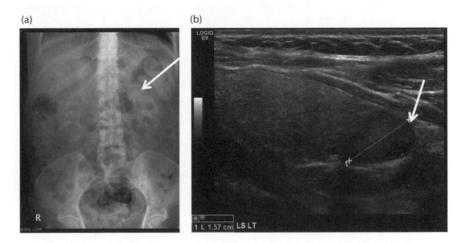

(a)   (b)

Figure 4.6 (a) Plain abdominal x-ray shows prominent, bilateral medullary nephrocalcinosis (white arrow). (b) Ultrasound of the thyroid gland (longitudinal view) shows a well-defined lesion at the base of the gland in keeping with a parathyroid adenoma (white arrow).

CT
- The pattern of calcification points to the underlying pathology—confluent calcification in renal tubular acidosis and punctate calcification in medullary sponge kidney.

CORTICAL

Most are due to cortical necrosis (e.g. from complicated pregnancy/shock or renal vein thrombosis), glomerulonephritis or hyperoxaluria.

US
- Echogenic (calcified) cortex

CT
- Characteristic tramline calcification suggests cortical necrosis.

ONCOCYTOMA

Benign tumour derived from epithelial cells—it is rare. Mostly asymptomatic. Difficult to differentiate from RCC based on imaging alone, so it is often excised.

US

- Mass with or without echogenic central scar.
- Vascularity tends to radiate out from the centre like spokes on a wheel.
- Usually >5 cm.

CT

- Poorly enhancing compared to adjacent renal parenchyma.
- Central, lower-density scar seen in up to a third of cases (could also be necrosis in a RCC).

PAPILLARY NECROSIS

Inflammation or ischaemic necrosis at the tip of the papilla that may then slough off and obstruct the collecting system. Causes include pyelonephritis, obstruction, sickle-cell, TB, cirrhosis, analgesic, renal vein thrombosis, diabetes.

CT

- Sloughed papilla appears as a filling defect in the collecting system
- The calyx appears clubbed due to loss of the papilla

PELVI-URETERIC JUNCTION OBSTRUCTION

Mostly congenital, often diagnosed in adulthood. Most unilateral. Varying aetiologies, including crossing vessels, abnormal collagen infiltration at the PUJ, kinks, etc.

US

- Hydronephrosis on prenatal/postnatal scan
- Marked ballooning of the renal pelvis with normal-calibre ureter

NUCLEAR MEDICINE

- MAG3 study used to assess renal function pre-operatively/to distinguish non-obstructive dilatation

POSTERIOR URETHRAL VALVES

Only occurs in males. It is due to a membrane in the posterior urethra causing near-complete obstruction to the flow of urine. Age of presentation depends on degree of obstruction. Mostly diagnosed after birth.

US

- Hydronephrosis
- Renal dysplasia
- Urinoma or urinary ascites

NUCLEAR MEDICINE

- Micturating cystourethrogram is the gold standard—calibre change in the posterior urethra.
- Reflux is also common.

PRUNE BELLY (EAGLE–BARRETT) SYNDROME

Congenital deficiency of abdominal musculature, urinary tract anomalies and cryptorchidism. Mostly affects males. Associated with cardiac anomalies in 10%.

US

- Grossly dilated collecting system, ureters, bladder (Note: Thin-walled) and urethra
- Check for cryptorchidism

PYONEPHROSIS

Infected urine in the context of an obstructed kidney. Needs urgent drainage (i.e. nephrostomy/ureteric stent) to preserve the kidney.

US

- Hydronephrosis, collecting system filled with echogenic debris (i.e. pus)
- Thickened urothelium may be seen

CT

- Useful to find cause of obstruction.
- Look for presence of gas in the pelvis (emphysematous pyelitis).
- Hyperdense 'urine' (i.e. pus).

REFLUX

Box 4.3 GRADING REFLUX	
I.	Ureters only
II.	Reaches pelvis, no dilatation
III.	Mild dilatation but no calcyeal clubbing
IV.	Moderate dilatation with calcyeal clubbing
V.	Severe dilatation with tortuous ureter

Vesico-ureteric reflux, usually diagnosed following workup after urinary tract infection (UTI) in a child. Thought to result from abnormal angulation of ureter insertion to the bladder. In adults due to e.g. neurogenic bladder or bladder outflow obstruction.

MICTURATING CYSTOURETHROGRAM

- Contrast instilled to the bladder refluxes to the ureter or kidney.

US

- Useful for staging the extent of pelvi-calyceal dilatation.

NUCLEAR MEDICINE

- MAG3 can be used to assess reflux at the end of a standard MAG3 (patient empties bladder in front of the γ-camera).

RENAL AGENESIS

Lethal to foetus if bilateral. Linked to genital tract anomalies (e.g. absence of ipsilateral vas/testis, partial agenesis of uterus, etc.).

US

- Expect to find contralateral renal hypertrophy.

RENAL CELL CARCINOMA (RCC)

Most common renal malignancy. Often incidental, more common in men and peaks from ages 50–70 years. In total, 70% are clear cell adenocarcinomas. Consider any solid mass in the kidney as RCC until proven otherwise. RCC metastasises to lung, liver, bone, adrenals and pancreas (Table 4.1).

Table 4.1 TNM staging of renal cell carcinoma

T	N	M

1. <7 cm size, confined to kidney (a <4 cm, b <7 cm)
 2. >7 cm, confined to kidney (a 7–10 cm, b >10 cm)
 3. Involves major veins or perinephric tissue; does not breach Gerota fascia
   a. Involves renal vein and perinephric fat
   b. Involves subdiaphragmatic inferior vena cava
   c. Involves supradiaphragmatic inferior vena cava
 4. Breach of Gerota fascia, may involve adrenal
	1. Tumour at regional nodes	1. Distant nodes or other organ involvement

Source: Edge, S.B. et al. 2010. *AJCC Cancer Staging Manual*. 7th edition. New York, NY: Springer-Verlag.

US

- Heterogeneous lobulated lesion, either hypo-reflective or mildly hyper-reflective.
- Cystic areas are haemorrhage/necrosis.
- Peripheral vascularity on colour Doppler.
- Check the inferior vena cava (IVC) and renal veins with Doppler—may show low flow or thrombus in lumen.

CT

- Look for a mass with heterogeneous enhancement (triple-phase CT).
- May appear cystic (i.e. Bosniak 3/4).
- A poorly enhancing solid mass could represent a papillary RCC (these are hypovascular).
- Areas of low density are likely to represent haemorrhage or necrosis.
- Nodules in perinephric fat suggest tumour spread (fat stranding does not).

- Invasion of renal veins or IVC indicates T3 disease—look for an enhancing filling defect with expansion of the vessel ('bland' thrombus does not enhance).
- Extension beyond Gerota fascia indicates T4 disease.
- Metastases may be hypervascular soft tissue lesions/destructive bone lesions.

RENAL TRANSPLANT

Preferred location is the right iliac fossa and it is extraperitoneal. Live donor grafts are usually given end-to-side arterial and venous anastomoses to the external iliac artery and vein.

EARLY COMPLICATIONS
Renal artery thrombosis
Rare complication, requires urgent surgical intervention to save the graft.

US
- No arterial or venous signal on Doppler

Acute tubular necrosis (ATN)
Most common cause of delayed graft function (i.e. need for dialysis in the first week post-transplant). Usually presents in cadaveric grafts. Rare late complication.

US
- Usually normal findings and normal Doppler flow
- May show reversed arterial flow in diastole

Venous thrombosis (Figure 4.7)
Expect a tender, swollen graft and sudden drop in renal function. Most occur in the first week post-transplant.

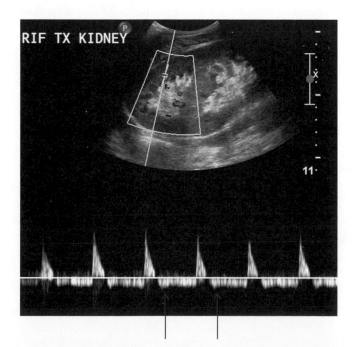

Figure 4.7 Doppler ultrasound scan of a renal transplant showing diastolic flow reversal (red arrows), in keeping with renal vein thrombosis (there is a differential).

US

- Enlarged with or without hypoechoic graft.
- Doppler shows no venous flow and arterial flow is reversed in diastole.

Peri-transplant haematoma

Small collections are common after surgery. Problematic if large or pressuring the graft.

US

- Hypoechoic crescent adjacent to the graft
- Free fluid in the abdomen with intraperitoneal grafts

LATE COMPLICATIONS

Rejection

In total, 90% show increased size of the kidney and large renal pyramids. Reduced corticomedullary differentiation. Most common cause of late graft loss.

US

- Reduction in central echoes
- Resistive index >0.7 (non-specific)
- Mild hydronephrosis

Nuclear medicine

- Reduced uptake of radiopharmaceutical

Renal artery stenosis

Affects up to 10%. Usually, stenosis occurs at the anastomosis/proximal graft artery. Segmental stenosis may occur in the setting of chronic rejection.

US

- Focal colour aliasing adjacent to stenotic segment
- Expect velocity >2 m/second, velocity gradient >2:1 across stenosis

Intervention

- Conventional angiography is reserved for stenosis confirmed on US or CT or clinical stenosis with normal US.
- May be treated with angioplasty/stent.

Pseudoaneurysm/arteriovenous fistula (AVF)

The result of biopsy, usually insignificant, unless large, when they may result in shunting and renal ischaemia.

US

- Focus of disorganised colour flow outside pattern of normal vasculature
- Draining vein may show arterialization (AVF)

Urinoma

Usually appears in the first month post-transplant, either from anastomotic failure or ischaemia.

US
- Non-specific fluid collection, fewer septations than haematoma

Nuclear medicine
- Persistent accumulation of radiotracer in the fluid collection

Abscess

Presents in the weeks post-transplant with fever and raised inflammatory markers.

US
- Complex fluid collection

Lymphocele

Usually presents between 1 and 4 months post-transplant in 10%–20% of recipients. Mostly inferomedial to the kidney. Mostly asymptomatic, but large collections may cause problems by direct pressure on the kidney/other structures.

US
- Rounded anechoic fluid collection, transplant hydronephrosis
- If leg swelling—check for deep vein thrombosis from pressure on external iliac vein.

Hydronephrosis

Mostly asymptomatic. Diagnosis made following deteriorating renal function. Mostly due to ischaemic stricture (usually at the vesico-ureteric junction [VUJ]—furthest from the transplanted renal artery).

US
- Dilated collecting system
- Echogenicity within the collecting system could be pus (pyonephrosis), blood, fungus balls or tumour
- Obstruction relieved with nephrostomy with or without stent

---

Box 4.4 RESISTIVE INDICES (RI)

Measurements are usually taken at the corticomedullary junction in the upper pole, interpolar region and lower pole (>0.80 = abnormal).

In native kidneys, high RIs predict progressive renal dysfunction and adverse cardiovascular events.

High RIs in transplanted kidneys have been linked to increased risk of graft loss and recipient death. However, a large prospective trial in 2013 showed RIs to be insufficiently accurate to be used in the management of renal allografts.

Read more:
Naesens, M. et al. 2013. Intrarenal resistive index after renal transplantation. *New England Journal of Medicine* 369:1797–1806.

STONES

All are seen on CT except indinavir calculi and some matrix calculi. About 50% of 5–mm stones will pass spontaneously. Recurrence is high without treatment. Complications are obstruction, infection and stricture. See Figures 4.8 and 4.9.

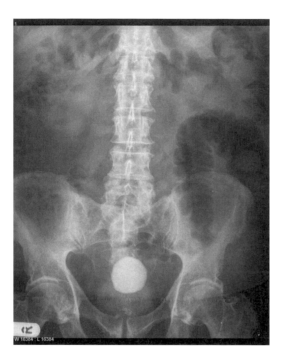

Figure 4.8 Plain abdominal x-ray shows a large opacity projected over the pelvis, in keeping with a bladder calculus.

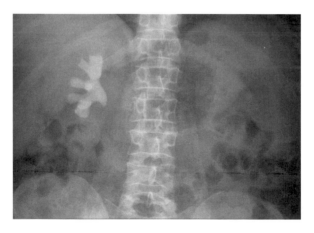

Figure 4.9 Plain abdominal x-ray shows a large right staghorn calculus. Even large staghorn calculi can be mistaken for renal sinus fat on ultrasound—look for loss of signal behind the stone.

CT

- Hyperdense calculus—commonly at a calyx, renal pelvis, PUJ, ureter or VUJ
- Hydronephrosis, hydroureter, perinephric stranding (fat oedema)
- Hypodense kidney (oedema)
- Perinephric fluid collection suggests ruptured fornix due to obstruction

- Beware false positives—phleboliths; parapelvic cyst and extra-renal pelvis mimic hydronephrosis

US

- Sensitivity is about 25%—normal renal sinus fat commonly mimics calculi
- Look for pelvi-calyceal dilatation, marked acoustic shadowing, speckle artefact with colour Doppler

TUBERCULOSIS

Kidneys involved by secondary spread, usually from the lungs (e.g. 10–15 years later). Kidneys involved first (papillae/renal mass), then ureters (strictures) and bladder (small, thickened). Consider TB with multifocal urinary tract disease. Urine is sterile, expect asymptomatic haematuria.

CT

- Small ill-defined cortical hypodensities on CT early on, then papillary necrosis and irregular 'moth-eaten' calyces
- Ureteral strictures may cause hydronephrosis
- Bladder is small volume and thickened
- Late on, small kidney (like in chronic kidney disease [CKD]) and heavy calcification

TUBEROUS SCLEROSIS

Rare, autosomal dominant inheritance and multi-system. Renal involvement is with multiple cysts, multiple angiomyolipoma and RCC.

CT (FIGURE 4.10)

- Multiple, bilateral angiomyolipoma (AML) strongly suggest TS (up to 90%).

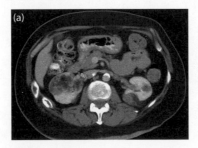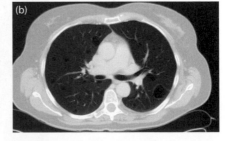

Figure 4.10 (a) Computed tomography image of an abdomen post-contrast shows fat-containing lesions in both kidneys in keeping with AML. (b) Computed tomography image of a thorax in the same patient shows multiple thin-walled lung cysts. The combination of findings is suggestive of tuberous sclerosis. The brain, bones and heart should also be assessed.

URACHAL ANOMALIES

Midline, fluid-filled structures lying somewhere between the bladder dome and umbilicus. They may be diagnosed *in utero* or present in adulthood (increased risk of infection and malignancy).

US

- Fluid-filled, midline lesions above the bladder.
- A direct connection to the bladder confirms 'patent urachus'—the most common anomaly.

URETERAL DUPLICATION

Incidence is up to 2%, mostly unilateral. Weigert–Meyer rule: upper pole ureter inserts low into the bladder, often has a ureterocele and tends to obstruct. The lower pole ureter tends to reflux. Upper renal pole is often non-functioning.

CT

- Ectopic ureter implanting to vagina/urethra/seminal vesicles, etc.
- Inferior displacement of the lower renal pole giving a 'drooping lily' appearance on IVU/coronal CT
- Dilated upper pole calyces

URETERAL STRICTURE

Differentials include infection (including TB), inflammation, calculus, iatrogenic conditions, tumour and extrinsic disease (e.g. tumour, retroperitoneal fibrosis, Crohn disease, endometriosis, etc.). See Figure 4.11.

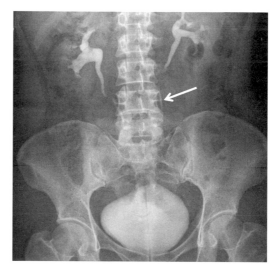

Figure 4.11 IVU shows medial deviation of the ureters (white arrow), suggestive of retroperitoneal fibrosis.

CT

● Focal narrowing with pre-stenotic dilatation

URETERITIS CYSTICA

Small, benign submucosal cysts that appear due to chronic infection. May also arise in the renal pelvis or bladder.

CT

● Small filling defects scalloping the margins of the ureter
● Mostly in the upper ureter

URETEROCELE

Distal ureter prolapses to the bladder lumen (orthotopic ureterocele). May be incidental or associated with obstruction, infection or stones. Ectopic ureterocele is associated with a duplex system. Always inserts above the external sphincter in males, but in females, it may insert to the vagina or uterus, resulting in incontinence.

US

● Mass in the bladder lumen adjacent to the VUJ (bladder base if ectopic).
● Look for obstructed upper pole if ectopic (i.e. duplex system).

CT

● 'Cobra's head' appearance on IVU (Figure 4.12)
● Soft tissue mass on CT, which opacifies in the excretory phase

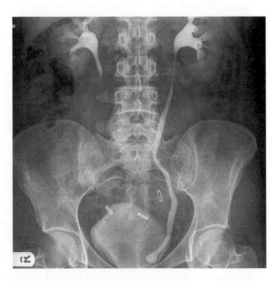

Figure 4.12 IVU showing the characteristic 'cobra's head' appearance of a left ureterocele.

URETHRAL STRICTURE

Most due to trauma or infection.

URETHROGRAM

- Antegrade and retrograde study to evaluate whole urethra.
- Post-traumatic strictures are short, post-infectious strictures tend to be long.

UROTHELIAL MALIGNANCY

In total, 90% of uroepithelial tumours are TCCs and 90% are found in the bladder. The remainder are SCCs, associated with chronic infection and strictures. Most TCCs are exophytic/polypoid (i.e. papillary TCC). Non-papillary is flat, aggressive and stricturing. About 30% with upper tract tumours will develop disease in the bladder (i.e. it drops down). Metastasises to local nodes, liver, lung and bone.

US

- Obstructed kidney
- Polypoid lesion in the bladder with or without vascularity

CT

- Intraluminal filling defect/mass showing arterial enhancement or thickening/ narrowing of the ureter/collecting system
- Infiltration of the renal parenchyma or renal sinus

MRI

- T1 useful for assessing extension into perivesical fat
- Tumour brighter on T2 than adjacent bladder wall

VON HIPPEL–LINDAU DISEASE

Rare, inherited, multi-system disease. Develops in the third decade.

US

- Multiple cysts (60%) and RCC (up to 45%) at a young age

XANTHOGRANULOMATOUS PYELONEPHRITIS (XGP)

Chronic inflammatory change, usually from an obstructing (staghorn) calculus. Begins within the kidney. When advanced, it may involve the retroperitoneum. Treatment with antibiotics/nephrectomy.

US

- Diffuse renal enlargement with central calculus
- Hydronephrosis/pyonephrosis
- Perinephric collection or soft tissue

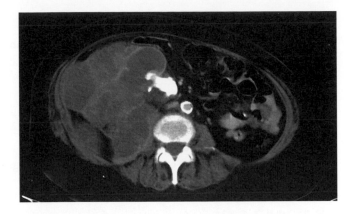

Figure 4.13 Post-contrast CT scan of the abdomen showing a large, mixed-density lesion arising from the right kidney. Note a large staghorn calculus on the medial side of the mass. The findings are in keeping with xanthogranulomatous pyelonephritis.

CT (FIGURE 4.13)

- Rim-enhancing hypodense renal masses, central calculus, little or no excretion of contrast.
- Look for aggressive perinephric and retroperitoneal extension.

ADRENAL GLANDS

ADRENOCORTICAL CARCINOMA (ACC)

Rare, presents when large and commonly (50%) associated with an endocrine syndrome (Li–Fraumeni syndrome or Beckwith–Wiedemann syndrome). More common in children. Also linked to hemihypertrophy and astrocytomas. Hormonally active—children present with virilisation/Cushing syndrome.

CT

- Central necrosis/haemorrhage typical.
- Delayed washout (like metastases).
- 30% calcify.
- Check the IVC and renal vein for thrombosis.
- Metastasises to the liver and lymph nodes.

POSITRON EMISSION TOMOGRAPHY (PET)/CT

- Useful for diagnosing ACC, recurrence and metastases

COLLISION TUMOUR

Rare occurrence of two tumours of differing pathologies in the same place. May be benign or malignant (e.g. adrenal metastasis within an adenoma).

HAEMORRHAGE

Due to e.g. trauma (more common), shock or tumour. Non-traumatic haemorrhage more likely bilateral. The neonatal adrenal is highly vascular and relatively large, so more prone to haemorrhage.

US

- Well-defined adrenal mass, appearances dependent on age of blood products—acute is hyper-reflective.
- Look for perinephric extension in large haemorrhage.

CT

- Well-defined foci of hyperdensity that do not enhance post-contrast
- Fat stranding
- May become cystic (most adrenal cysts are from a previous haemorrhage) and calcify with time

HYPERPLASIA

Diffuse thickening (>10 mm) of the adrenal limbs (normal 5–7 mm). Needs clinical and biochemical correlation—may be normal at time of physiological stress.

METASTASES

Common, mostly from the lungs, breast, melanoma, gastrointestinal tract and renal. Lymphoma (mostly non-Hodgkin) may also spread to the adrenals.

CT

- Small lesions that are difficult to distinguish from benign adenoma; stability over 6 months suggests benignity.
- Expect delayed washout on adrenal CT.
- Large masses with a heterogeneous appearance (e.g. central necrosis, haemorrhage) and irregular borders suggest frank malignancy.

NUCLEAR MEDICINE

- PET/CT is useful for assessing indeterminate lesions—sensitive and specific for differentiating benign from malignant disease.

MYELOLIPOMA

Rare, benign, non-functioning tumour commonly with punctate calcification. Small risk of haemorrhage with large lesions.

CT

- Low-density lesion, fat density (i.e. −30 to −90 HU) is diagnostic.

MRI

- Hyperintense on T1 with loss of signal on fat suppression/out-of-phase imaging

NODULES

If there is malignancy elsewhere, there is up to a 50% risk of the nodule being a metastasis. Masses >4 cm may be resected, while benign-appearing lesions <1 cm do not require follow-up.

CT

- HU ≤10 (lipid rich) is an adenoma; if HU >10 (lipid poor), then the lesion is indeterminate so proceed with contrast.
- Dedicated adrenal assessment with a triple-phase (pre- and post-contrast, then delayed at 15 minutes) scan to allow you to calculate the absolute percentage washout (APW)
- APW = ([HU enhanced – HU delayed]/[HU enhanced – HU unenhanced]). Use thin slices and region of interest (ROI) >50% of the size of the nodule.
- APW >60% = likely adenoma (i.e. rapid enhancement and washout)
- APW <60% and delayed HU >35 = indeterminate—could be a metastasis!

These patients may get a biopsy if there is a history of malignancy or it is a new mass; otherwise, follow-up is recommended.

Box 4.5 POSITRON EMISSION TOMOGRAPHY (PET)/COMPUTED TOMOGRAPHY (CT) FOR ADRENAL MASSES

PET/CT is sensitive (97%) and specific (91%) for differentiating benign from malignant nodules. Useful in high-risk patients (i.e. with a known cancer).

Read more:
Boland, G.W. et al. 2011. Characterization of adrenal masses by using FDG PET: A systematic review and meta-analysis of diagnostic test performance. *Radiology* 259:117–126.

PHEOCHROMOCYTOMA

Rare catecholamine-secreting tumour, a type of paraganglioma (same as glomus tumours). More common in children, associated with syndromes (Von Hippel–Lindau disease, multiple endocrine neoplasia type-2 and neurofibromatosis type 1). Bilateral in up to a third, extra-adrenal in 10% (e.g. bladder and organ of Zuckerkandl—near aortic bifurcation). Beware biopsy, which may induce a hypertensive crisis!

CT (FIGURE 4.14a,b)

- Soft tissue adrenal mass, homogeneous enhancement, prone to haemorrhage (then appears heterogeneous)
- May have peripheral calcification

MRI

- Hyperintense on T2, may have areas of T1 hyperintensity from previous haemorrhage
- Enhancement as for CT (however, flow voids may be apparent—salt and pepper appearance)

NUCLEAR MEDICINE

- MIBG is most sensitive for the detection of extra-adrenal disease and metastases.

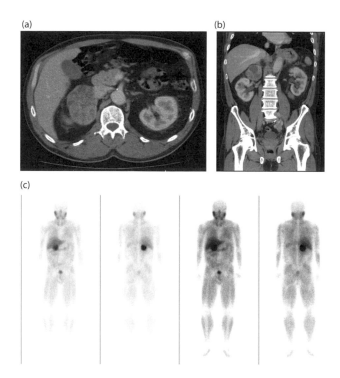

Figure 4.14 Axial (a) and coronal (b) post-contrast computed tomography scan of the abdomen shows an enhancing soft tissue mass arising from the right adrenal. There is intense, increased activity on the iodine-123-meta-iodobenzylguanidine (MIBG) scan (c) in keeping with a pheochromocytoma.

TRAUMA

Adrenal injury is rare. It is seen in only 2% of adults with severe trauma. The right adrenal is most commonly injured (90%) due to the compression of the gland between the liver and spine.

CT

- Unilateral adrenal haemorrhage (bilateral haemorrhage is more commonly due to physiological stress; e.g. sepsis, major surgery, etc.).

GYNAECOLOGY

ADENOMYOSIS OF THE UTERUS

Benign, ectopic endometrial glands in the myometrium that cause myometrial hypertrophy. The symptoms are dysmenorrhoea/menorrhagia.

MRI (FIGURE 4.15)

- Ill-defined thickening of the junctional zone (>12 mm), fibrotic with low signal on T1 and T2.
- Small foci of high signal on susceptibility sequences indicate blood products.

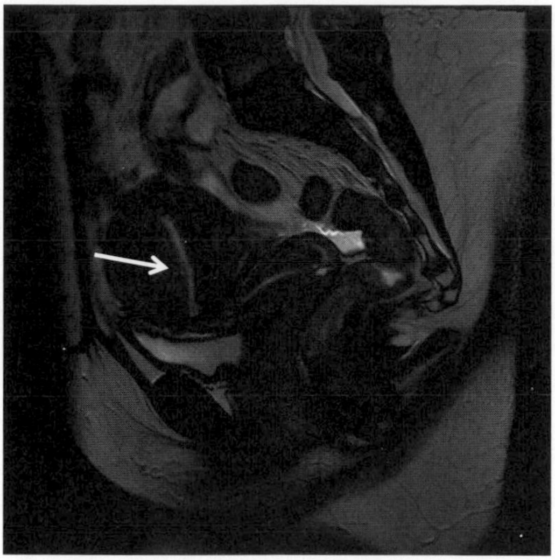

Figure 4.15 Sagittal T2-weighted image of the pelvis showing thickening of the junctional zone and multiple small foci of T2 hyperintensity in the myometrium (white arrow), in keeping with adenomyosis.

- The uterus is diffusely enlarged, but no discrete mass and outer contours are preserved (unlike fibroids).
- May also appear as focal disease.

CERVICAL CANCER

Second most common malignancy in women after breast cancer, peaks in the fifth decade. Mostly SCC and spreads by direct invasion to the vagina, paracervical/parametrial tissue, bladder and rectum. Frequently causes hydronephrosis as it progresses. Metastases to the lungs, bones, brain and liver.

CT
- Used for staging disease
- Check pelvic, inguinal, retroperitoneal and para-aortic nodes—nodes may be involved without enlargement.

MRI
- Tumour is intermediate signal on T2, which stands out next to the normal low-signal cervical stroma.

NUCLEAR MEDICINE
- PET/CT is useful for demonstrating metastatic disease.

Box 4.6 THE BASICS OF STAGING CERVICAL CARCINOMA
T1: confined to cervix T2: beyond uterus, not pelvic side wall or lower third of the vagina T3: involves pelvic wall or lower third of the vagina or ureteral obstruction T4: adjacent organs involved

DERMOID CYST (MATURE TERATOMA)

Most common germ cell tumour of the ovary. An age of 30 years is typical at diagnosis. Most are asymptomatic. Dermoids grow slowly and, if <6 cm, non-surgical management is preferred. It is a thick-walled cyst containing fat and the three germ layers (the Rokitansky nodule). Dermoid cysts may rupture or cause ovarian torsion (higher risk if large). Small malignant potential.

US

- Variable appearance from solid to cystic, depending on the contents of the dermoid

PLAIN FILM

- Tooth-shaped focus of calcification projected over the pelvis—classic

CT (FIGURE 4.16)

- Fat-containing lesion is diagnostic, may also see calcification (e.g. tooth).
- Solid components may enhance.
- Look for a thick-walled tube and uterus deviating towards the affected side in suspected torsion.

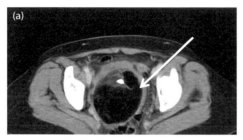 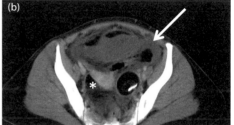

Figure 4.16 (a) Post-contrast axial computed tomography scan of the pelvis showing a lesion in the inferior pelvis (white arrow) containing fat and enhancing soft tissue components. The tooth-shaped focus of calcification is characteristic of a dermoid cyst. (b) A follow-up computed tomography scan shows the dermoid to have ruptured. The dermoid has decreased in size and there is now free fluid (white arrow) and free fatty locules (asterisk).

MRI

- Signal loss on fat-suppressed sequences/out-of-phase imaging
- Restriction of diffusion on diffusion-weighted imaging.

ENDOMETRIAL CANCER

Peaks in the fifth decade. Typically, it presents with postmenopausal bleeding. The vast majority are adenocarcinomas. It metastasises to the lungs, bones, liver and brain.

US

- Transvaginal US is the mainstay initial examination; the endometrium is abnormal if >4 mm postmenopause, >8 mm postmenopause on hormone replacement theraphy (HRT) or >14 mm premenopause.

CT

- Useful for demonstrating lymph node involvement, peritoneal disease and metastases

MRI

- Optimal for local staging: the tumour is best demonstrated on T1 post-contrast, where it enhances poorly compared to adjacent myometrium.
- The cervical canal commonly becomes obstructed, filling the uterine cavity with debris.

NUCLEAR MEDICINE

- PET/CT is useful for demonstrating metastases and disease recurrence.

Box 4.7 THE BASICS OF STAGING ENDOMETRIAL CARCINOMA
T1: confined to uterus T2: involves cervix T3a: adnexal involvement T3b: vaginal involvement T3c: pelvic/para-aortic nodes T4: adjacent organs

ENDOMETRIOSIS

Endometrial tissue outside the uterus responds to hormonal signals from the menstrual cycle. This results in bleeding, inflammation and fibrosis. Deposits of <3 mm are impossible to detect with imaging. Larger deposits (endometrioma/chocolate cyst) are diagnostic. Typically located in the pelvis (e.g. 'cul de sac'), abdomen and also extra-abdominal sites, including the lungs (catamenial pneumothorax) and even the central nervous system.

CT

- Complex, heterogeneous cyst with or without extension to adjacent pelvic viscera

MRI

- Large mass, containing blood products of differing ages
- Tend to be multiple and bilateral
- Typically low signal on T2 with high-signal foci on T1 and T2 (blood products of different ages)
- May cause haematosalpinx (tubal endometriosis) or hydrosalpinx from obstruction

Box 4.8 UNINTENDED FOETAL RADIATION EXPOSURE: DUTIES OF THE RADIOLOGIST
1. Discuss the case with the responsible radiographer and referring team to establish the circumstances of the incident. 2. Contact the medical physics department to advise them of the incident. They should begin an investigation into the circumstances of the event and likely foetal dose. 3. Discuss the case with the referring team and offer to counsel the patient regarding risks to the foetus. **Note** 1. Foetal risk is highest in the first trimester.

> **2.** In most cases, a dose <100 mGy is unlikely to have an adverse effect on the foetus. Above this, there is an increased risk of learning disability or induction of malignancy.
> **3.** In normal circumstances, diagnostic scans are well below the threshold. Exposure for an interventional procedure could exceed 100 mGy.

FIBROTIC OVARIAN TUMOURS

Theses consist of thecoma, fibroma and fibrothecoma (most common). Usually large and benign, they look like fibroids, but on the ovary. Meig syndrome is a combination of fibroma, effusion and ascites, mimicking malignancy.

US

- Solid mass, hypo-reflective with acoustic shadow

MRI

- Similar appearance to fibroids—low signal on T2, may have cystic areas (i.e. T2 hyperintense)

LEIOMYOMA (FIBROIDS)

Common, benign uterine tumour. In total, 50% of women of reproductive age are affected. Most are asymptomatic, others have menorrhagia, pelvic pain/mass and subfertility. Rarely malignant transformation (leiomyosarcoma). Defined as intramural (most common), submucosal, subserosal and pedunculated (may tort).

US

- Focal uterine masses, hypo-reflective compared to myometrium and cast an acoustic shadow

MRI

- Low signal on T2 compared to adjacent myometrium.
- Variable signal on T1, high if blood products present.
- Varying degrees of enhancement depending on whether they have started to degenerate.
- Rapid growth, ill-defined margins and invasion are red flags for sarcomatous transformation.

INTERVENTION

- Uterine artery embolisation is a popular alternative to surgery in selected patients.
- Overall clinical success rates are about 85% at 6 years.
- Pedunculated/subserosal fibroids are a relative contraindication (greater risk of detachment).

NABOTHIAN CYST

Very common, benign superficial cyst of the mucus-secreting glands of the cervix. Rarely of any clinical significance.

MRI

- Well-marginated T2 hyperintensity located in the superficial cervix

OVARIAN CANCER

About 40% of ovarian tumours are malignant, mostly advanced (i.e. peritoneal disease) at presentation. Ca-125 elevated in 80%, but in early disease, the specificity of this is only 50%. Most are epithelial in origin, and the serous type is most common (i.e. serous cystadenocarcinoma). Metastasises to the lungs and bone.

CT (FIGURE 4.17)

- Preferred for initial staging (formal staging with the International Federation of Gynaecology and Obstetrics [FIGO] system at laparotomy).
- Enhancing ovarian nodules with large cystic component, hyperdense ascites, peritoneal nodules.
- Check pelvic and retroperitoneal lymph nodes.
- Thick-walled bowel indicates gut serosal infiltration.
- Liver deposits tend to be subcapsular.

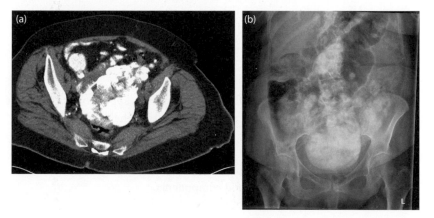

Figure 4.17 (a) Unenhanced axial computed tomography scan of the pelvis shows a large, densely calcified mass in the inferior pelvis with soft tissue elements. The diagnosis proved to be serous cystadenocarcinoma of the ovary. (b) The abnormality is clearly demonstrated on a plain abdominal film.

OVARIAN METASTASES

Up to 15% of ovarian malignancies are secondary via peritoneal spread, direct invasion or haematogenous dissemination. Gastrointestinal tumours are the most likely source. Krukenberg tumour refers specifically to an ovarian secondary made up of mucin-producing cells, commonly from a gastric primary.

CT

- Large, solid ovarian masses.
- Areas of low attenuation are likely to represent necrosis.

OVARIAN CYST

Normal ovarian follicles contain cysts. Cysts <3 cm are physiological (follicular cyst). Cysts larger than 4 cm are more likely to tort. Best assessed with transvaginal US first.

US

- Thin-walled cyst with no Doppler flow (first half of menstrual cycle).
- Marked peripheral vascularity is seen later in the menstrual cycle, when the cyst may become thick-walled and contain hyperechoic material (haemorrhage; i.e. corpus luteum cyst).
- Indeterminate lesions are followed up at 4–8 weeks when the cyst should have decreased in size (due to different phase of the menstrual cycle).

PERITONEAL INCLUSION CYST

Occur in women with functioning ovaries and a history of abdominal surgery/adhesions. Adhesions are thought to prevent normal absorption of ovarian fluid leading to a build-up that surrounds the ovary.

US

- Septated fluid collection associated with the ovary
- Ovary may have a normal appearance

CT

- Multi-loculated fluid collection (may appear hyperdense due to blood products)
- Enhancing soft tissue (ovary) within the fluid collection

MRI

- Used for problem-solving to exclude malignancy
- No enhancing solid components

UTERINE ANOMALIES

Arise from abnormal fusion of the Mullerian ducts during foetal life. Best assessed with MRI. All are associated with renal anomalies. See Figure 4.18.

UTERINE SARCOMA

Rare, aggressive tumour. Presents with dysmenorrhoea. Tends to affect a younger age group than endometrial cancer. Most common subtype is leiomyosarcoma (beware rapidly enlarging fibroid with ill-defined margins).

CT

- Useful for demonstrating lymph node involvement, peritoneal disease and metastases

MRI

- On T1 post-contrast, the mass enhances less than the adjacent myometrium and cervix.

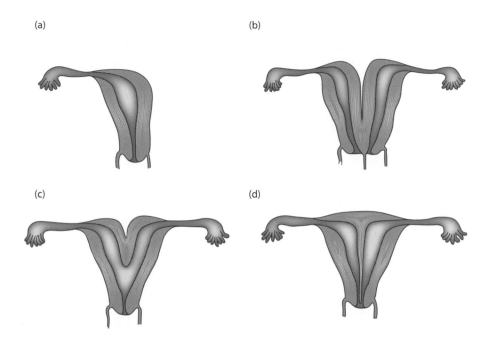

Figure 4.18 Abnormalities of uterine fusion. (a) Unicornuate. (b) Didelphys (75% have a vaginal septum, which may cause an obstruction). (c) Bicornuate (either unicollisor bicollis). (d) Septateuterus (septum may extend to the vagina, associated with subfertility).

- Heterogeneous appearance to the lesion.
- Large mass with a greater myometrial component than other endometrial cancers.
- Leiomyosarcoma contains foci of haemorrhage and calcification.

VAGINAL MALIGNANCY

More commonly involved by direct invasion from cervical, uterine or rectal tumours. Primary vaginal cancer is rare and mostly SCC, with a minority being adenocarcinoma. Tends to affect postmenopausal women.

MRI

- Exophytic intermediate signal mass, disrupts normal low T2 signal vaginal wall.
- Tends to arise from the upper posterior wall.
- Look for fistulation to the bladder.

MALE GENITAL TRACT

BENIGN PROSTATIC HYPERTROPHY

Increasingly common with age, 80% by 80 years of age. Nodular fibromyoadenomatous hyperplasia, mostly affecting the central zone of the prostate. Complications when severe include bladder outflow obstruction, infection, hydronephrosis, infection and haematuria.

US

- Enlarged prostate (>30 mL), signs of bladder outflow obstruction (BOO) (e.g. trabeculated bladder, post-micturition residual bladder volume)

CT

- Enlarged gland, may be calcified or have areas of cystic degeneration
- Thickened, trabeculated bladder

MRI

- Small foci of T2 hyperintensity in the central zone
- Large gland

INTERVENTION

- Prostate artery embolisation increasingly considered for selected patients not suitable for surgery

---

Box 4.9 PROSTATE IMAGING AND REPORTING AND DATA SYSTEM (PIRADS)

Increasingly, magnetic resonance imaging (MRI) is used for diagnosis, risk stratification, surveillance, etc. PIRADS is a scoring system designed to standardise reporting of prostate MRI in order to improve performance and facilitate multi-centre comparison.

PIRADS 1—very low (clinically significant cancer is highly unlikely to be present)
PIRADS 2—low (clinically significant cancer is unlikely to be present)
PIRADS 3—intermediate (the presence of clinically significant cancer is equivocal)
PIRADS 4—high (clinically significant cancer is likely to be present)
PIRADS 5—very high (clinically significant cancer is highly likely to be present)

Read more:
http://www.acr.org/~/media/ACR/Documents/PDF/QualitySafety/Resources/PIRADS/PIRADS%20V2.pdf

---

EPIDIDYMITIS/ORCHITIS

Most common in sexually active young men. Bacteria spreads from the genitourinary (GU) tract, most commonly *Chlamydia*, *E. coli*, *Pseudomonas*, etc. Epididymitis occurs first, which may progress to orchitis. Note that 10% of testicular tumours present with orchitis—follow all hypoechoic testicular lesions until resolution.

US

- Enlarged, hyperaemic epididymis with or without spermatic cord.
- Hypo-reflective bands and hyperaemia in orchitis (avascular areas could represent infarction in severe cases).
- Low-resistance flow pattern on Doppler (resistive index <0.50).
- Hydrocele commonly (may be septated).
- Thickened scrotal skin.

ERECTILE DYSFUNCTION

May be due to a cord injury/tumour. Peyronie disease can also cause erectile dysfunction, and it results from focal fibrosis of the penile fascia (tunica albuginea).

US

- Echogenic plaques seen on the dorsal aspect of the penis with Peyronie disease

PENILE CANCER

Most malignancies affecting the penis are either urethral (SCC, commonly bulbomembranous urethra) or soft tissue (epithelioid sarcoma).

PROSTATE CANCER

Present in 10% of men aged >50 years. Gleason score indicates degree of differentiation: 1 = well differentiated → 5 = anaplastic. Capsular penetration indicates poor prognosis. In total, 95% of cases are adenocarcinomas and 70% are in the peripheral zone. Metastasises to the lungs, liver, kidneys and bones (sclerotic).

CT (FIGURE 4.19)

- Used to screen for metastases and local invasion
- Affects pelvic nodes, then para-aortic and inguinal

MRI

- Optimal images are obtained with an endorectal coil.
- Tumour is low signal on T2 with matched area of restriction on diffusion-weighted imaging.
- Haemorrhage from recent biopsy may mimic tumour on T2.

NUCLEAR MEDICINE

- Whole-body bone scan is most sensitive (though not specific) for detecting of bone metastases—offered routinely with prostate-specific antigen >10 ng/mL.

TESTICULAR TORSION

Mostly unilateral and intravaginal ('bell-clapper'). The extra-vaginal variant is more common in newborns. Salvation rate depends on the extent and duration of torsion—not salvageable after 24 hours.

US

- Absent or decreased colour flow (compare to normal contralateral side), may have normal B-mode appearance.
- Later on, the testis has a heterogeneous appearance on B-mode (poor prognostic indicator).
- Hydrocele is common.
- There may be increased Doppler flow to the spermatic cord and epididymis in the chronic setting.

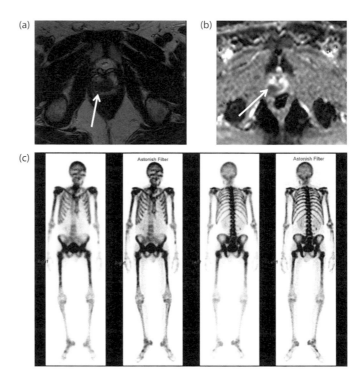

Figure 4.19 (a) Axial T2 of the prostate shows a focus of low signal in the right prostate (white arrow). Note the lesion has not penetrated the capsule and is therefore staged T2. (b) A corresponding area of low signal is seen on the ADC map (white arrow), in keeping with malignancy. (c) Technetium-99m bone scan shows diffuse increased uptake of tracer in the skeleton (different patient). Note that the renal parenchyma is not demonstrated. This appearance is called the 'superscan' and may be seen with extensive bone activity, in this case due to metastatic prostate cancer.

TESTICULAR TRAUMA

Commonly either haematocele or testicular rupture.

US

- Blood products surrounding the testicle, septated if chronic in haematocele.
- Look for break in contour of the testis, heterogeneous appearance and reduced vascularity with testis rupture.

TESTICULAR TUMOURS (FIGURE 4.20)

Either germ cell, non-germ cell, lymphoma or a secondary tumour. Most are germ cell tumours, typically teratoma in those age <40 years and seminoma in those aged >40 years. Lymphoma more common in those aged >70 years.

US

- Discrete intratesticular mass(es), variable reflectivity and size.
- Any intratesticular mass should be considered a malignancy.

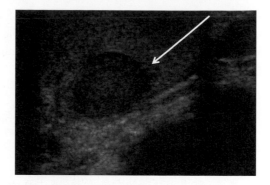

Figure 4.20 Cropped US imaging showing a hypoechoic lesion at the periphery of the testis (white arrow). Teratoma, seminoma and lymphoma are differentials. The age of the patient helps to steer the diagnosis. This lesion was a seminoma.

CT

- Used to screen for metastases.
- Lung metastases tend to follow retroperitoneal lymph node disease.
- Metastases to retroperitoneal lymph nodes and lungs.

VARICOCELE

Retrograde flow in the spermatic vein causes dilatation of the pampiniform plexus. It is the most common cause of infertility in men. Mostly left-sided.

US

- Dilated veins found behind the upper pole of the testis, diameter >3 mm
- Augmentation on Valsalva
- Consider renal/adrenal tumour in the elderly, from obstruction to the left renal vein

INTERVENTION

- Embolisation of the testicular vein(s)—associated with improved sperm quality post-procedure

BREAST

Box 4.10 TRIPLE ASSESSMENT OF BREAST LESIONS
All breast lesions are investigated with triple assessment: clinical exam, imaging and biopsy. • Imaging usually involves ultrasound, mammography (if aged >35 years) and magnetic resonance imaging in selected cases (Box 4.15). • Contrast-enhanced mammography is useful to characterise indeterminate lesions.

BREAST CYSTS

A mass in the female breast is most likely a cyst. The peak age group approximately 40 years. Size waxes and wanes premenopause. Simple cysts have no risk of malignancy, complex cysts are rarely (<2%) malignant.

US

- Well-defined, imperceptible wall, anechoic contents and posterior acoustic enhancement (i.e. classic cyst).
- Aspirated for symptom relief.
- Complex cysts contain echogenic debris (not nodules)—send sample to cytology.

MAMMOGRAM

- Well-defined round/oval lucency

Box 4.11 PATTERNS OF CALCIFICATION IN BREAST DISEASE

Benign
Tram-line: vascular
Broken needle: ductal, may extrude into the breast parenchyma → local reaction → fat necrosis and lead pipe calcification
Eggshell: fat necrosis
Tea cup: due to fibrocystic change, calcium deposition within a tiny cyst at dependent margin
Plasma cell mastitis: rod-shaped, thick, point to the nipple
Popcorn: degenerating fibroadenoma in postmenopausal woman

Malignant
Clustered microcalcification
Variable size and shape
Linear distribution, rod-shaped or branching

CANCER

Most common malignancy in females. About 1% occurs in males. Age, oestrogen exposure, family history and genetics (e.g. *BRCA*, Li–Fraumeni syndrome and *TP-53* mutation) are risk factors in women.

The taxonomy of the underlying pathology is complex. The vast majority (99%) of tumours are carcinomas (i.e. they arise from epithelial components of the ducts) rather than sarcomas (connective tissue origin). In total, 80% of carcinomas are invasive ductal carcinomas, and a further 10%–15% are invasive lobular carcinomas. Metastases occur anywhere, but preference is for the axillary nodes, internal mammary nodes, bones and liver.

MAMMOGRAM

- Often ill-defined mass with or without spiculate margins (implies desmoplasia)
- Microcalcification if ductal carcinoma *in situ*

US

- Expect a hypo-reflective lesion distorting the normal breast architecture with posterior acoustic shadowing.

Box 4.12 BREAST IMAGING REPORTING AND DATA SYSTEM (BIRADS)

This schema is used to standardise and optimise mammography, ultrasound and magnetic resonance imaging reports for diagnosis in breast disease.

1. Inadequate imaging
2. Normal appearances
3. Definitely benign disease
4. Probably benign—follow-up
5. Suspicious for malignancy—biopsy
6. Likely malignancy—biopsy
7. Confirmed malignancy

- There may be central vascularity on Doppler.
- Suspicious lymph nodes tend to be rounded with a cortex >2 mm thick.

FAT NECROSIS

Results from damage to adipocytes from trauma, iatrogenic, inflammation, etc. Tends to occur in the superficial breast (most susceptible to trauma). Appearance depends on the age of the lesion—oedema initially, then a fluid collection and finally a more solid-appearing mass (may need biopsy to exclude malignancy).

US

- Oedema within the affected area, a cyst develops within this after days to months.
- Eventually, the cyst wall calcifies and may appear as a spiculated mass (due to desmoplasia).

MAMMOGRAM

- Lucent mass; if round, then it represents an oil cyst.
- Rim calcification (takes 18 months to appear after the insult).
- Desmoplastic reaction may give the appearance of a spiculated mass.

FIBROADENOMA

Overall, this is the most common solid breast lesion. They are benign, feel smooth and are mobile. Peak in the third decade. They are usually solitary. Typical fibroadenomas in patients aged <25 years are not routinely biopsied.

US

- Well-defined, slightly hypoechoic lesion with internal echo
- May show posterior acoustic enhancement and vascularity with Doppler
- Small cysts may be seen within the mass, may represent complex fibroadenoma (need to exclude malignancy—phyllodes tumour)

MAMMOGRAM

- Rounded mass with density similar to adjacent breast tissue
- Common to see popcorn calcification when degenerating

FIBROADENOLIPOMA

This is a hamartoma, a benign mass made up of various elements of normal breast tissue. Occurs in all age groups.

US

- Oval-shaped, may have ill-defined edges, mix of echogenic glandular tissue and fat

MAMMOGRAM

- Well-defined lesion, 'breast within breast' appearance

GYNAECOMASTIA

Often a normal finding in adolescent boys. In adults, it is linked to drugs (e.g. spironolactone and digoxin), testicular tumours, cirrhotic liver disease, Klinefelter syndrome, cryptorchidism, etc. Usually affects one side more than the other.

US

- Breast tissue in the retroareolar region may show increased vascularity on Doppler.
- US is useful to rule out a focal mass.

MAMMOGRAM

- Retroareolar breast tissue, compare to the contralateral side

IMPLANT RUPTURE

Implant ruptures are either intracapsular (within the fibrous capsule that forms after implant placement) or extracapsular. Material from the implant may leak outside the breast in an extracapsular rupture to cause e.g. silicone adenitis.

US

- May be first-line investigation depending on availability of MRI.
- Look for the 'linguine sign'.
- Silicone-filled lymph nodes produce a 'snowstorm' appearance.

MRI

- Most sensitive and specific for implant rupture.
- Look for linguine, keyhole, salad oil or subcapsular line signs.
- Review axillary nodes for evidence of adenitis.

Box 4.13 MAMMOGRAPHY

Mediolateral oblique (MLO) and craniocaudal (CC) views are standard. MLO view should show all breast tissue. CC view will miss off the axillary tail. Supplementary views—paddle, focal compression to spot of interest to displace overlying tissue; magnification view to examine areas of microcalcification, typically CC or true lateral.

METASTASES TO THE BREAST

Rarely other primaries metastasise to the breast. Most common primaries to do so are lymphoma and prostate cancer in men; also, choriocarcinoma, melanoma and RCC.

MAMMOGRAM

- Lesions tend to be multiple, bilateral and more well defined than primary breast cancer.
- Unlikely to calcify.

US

- Usually well defined, more likely multiple and bilateral
- Vascularity on Doppler

Box 4.14 MAGNETIC RESONANCE IMAGING (MRI) IN BREAST DISEASE (FIGURE 4.21)

Contrast-enhanced MRI is nearly 100% sensitive for invasive breast carcinoma; specificity is <100%. The patient is scanned prone with a breast coil. Fat suppression is key, then the enhancing lesion stands out against suppressed breast fat on T1.
  Used as a problem-solving tool, namely:

1. **In response assessment following chemotherapy** (neoadjuvant chemotherapy is routinely given for tumours >2 cm). Assessment is done pre-treatment, mid-treatment and on completion of treatment prior to surgery.
2. **Invasive lobular carcinoma**—more sensitive than mammography (93% compared to 71%), and useful for assessing multifocality/bilaterality (more common in lobular).
3. **Ductal carcinoma *in situ***—non-calcified or if being considered for breast conserving surgery.
4. **For screening high-risk groups** (*BRCA* mutation, Li–Fraumeni syndrome, previous lymphoma [risk of late breast cancer], *TP-53* mutation).
5. **To assess breast implant integrity**.
6. **Dense breasts in the context of a proven cancer** (e.g. young patient or on hormone-replacement therapy).

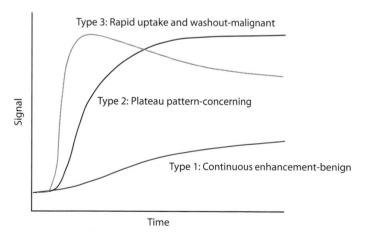

Figure 4.21 Breast lesions can be characterised with dynamic magnetic resonance imaging post-contrast: the Kuhl enhancement curves. Lesions that enhance rapidly and wash out rapidly are at highest risk for malignancy (type 3).

PAPILLOMA

More common in those aged 40–50 years. Typically present with spontaneous nipple discharge (often bloody). It is a benign lesion, although there is a slightly increased risk of later breast cancer.

US

- Look for a dilated duct in the retroareolar region containing a filling defect.
- US-guided core biopsy or vacuum-assisted biopsy to exclude papillary carcinoma.

PHYLLODES

Rapidly growing mass. The majority are benign, but up to 25% are malignant. Typically affects middle-aged women (fibroadenoma tends to present at a younger age).

US

- Well-defined solid lesion with posterior acoustic enhancement.
- Cystic spaces are characteristic.
- Vascularity on Doppler.

MAMMOGRAM

- Dense, rounded lesion with well-defined margins
- Rarely calcification

RADIAL SCAR

Incidental finding, not related to previous surgery or trauma. Small risk of malignancy, usually in the periphery of the scar, so may be excised.

MAMMOGRAM

- Irregular mass, 'hub and spoke' appearance is typical (central lucency, opaque bands radiating out from centre).

Box 4.15 U.K. BREAST SCREENING PROGRAMME
Women are invited for a mammogram at 47 years of age, then every 3 years until aged 73 years. The aim is to reduce mortality from breast cancer by 25%–30%. For every false positive, 2–2.5 lives are saved from breast cancer.

CHAPTER 5

Paediatrics

CENTRAL NERVOUS SYSTEM (CNS)

Box 5.1 IMAGING THE PAEDIATRIC BRAIN
Computed tomography is regularly used for trauma and to investigate calcification and the calvarium. In patients aged <6 years, sedation is usually needed for magnetic resonance imaging. Neonates are usually scanned when asleep without difficulty.

ACUTE DISSEMINATED ENCEPHALITIS

This is an acute autoimmune encephalomyelitis that is usually triggered by an inflammatory response to e.g. a viral infection or a vaccination. It gives rise to multi-focal neurology.

MAGNETIC RESONANCE IMAGING (MRI)
- Demyelination in a perivenous pattern is a hallmark.
- Multiple, large and confluent/punctate foci of high T2 signal in the subcortical white matter, cerebellum and grey matter.
- The appearance is indistinguishable from multiple sclerosis (MS) (settled with clinical correlation).
- Hurst disease is a haemorrhagic hyperacute variant that causes a marked generalised mass effect and is fatal in a matter of days.

ARACHNOID CYST

The most common congenital intracranial cystic abnormality. Found most commonly in the middle cranial fossa (60%), cerebellopontine angle (10%) or suprasellar (10%).

COMPUTED TOMOGRAPHY (CT)
- Paramedian cystic lesion, may compress adjacent brain and scallop the adjacent bone

MRI
- Behaves like cerebrospinal fluid (CSF) on all sequences.
- No restriction of diffusion (unlike an epidermoid cyst).

AQUEDUCTAL STENOSIS

Congenital or acquired (e.g. tumour). Aqueductal stenosis is the most common cause of congenital hydrocephalus.

MRI

- Hydrocephalus (may be extreme)—very dilated third ventricle with normal fourth ventricle.
- The corpus callosum appears stretched and thinned.
- The aqueduct has a funnel shape on a midline sagittal slice.
- Expect a normal posterior fossa (distinguishes from e.g. Chiari and Dandy–Walker malformations).
- The choroid plexus may be seen suspended in the ventricle ('dangling choroid sign').

ATAXIA TELANGIECTASIA

This is a rare, autosomal recessive disorder characterised by telangiectasia, cerebellar ataxia and immunodeficiency due to a lack of lymphoid tissue (spleen, thymus and lymph nodes). It gives rise to recurrent sinusitis, pneumonia and an increased risk of malignancy (10% develop lymphoma and leukaemia).

ULTRASOUND (US)

- Check for congenital asplenia.

CT

- Check for pulmonary vascular malformations.
- Ruptured teleangiectatic intracerebral vessels may cause intracerebral haemorrhage.

MRI

- Check for high signal on diffusion-weighted imaging (DWI) in keeping with infarcts (emboli shunted through pulmonary arteriovenous malformations [AVMs]).
- Expect a small cerebellum with atrophy of the anterior vermis and compensatory enlargement of the fourth ventricle.

Box 5.2 PATTERNS OF PAEDIATRIC INTRACEREBRAL CALCIFICATION

- Pathological ('Pit MITCH')
  - **Pit**uitary fossa
  - **M**ammillary bodies
  - **I**ntrasellar or parasellar regions (consider craniopharyngioma)
  - **T**ectal plate
  - **C**orpus callosum
  - **H**abenular commissure
- Normal ('ABCD')
  - **A** pineal calcification <1 cm
  - **B**asal ganglia
  - **C**horoid plexus
  - **D**ural

CHIARI I MALFORMATION

This is typically an incidental finding in adults. It may be acquired secondary to increased intracranial pressure, decreased intraspinal pressure or decreased posterior fossa volume. May cause chronic headache or cranial nerve palsy. It is the commonest cause of a syrinx (not associated with myelomeningocele). Syndrome associations include craniosynostosis, Klippel–Feil syndrome and Sprengel deformity.

MRI

- Sagittal reformats of the craniovertebral junction are most useful.
- Expect an isolated hindbrain abnormality, normal cortex.
- Look for pointed, peg-shaped cerebellar tonsils protruding ≥5 mm below the foramen magnum (opisthion–basion line).
- Normal appearance of the fourth ventricle.
- Additional findings may include: hydrocephalus (up to 40%), syrinx (up to 75%), tethered cord, craniovertebral segmentation anomalies.

CHIARI II MALFORMATION

This is the most commonly diagnosed Chiari malformation. Usually prenatal or neonatal diagnosis with myelomeningocele, enlarging head and neurological signs. Folate supplementation has reduced incidence. Overall problem is a small posterior fossa with herniation of the hindbrain.

MRI

- Thoracolumbar myelomeningocele (95%), obstructive hydrocephalus (90%), callosal dysgenesis (85%), tectal beaking, low-lying 'towering' cerebellar tonsils, small posterior fossa, elongated fourth ventricle.
- Other findings include an absent septum pellucidum, excessive cortical gyration and wrapping of the cerebellum around the brainstem ('banana sign').

CHIARI III MALFORMATION

Very rare. The features are the same as for Chiari II malformation with the addition of encephalocele (posterior fossa contents herniate into a high cervical or occipital meningocele).

CHOROID PLEXUS PAPILLOMA

More common in children aged <5 years, mostly found in the lateral ventricles adjacent to the trigone. CSF production is increased, resulting in hydrocephalus. These are benign tumours; however, up to 20% become malignant.

CT

- Smooth, lobulated, iso-hyperdense mass with small calcified foci
- Intense enhancement with contrast

MRI
- Low signal on both T1 and T2, avid contrast enhancement

CONGENITAL INFECTION

CYTOMEGALOVIRUS (CMV)

This is the most common cause of intrauterine infection. It causes irreversible brain damage.

US
- Hyperechoic foci in a periventricular and cerebral distribution (i.e. calcification)
- Hydrocephalus

CT
- Expect low-attenuation white matter and periventricular/cerebral calcifications

TOXOPLASMOSIS

US
- The findings on US are characteristic—basal ganglia and periventricular calcification with or without choroid plexus calcification.
- The calcifications may be lobulated or curvilinear.

CORPUS CALLOSUM MALFORMATION

Brain function is normal with isolated callosal agenesis. Partial agenesis always affects the splenium or rostrum (the posterior callosum develops last). In total, 60% have developmental anomalies elsewhere in the body and 50% have other neurological anomalies (e.g. holoprosencephaly [not lobar], Chiari II malformation, Dandy–Walker syndrome, encephalocele, etc.).

US
- Can be diagnosed on the 20–week scan
- Colpocephaly (i.e. dilated trigones, occipital horns and posterior temporal horns)
- Absent splenium
- Dilated and elevated third ventricle

MRI
- Lateral ventricles have a 'steerhorn' appearance on the coronals.
- Look for an absent cavum septum pellucidum/cingulate gyrus, high-riding third ventricle and colpocephaly.

CORTICAL MALFORMATION

LISSENCEPHALY

Means 'smooth', same as agyria (pachygyria = broad, flat gyri). Due to arrested neuronal migration. The brain looks as it should at 18–20 weeks of gestation. It is the most severe malformation of cortical development.

MRI

- Thickened, smooth cortex with slight indentation at the Sylvian fissures.
- May be localised to a single lobe and usually the cerebellum is spared.
- Dilated occipital horns of the lateral ventricles (i.e. colpocephaly).

POLYMICROGYRIA

This is the most common cortical developmental anomaly arising from a problem in late neuronal migration. May follow 'toxoplasmosis, other (syphilis, varicella-zoster, parvovirus B19), rubella, cytomegalovirus (CMV), and herpes (TORCH)' infection. Developmental delay and seizures are common.

MRI

- Numerous small, undulating gyri, mostly in the perisylvian cortex (may involve a small part of the brain or the whole brain).
- High-resolution MRI improves sensitivity in subtle cases.

SCHIZENCEPHALY

Abnormal cleft lined with polymicrogyric grey matter linking the pial and ependymal surfaces. May communicate openly with the ventricular system. In total, 90% have an absent septum pellucidum. Linked to polymicrogyria and septo-optic dysplasia.

MRI

- Cleft lined by grey matter; if there is CSF in the cleft it is known as 'open lipped', if there is not it is 'close lipped'.
- Note: A porencephalic cleft (i.e. old hypoxic ischaemic injury [HII]) can appear similar but is lined by white matter.

HETEROTOPIA

This anomaly is inherited. It is due to migrational failure that leaves grey matter trapped in white matter. It presents with seizures.

CT–MRI

- Non-enhancing white matter nodules appearing like grey matter on CT and all MRI sequences.
- Tuberous sclerosis tubers look similar but commonly calcify.

BAND HETEROTOPIA

Early arrest of neuronal migration leads to a circumferential band of heterotopic grey matter.

MRI

- Look for a band of grey matter giving the appearance of a double cortex.

COWDEN SYNDROME

This is a multiple hamartoma syndrome. The hallmark is Lhermitte–Duclos disease (dysplastic cerebellar gangliocytoma). It is a rare phakomatosis.

CRANIOPHARYNGIOMA

Think of this if you see a suprasellar mass in a child—it is the most likely diagnosis. There is a bimodal incidence peak (from ages 5–10 years and 50–60 years). It is more common in males. Clinical presentation is with visual field defects and/or diabetes insipidus. The tumour contains calcium, keratin and epithelium due to its origin from squamous epithelial rest metaplasia (see Figure 6.19).

CT

- Irregular outline, up to 90% in the suprasellar cistern
- Appearance ranges from solid to cystic, or a mix of the two
- Commonly calcified (90%—especially in children)
- Associated with bone destruction in up to 75%

MRI

- Typically high signal on both T1 (due to proteinaceous debris) and T2 with contrast enhancement of the solid component

CRANIOSYNOSTOSIS

This is the premature bony fusion of one or more cranial sutures (normally open until about 18 months, except for the metopic suture). The posterior fontanelle closes at 6 months, whilst the anterior fontanelle closes at 12 months. Presents with a deformed head and raised intracranial pressure, see Figure 5.1.

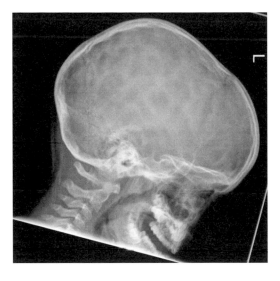

Figure 5.1 Lateral skull x-ray showing the 'copper-beaten skull' appearance. In children, this is a sign of raised intracranial pressure.

Causes classified as primary (idiopathic) or secondary. Secondary causes are syndromic: metabolic (rickets, hypercalcaemia, hyperthyroidism or hypervitaminosis D), haematological (thalassaemia or sickle cell) or bone dysplasias (achondroplasia or metaphyseal dysplasia), as well as Crouzon, Apert and Treacher–Collins syndromes.

Best assessed with a skull x-ray: Towne's view (for lambdoid and sagittal sutures), AP and lateral projections.

SCAPHOCEPHALY

Premature fusion of the sagittal suture. Most common (60%), causes a long and thin head.

BRACHYCEPHALY

Bilateral lambdoid or coronal synostosis giving a short, wide head. Accounts for 20% of synostoses. May cause a Harlequin eye deformity. Associated with a higher incidence of neurological abnormalities compared to scaphocephaly. See Figure 5.2.

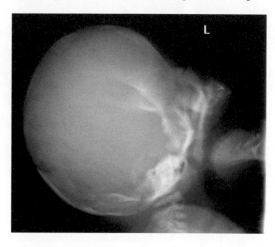

Figure 5.2 Lateral skull x-ray showing enlargement of the skull with fusion of the coronal sutures and frontal bossing. This form of craniosynostosis is known as brachycephaly.

PLAGIOCEPHALY

Unilateral fusion of the coronal or lambdoid suture producing a lopsided skull, described as either anterior (unilateral coronal synostosis) or posterior (unilateral lambdoid synostosis).

TRIGONOCEPHALY

Metopic synostosis, skull has a forward-pointing appearance.

KLEEBLATTSCHÄDEL

Severe craniosynostosis due to intrauterine sagittal, coronal and lambdoid synostosis. Skull adopts a clover leaf appearance. Associated with thanatophoric dysplasia.

DANDY–WALKER SPECTRUM

This is a spectrum of abnormalities ranging from the least severe megacisterna magna to the classic Dandy–Walker malformation.

MEGACISTERNA MAGNA

Enlarged cisterna magna crosses beneath the tentorium cerebelli. The posterior fossa may be enlarged. Note: Fourth ventricle, cerebellar vermis and tentorium normal.

HYPOPLASTIC VERMIS WITH ROTATION (ALSO KNOWN AS DANDY–WALKER VARIANT)

This is more common than Dandy–Walker syndrome. There is a small posterior fossa cyst. The cerebellar vermis is present but hypoplastic, the brainstem is normal and the posterior fossa is not enlarged.

DANDY–WALKER MALFORMATION (FIGURE 5.3)

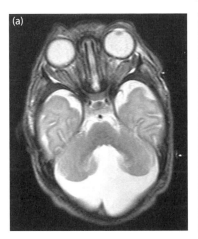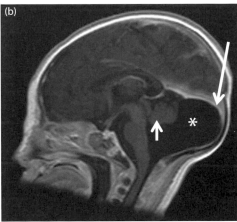

Figure 5.3 (a) Axial T2-weighted magnetic resonance image of the brain showing gross enlargement of the fourth ventricle and cerebellar hypoplasia. (b) Sagittal T1-weighted image in the same patient shows enlargement of the fourth ventricle, enlargement of the posterior fossa (asterisk) and cerebellar hypoplasia (short arrow). The torcula is elevated (long arrow). The appearance is in keeping with a Dandy–Walker malformation.

This is a congenital anomaly that is thought to arise from an *in utero* insult to the fourth ventricle. Associated with callosal dysgenesis or agenesis (25%), holoprosencephaly (25%) or polymicrogyria (25%).

CT/MRI

- Enlarged posterior fossa
- Elevated torcula
- Cystic enlargement of fourth ventricle
- Hypoplastic cerebellum (with or without hypoplastic tentorium)
- 80% have hydrocephalus

THE DEVELOPING BRAIN

SULCATION

From 18 weeks to term, the main change is cortical infolding. An adult pattern of sulcation is reached by 38 weeks. The mainstay of imaging is US at this stage.

MYELINATION

In the first year of life, T1-weighted MRI provides the best view of the myelinating structures—active myelination is high signal on T1. From 1–1.5 years of age, T2 is better.

- Myelination occurs from caudal to cranial and from posterior to anterior.
- The brain has an adult appearance on T1 at 8 months, and on T2 at 18 months.

DIASTEMATOMYELIA

Congenital sagittal division of the spinal cord into two hemichords, each containing a central canal, dorsal horn and ventral horn. Each hemicord has its own blood supply and the hemicords reunite caudally. More common in females (see Figure 6.31).

SPINE X-RAY

- Segmentation anomalies are common, 50%–75% have a scoliosis.
- Look for spina bifida at multiple levels, anteroposterior vertebral body narrowing and fusion/thickening of the laminae.

MRI

- Dual cords (may be of unequal size), most common between T9 and S1.
- In 75%, the conus lies below L2 (i.e. tethered cord).
- About 40% have separate dural sheaths.
- Myelomeningocele is present in up to 30%, syringohydromyelia in 50%.
- Also associated with Chiari II malformations and dermoid cysts.

FRIEDREICH ATAXIA

This is the most common inherited progressive ataxia. It is due to a loss of myelinated fibres and gliosis of the posterior and lateral spinal columns.

MRI

- Thinned cervical cord and medulla with associated mild cerebral atrophy.
- The cerebellum is spared.

GERMINAL MATRIX HAEMORRHAGE

The germinal matrix is highly vascular tissue present at 24–32 weeks of gestation located anterior to the caudothalamic groove and inferior to the lateral ventricles. It produces the neurons that later migrate to the cortex. Ischaemia causes a loss of vessel integrity and haemorrhage.

US

- Non-shadowing hyperechoic material lying anterior to the caudothalamic groove

Box 5.3 GERMINAL MATRIX HAEMORRHAGE IN PREMATURE NEONATES
The risk of haemorrhage is linked to birth weight, trauma at birth and coagulopathy. The lower the birth weight, the greater the risk of haemorrhage. At 2 kg, the risk of haemorrhage is 25%.

> **Box 5.4 GERMINAL MATRIX HAEMORRHAGE GRADING**
>
> Grade I: subependymal haemorrhage, usually has no long-term consequences
> Grade II: intraventricular haemorrhage without ventricular dilatation, 10% mortality
> Grade III: intraventricular haemorrhage with ventricular dilatation, 20% mortality
> Grade IV: intraparenchymal haemorrhage, >50% mortality

HERPES SIMPLEX ENCEPHALITIS

Most commonly affects the temporal lobe, with a propensity for the limbic system and inferolateral frontal lobes. CT scan may be negative for 3 days. MRI should be positive in 2 days.

MRI

- Non-specific high T2 and low T1 signal in the medial temporal lobes/inferior frontal lobes.
- Lesions restrict on DWI.
- Small focal haemorrhages are common.

HOLOPROSENCEPHALY

Range of presentations, from silent to fatal. It arises from a failure of cleavage of the developing forebrain. 'Face predicts the brain'—the extent of facial cleavage correlates to the extent of intracranial abnormality.

ALOBAR

Most severe type, commonly there is a facial deformity. No cleavage occurs, so there is fusion of the cerebral hemispheres and a monoventricle communicating with a posterior cyst. Midline structures (e.g. falx and third ventricle) are absent and thalami are fused.

SEMILOBAR

Extent of cleavage is variable. Typically, the frontal cortices are fused and midline structures deficient anteriorly but present posteriorly. The third ventricle is rudimentary and there is an anterior monoventricle (Figure 5.4).

LOBAR

There is a mild degree of fusion affecting the frontal brain only. The septum pellucidum is absent (as in all forms). May appear identical to septo-optic dysplasia.

HYPOTHALAMIC GLIOMA

These are the most common hypothalamic masses and account for 10%–15% of supratentorial tumours. Typical presentation is at 2–4 years of age with visual deficits and diencephalic syndrome (i.e. hypothalamic and thalamic dysfunction).

CT

- Mass in suprasellar region extending into the optic chiasm

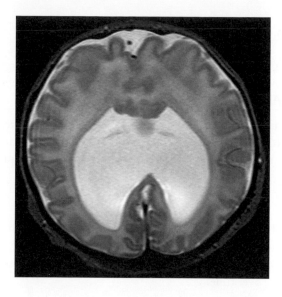

Figure 5.4 T2-weighted axial magnetic resonance imaging scan of a neonate shows a large monoventricle and fusion of the frontal cortices, in keeping with semi-lobar holoprosencephaly.

- Mixed enhancement due to tumour necrosis
- Cystic areas and calcifications

HYPOTHALAMIC HAMARTOMA

This is a tumour of the tuber cinerium that affects patients aged less than 2 years. It presents with precocious puberty and gelastic ('laughing') seizures.

CT

- Well-defined homogeneous mass with no enhancement located in the hypothalamus (i.e. floor of the third ventricle)

MRI

- Isointense on both T1 and T2

HYPOXIC ISCHAEMIC INJURY IN INFANCY

After about 2 years of age, the pattern of injury is the same as that seen in an adult. There is relative sparing of the thalamic nuclei from ages 1–2 years. The corpora striata, hippocampi and cortex are most affected.

CT

- Bilateral low-density basal ganglia, cerebral oedema.
- Occasionally, there is reversal of the normal pattern of grey and white matter attenuation (white matter appears more dense than the grey matter)—the 'reversal sign'.
- Diffuse cortical oedema with sparing of the cerebellum causes the 'white cerebellum sign'.

MRI

- DWI most sensitive acutely, usually abnormal by 24 hours
- T2 abnormalities appear by 2 days

HYPOXIC ISCHAEMIC INJURY IN PREMATURITY

More common than term HII—due to more risk factors and impaired cerebral autoregulation. Severe HII affects deep grey matter structures and the brain stem. Less severe injury tends to cause germinal matrix haemorrhage or periventricular leukomalacia (PVL).

US

- Often normal in the first 2 days, look for areas of increased echogenicity.
- The thalami are more commonly spared than in term HII.
- Periventricular echogenicity suggests acute PVL; after 2 weeks, these areas become cystic (these resolve over time).

MRI

- As with term HII, DWI most sensitive acutely at 3–5 days.
- T2 hyperintensity develops at 1 week.
- Ischaemic lesions adjacent to the ventricular trigone suggest PVL.

HYPOXIC ISCHAEMIC INJURY AT TERM

Due to an ischaemic injury in the term neonate. Affects <0.5% of live births. Severe ischaemia affects the deep grey matter (putamen, thalami, hippocampi, dorsal brainstem and lateral geniculate nuclei) predominantly, due to its energy demands. Mild to moderate ischaemia tends to spare deep grey matter at the expense of the cortex and white matter. See Figure 5.5.

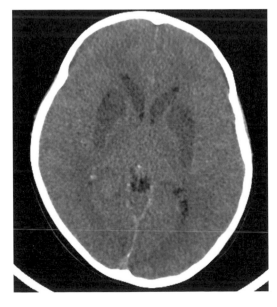

Figure 5.5 Unenhanced axial CT scan of a term neonate showing diffuse cerebral oedema and loss of grey–white matter differentiation. There are bilateral symmetrical infarcts of the putamen, consistent with hypoxic ischaemic brain injury.

US

- Most sensitive 1 week post-injury.
- Look for diffusely increased echogenicity, effaced CSF spaces (i.e. oedema) and increased echogenicity in the deep grey matter.
- Look for multiple cysts following devastating HII—'multicystic encephalomalacia'.

MRI

- DWI is most sensitive for detecting areas of acute (i.e. 3–5 days) ischaemia—sensitivity recedes after 1 week.
- T1 and T2 imaging most useful 1 week after injury (look for foci of T2 hyperintensity)—before 1 week, expect foci of high T1 and high T2 signal.
- Expect a thinned cortex and white matter loss long term.

Box 5.5 READ MORE

Huang, B., Castillo, M. 2008. Hypoxic–ischemic brain injury: Imaging findings from birth to adulthood. *Radiographics* 28:417–439.

LACUNAR SKULL

This is a bone deformity of the skull due to hydrocephalus. There is defective ossification of the inner table of the skull. Also known as Lückenschädel skull. Associated with Chiari II malformation, encephalocele and myelomeningocele. See Figure 5.1.

PLAIN FILM

- Multiple ovoid lucencies (present at birth, disappear by 5 months of age)
- Thinning of the inner table of the calvarium

LEPTOMENINGEAL CYST

Occurs following a paediatric skull fracture in about 1%, known as a 'growing' fracture. Fracture diastasis occurs due to adjacent CSF pulsation and dural tears with arachnoid herniation. A pulsatile mass overlying the bone defect is found clinically.

CT

- Smooth-edged defect in the calvarium and overlying soft-tissue mass
- Gliosis of the adjacent brain parenchyma

LIPOMA

Intracranial lipomas are mostly found in the midline—corpus callosum, quadrigeminal plate and suprasellar cisterns.

MRI

- Midline mass, high signal on T1.
- Mass signal suppresses on fat-saturated sequences and shows chemical shift artefact.
- No mass effect, vessels may pass through it.

MEDULLOBLASTOMA

This is the most common malignant posterior fossa tumour in children. Most present at <5 years of age. They tend to seed along the neuraxis (up to 30% at presentation). In total, 5% have metastases outside the CNS, mostly to the bone. Treatment is with surgery and radiotherapy to the whole neuraxis. Without metastases, 5–year survival is 80%.

CT

- Hyperdense midline posterior fossa mass on pre-contrast scan, arising from the cerebellar vermis or floor of the fourth ventricle (Figure 5.6)
- Homogeneous enhancement post-contrast, variable surrounding oedema
- Hydrocephalus in 90%
- Foci of haemorrhage, cystic change, necrosis and calcification may be seen

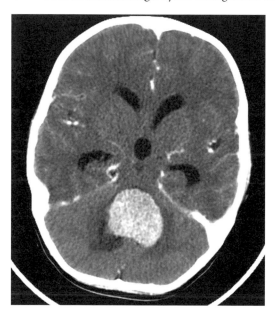

Figure 5.6 Post-contrast axial computed tomography scan of the brain of a child showing a large lesion in the posterior fossa that enhances uniformly. There is perilesional oedema and hydrocephalus due to obstruction of the fourth ventricle. The appearance is in keeping with medulloblastoma.

MRI

- Low to intermediate T1 signal with intermediate to high signal on T2.
- Enhancement more heterogeneous than on CT (more sensitive).
- Whole neuraxis must be imaged—check for foci of high T1 signal post-contrast, may be intra-dural, extra-dural or sub-pial.

MENINGITIS

Life-threatening illness due to infection of the subarachnoid space. In neonates, the most common source of infection is the mother's urogenital tract; causative pathogens are therefore group B *Streptococcus*, Gram-negative rods, etc. After the neonatal period, the most common pathogens are *Streptococcus pneumoniae* (most common between 1 and 23 months of age).

US

- Look for evidence of ventriculitis (up to 90% affected; e.g. hydrocephalus, echogenic debris/septations in the ventricles, thickened ependymal surface)
- Subdural effusion (common) or empyema (rare)

CT

- Consider post-contrast imaging.
- Hydrocephalus, subdural effusion or empyema and intracerebral abscess.
- Check for sinusitis.

MRI

- Most useful for diagnosis and detection of complications
- CSF spaces not as low signal on T1 as usual—CSF spaces may be effaced due to oedema
- Enhancement of the leptomeninges—seen on T1 post-contrast or fluid attenuated inversion recovery (FLAIR) post-contrast (non-specific)
- Subdural empyema—collection in the subdural space high signal on both T1 and T2

Box 5.6 CAUSES OF LEPTOMENINGEAL ENHANCEMENT ('MIRCI')

Malignancy
Infection
Reactive (e.g. surgery, shunt, trauma)
Chemical (e.g. cyst rupture, intra-thecal treatment)
Inflammatory (e.g. sarcoid)

NEUROFIBROMATOSIS TYPE 1 (NF1, VON RECKLINGHAUSEN DISEASE)

Autosomal dominant inheritance, 50% spontaneous (long arm mutation on chromosome 17). Fifteen-times more common than neurofibromatosis type 2 (NF2). It is a dynamic, slow-growing disease with features that peak at 10 years of age before regressing. CNS, spine, musculoskeletal (MSK) and renal systems are most commonly affected.

Box 5.7 THE PHAKOMATOSES (I.E. NEUROCUTANEOUS DISORDERS)

Neurofibromatosis
Tuberous sclerosis
Von Hippel–Lindau disease
Sturge–Weber syndrome
PHACE syndrome
Cowden syndrome

MRI

- Optic nerve glioma (astrocytoma) is the most common intracranial abnormality (30%); look for a diffusely thickened optic nerve with avid enhancement (may extend into the subarachnoid space) and enlargement of the optic nerve foramina.
- Foci of abnormal signal intensity (or unidentified bright objects) on T2/FLAIR, typically in the basal ganglia and thalami, deep white matter and cerebellum.
- No mass effect or enhancement and no restriction on DWI.
- Check for flow voids—Moyamoya disease—due to bilateral internal carotid artery stenosis.

SPINE MRI (FIGURE 5.7)

(a)   (b)

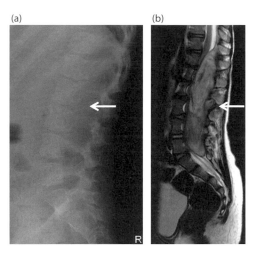

Figure 5.7 (a) Lateral x-ray of the lumbar spine showing scalloping of the posterior vertebral bodies (white arrow) and pedicles and widening of the spinal canal. (b) Sagittal T2-weighted magnetic resonance image showing a large mass filling and expanding the spinal canal and moulding between the spinous processes (white arrow). The diagnosis is a spinal neurofibroma.

- Neurofibromas cause bony abnormalities in 60%: kyphosis, scoliosis, posterior vertebral scalloping, enlargement of the neural foramina
- Also lateral thoracic meningoceles and dural ectasia

Box 5.8 CAFÉ SPOT—NF1 FEATURES

Café au lait spots
Axillary freckles
Fibromatosis
Eye (iris hamartomas)
Sphenoid wing hypoplasia/scoliosis
Pilocytic astrocytoma
Optic **t**umours

NEUROFIBROMATOSIS TYPE 2

Tends to present with hearing loss with or without vertigo in patients aged between 20 and 40 years. Accounts for about 10% of NF, inherited by autosomal dominance (deletion on chromosome 22).

Box 5.9 NF2, 'MISME'

Multiple
Inherited (autosomal dominant)
Schwannomas
Meningiomas (often intraventricular)
Ependymomas
Note: Think of NF2 if you see meningioma in a child.

MRI

- Bilateral acoustic schwannoma with or without enlargement of the internal acoustic meatus, may contain foci of calcification, rarely cystic.
- There are schwannomas on spinal roots in up to 90% and other cranial nerves in up to 50%.
- Associated with cord/brain ependymoma in up to 10%.
- Diffuse enhancement of schwannoma.

PHACE SYNDROME

This is a combination of a posterior fossa malformation, segmental haemangioma, arterial anomalies (affecting the aorta and circle of Willis), cardiac defects, eye defects and sternal defects. This is a rare phakomatosis.

PILOCYTIC ASTROCYTOMA

This is the most common intracranial tumour in children. Most present at <9 years of age. It is associated with NF1.

CT

- Well-circumscribed unilocular cyst, two-thirds are found in the posterior fossa (typically cerebellar vermis) with an enhancing solid mural nodule (low-grade tumours show no/poor enhancement).
- Commonly calcify.
- The wall of the cyst does not usually enhance.
- Complicated by hydrocephalus.

MRI

- T2—well-circumscribed, hyperintense lesion with a rim of low signal containing multiple cysts

PORENCEPHALY

Also known as a porencephalic cyst—these are congenital or acquired cavities that usually communicate with the subarachnoid space. Due to developmental insult, infection, trauma, vascular event, etc.

MRI

- Asymmetric, CSF-filled cystic space communicating with an enlarged ventricle
- May be seen in a vascular or watershed distribution

SEPTO-OPTIC DYSPLASIA

Mild holoprosencephaly (very similar to lobar type). It is a combination of a hypoplastic optic nerve, an absent septum pellucidum and a hypoplastic pituitary. Presents with a visual defect, pituitary dysfunction (45%) and seizures.

MRI

- Small optic chiasm and nerves
- Absent septum pellucidum
- Ectopic posterior pituitary
- Associated with cortical abnormalities in up to 90%, most commonly schizencephaly

STURGE–WEBER SYNDROME

Spontaneous disorder due to disrupted development of the cortical veins. The face is affected (port wine stain in the distribution of the trigeminal nerve) and there are ipsilateral leptomeningeal venous angiomas. In total, 90% have seizures; these are contralateral to the facial naevus.

CT

- Gyral/subcortical white matter calcification is pathognomic—these are like phleboliths and arise from venous stasis (apparent from 1 year of age).
- Choroid plexus hypertrophy, engorgement and enhancement, ipsilateral to the stain on the face.
- Long term—cortical atrophy on the affected side.
- Check for a choroidal angioma (eye)—leads to glaucoma.

MRI (FIGURE 5.8)

- Check for focal areas of restricted diffusion due to acute ischaemia.

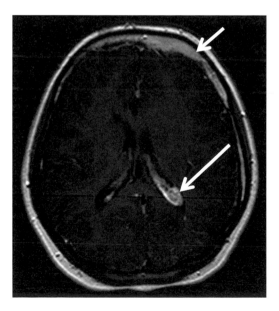

Figure 5.8 Axial T1 post-contrast magnetic resonance image of the brain showing a large venous angioma (short arrow) and ipsilateral hypertrophy and enhancement of the choroid plexus (long arrow). The appearance is in keeping with Sturge–Weber syndrome.

Box 5.10 SUTURE WIDTHS
10 mm at birth 3 mm at 2 years 2 mm at 3 years Rickets is a recognised cause of widened sutures.

TEMPORAL LOBE EPILEPSY

The temporal lobe is the most epileptogenic part of the brain. About two-thirds of those with temporal lobe seizures have hippocampal sclerosis (and atrophy of the amygdala, maxillary bodies and fornix), termed 'mesial temporal sclerosis' on neuroimaging.

MRI

- Thin-section coronal oblique T2 is most useful.
- Imaging shows hippocampal atrophy (bilateral in up to 20%) and focal hippocampal high signal on FLAIR.
- *Ex vacuo* dilatation of the adjacent temporal horn.

NUCLEAR MEDICINE

- Positron emission tomography (PET) or SPECT performed between seizures (i.e. inter-ictal) show a focus of reduced radiotracer uptake at the seizure focus.
- Ictal SPECT using hexamethylpropyleneamine oxime will show increased tracer uptake at the seizure focus—rarely used clinically.

TETHERED CORD

Suspected in patients presenting with lower-extremity motor or sensory dysfunction, urinary dysfunction and scoliosis or foot deformity (e.g. club foot, hammer toes, etc.). It is a developmental anomaly due to obstruction to the normal ascent of the cord. Associated with e.g. spinal lipoma, diastematomyelia, thickened filum terminale, Chiari malformation, syrinx, myelomeningocele and dermal sinus.

MRI

- Conus lies lower than normal (i.e. below L2).
- Look for a cause (e.g. spinal lipoma [high signal on T1 and T2], diastematomyelia, thickened filum terminale [>2 mm at L5–S1]).

TUBEROUS SCLEROSIS

Autosomal dominant inheritance. The main feature is multi-organ hamartomas (brain, lung, skin, kidneys and heart). Classic clinical triad in <50%: (1) facial angiofibroma; (2) seizures; and (3) learning disability. Multidisciplinary management, work-up with brain MRI, renal US and cardiac echo. See Figure 6.16.

Apart from the CNS abnormalities, look for:

- **Cardiac/chest:** lung cysts, spontaneous pneumothorax, chylothorax and cardiac rhabdomyoma

- **Renal**: multiple angiomyolipoma (may be large and bleed), renal cysts and increased risk of renal cell carcinoma
- **Skin**: adenoma sebaceum, shagreen patches and subungual fibrosis
- **Bones**: multiple bone islands

MRI

- 95% have a subependymal hamartoma (slow enhancement), these are often calcified (especially in those age >10 years) and protrude into the lateral ventricles; they are high signal on T2.
- Ventriculomegaly.
- Hamartomas may degenerate into subependymal giant cell astrocytomas: cystic and typically found near the foramen of Monro (differential is colloid cyst). May obstruct or show malignant change.
- Broadened gyri, curvilinear calcification and heterotopic grey matter are also features.

VEIN OF GALEN MALFORMATION

Malformation detected either *in utero*, with a neonatal pattern (<1 month), with an infantile pattern or with an adult pattern (>1 years—low flow). *In utero* and neonatal manifestations are due to either direct mass effect of the vein of Galen aneurysm (commonly hydrocephalus due to pressure on the aqueduct) or secondary high-output cardiac failure (cardiomegaly).

Three types:

- I: Arteriovenous (AV) fistula
- II: Angiomatous malformation of the basal ganglia, thalalmi and midbrain
- III: Both features

PLAIN FILM
- Chest x-ray shows cardiomegaly.

US
- Midline cystic mass posterior to the third ventricle containing mobile echogenic sparkles
- With or without hydrocephalus

MRI
- Vein of Galen aneurysms may bleed or cause infarction by a steal mechanism.

VON HIPPEL–LINDAU (VHL) DISEASE

Autosomal dominant inheritance. Rare syndrome giving rise to multiple benign and malignant tumours affecting multiple systems. Associated with renal cell carcinoma (most common cause of mortality), pancreatic cancer, pheochromocytoma, benign cysts and renal/hepatic angiomas. Haemangioblastomas are characteristic in the nervous system.

> **Box 5.11 DIAGNOSTIC CRITERIA FOR VON HIPPEL–LINDAU (VHL) DISEASE**
>
> >1 central nervous system haemangioblastoma
>
> OR
>
> 1 central nervous system haemangioblastoma and any of the visceral features of VHL
>
> OR
>
> Any of the features of VHL with a positive family history

MRI

- Look for haemangioblastoma (cerebellar—70%, retinal—50%, spinal—10%), a cystic lesion with an enhancing mural nodule. They can be solid.
- These are highly vascular tumours at risk of haemorrhage.

ENT AND ORBITS

BRANCHIAL CLEFT CYST

In total, 95% arise from the second branchial cleft, found lying along the anterior border of the sternocleidomastoid muscle (SCM), displacing the SCM posteriorly. The carotid and internal jugular vessels are displaced posteromedially. They typically enlarge with an upper respiratory tract infection.

> **Box 5.12 BAILEY CLASSIFICATION OF BRANCHIAL CLEFT CYSTS (TYPE II IS MOST COMMON)**
>
> **I.**   Along anterior surface of the sternocleidomastoid muscle, just deep to the platysma
> **II.** Along anterior surface of sternocleidomastoid muscle, lateral to carotid space, posterior to submandibular gland and adherent to vessels
> **III.** Extends medially between the internal and external carotid arteries to the lateral pharyngeal wall
> **IV.** Within pharyngeal mucosal space

US

- Cystic lesion with internal debris
- Well circumscribed, compressible, has internal structure and extends beyond the bifurcation of the internal and external carotid artery

CT

- Cystic lesion.
- A beak of tissue pointing between the internal and external carotid arteries is pathognomonic (type II cyst).

CHOLESTEATOMA

Due to squamous epithelium trapped in the skull base. It behaves in an aggressive way, destroying temporal bone structures. Associated with a conductive hearing loss. CNS complications are rare but include sinus thrombosis, epidural abscess and meningitis. There are congenital, primary and secondary types. The congenital type is unique in that it is found behind an intact tympanic membrane.

MRI

- Middle ear mass, isointense on T1 and hyperintense on T2
- May contain non-enhancing cystic foci
- Granuloma is hyperintense on T1

EPIGLOTTITIS

Caused by *Haemophilus influenzae*, now less common since the implementation of a vaccination programme. Causes abrupt stridor. Typical onset at 3–6 years of age, older than croup (3.5 years of age).

PLAIN FILM

- Soft tissue lateral neck—check for marked enlargement of the epiglottis and thickening of the aryepiglottic folds.
- With or without prevertebral soft tissue thickening.

JUVENILE ANGIOFIBROMA

Commonest nasopharyngeal benign tumour, but rare overall. Most are seen in adolescent males. Diagnosis is made with imaging biopsy is contraindicated due to bleeding risk. Treatment is with surgery with or without pre-operative embolisation.

CT/MRI

- Widening of the pterygopalatine fossa in 90%—pathognomonic
- Characteristic erosion of the medial pterygoid plate
- Anterior bowing of the posterior wall of the maxillary sinus (Holman–Miller sign)
- Invasion of the sphenoid sinus in two-thirds of cases
- Early, homogeneous enhancement post-contrast

HIV PAROTITIS

HIV parotitis is much more common in children with HIV than adults. The parotid glands are chronically enlarged, firm and non-tender. It does not usually require specific treatment. Thought to be associated with an improved prognosis.

US

- Enlarged, non-tender gland
- Multiple anechoic areas without associated posterior acoustic enhancement

PERSISTENT HYPERPLASTIC PRIMARY VITREOUS

Considered in newborns with leukocoria (i.e. absent light reflex). Most common cause of is retinoblastoma; however, when there is microphthalmia, the diagnosis is most likely persistent hyperplastic primary vitreous. Caused by arrest of the usual regression of connective tissue within the globe. Usually affects one eye only.

US

- Band from the retina to the posterior surface of the lens
- No calcification

CT

- Unilateral microphthalmia
- Hyperdense vitreous (previous haemorrhage)
- No calcification

RETINOBLASTOMA

About 50% of childhood leukokorias (i.e. absent light reflex) are caused by retinoblastomas. Rare, but it is the most common primary malignant orbital tumour. The mean age of presentation is 18 months. Unilateral in two-thirds. Inherited tumours are more commonly bilateral. If there is a pineoblastoma as well, it is known as a 'trilateral retinoblastoma'.

US

- Heterogeneous, hyperechoic, cystic intra-ocular mass with retinal detachment
- Cysts due to tumour necrosis
- Acoustic shadowing present in 75% (calcification)

CT

- Calcification in an ocular mass in a child <3 years of age is a retinoblastoma until proven otherwise.
- Smooth, solid intraorbital hyperdense lesions (nodular calcification).
- Enhances poorly.

RHABDOMYOSARCOMA

Rare—however, this is the most common extraocular orbital tumour of childhood (typically presents at <10 years of age). Presents with painless, rapidly progressive proptosis. It is unilateral and originates from the orbit, not the globe. Commonly, it has invaded adjacent bone at presentation. There is >90% survival at 5 years with surgery, radiotherapy and chemotherapy.

CT

- Useful to assess bone involvement
- Well-circumscribed, muscle-density extraconal mass
- Moderate—marked enhancement post-contrast

MRI

- Enhancing soft tissue mass that may extend to involve the eyelid (expect a thickened eyelid whether or not it is involved)
- Often continuous with the extra-ocular muscles
- Low/intermediate T1 with or without areas of haemorrhage
- High signal on T2

CARDIOVASCULAR

Table 5.1 Congenital heart disease

Blue baby	Heart size	Diagnosis	Chest x-ray
Decreased flow	Normal heart size	Tetralogy of Fallot	Normal heart size Decreased pulmonary blood flow Uplifting of the cardiac apex due to RV hypertrophy
	Giant heart size	Ebstein anomaly	Massive heart Decreased blood flow Hypoplastic aorta and pulmonary trunk
		Pulmonary atresia with intact ventricular septum	
Increased flow Patients who are cyanotic with increased flow have a mixture of lesions		Truncus arteriosus	Forked ribs Increased blood flow Cardiomegaly Right arch Wide mediastinum
		TAPVR	Normal heart Plethora Snowman appearance with a supracardiac type I
Variable flow		D-transposition of the great arteries Most common CHD presenting with cyanosis at birth	Most common finding is normal Narrowed superior mediastinum Small aortic arch Plethora Egg on a string
		Tricuspid atresia second most common CHD presenting with cyanosis in the neonatal period	Marked cardiomegaly plethora

Pink baby			Chest x-ray
Increased pulmonary arterial flow and left-to-right shunt		VSD	Acyanotic Pulmonary plethora Cardiomegaly Normal aorta

continued ❯

Table 5.1(*Continued*) Congenital heart disease

Pink baby			Chest x-ray
		PDA	Acyanotic
			Pulmonary plethora
			Cardiomegaly
			Enlarged aorta
		ASD	
		AVC	
Increased pulmonary venous flow		CHF in the newborn	
Normal pulmonary flow	Obstructive lesion	Coarctation	
		Aortic stenosis	
		Pulmonary artery stenosis	

Note: To narrow the differential diagnosis, consider first whether the baby is cyanotic, then whether there is pulmonary plethora.

Abbreviations: ASD: atrial septal defect; VSD: ventricular septal defect; PDA: persistent ductus arteriosus; RA: right atrium; RV: right ventricle; LA: left atrium; LV: left ventricle; AO: aorta; PV: pulmonary vasculature; TAPVR: total anomalous pulmonary venous return; CHD: congenital heart disease; CHF: congestive heart failure; AVC: atrioventricular canal.

ABERRANT RIGHT SUBCLAVIAN ARTERY

This is the most common arch anomaly. Ordinarily, the right subclavian artery arises with the right common carotid artery from the brachiocephalic trunk. An anomalous right subclavian arises directly from the aortic arch after the left subclavian and in 80% passes posterior to the oesophagus. It is mostly asymptomatic; occasionally, it causes dysphagia due to compression on the oesophagus.

WATER SOLUBLE SWALLOW

● Posterior oesophageal impression on the mid-oesophagus

ABERRANT LEFT PULMONARY ARTERY

Commonly described as a pulmonary sling, the aberrant left pulmonary artery arises from the right pulmonary artery. It then passes around distal trachea and between the trachea and oesophagus to reach the left lung. It therefore causes an impression on the anterior oesophageal wall. It presents in infancy with stridor and respiratory distress due to compression of the right main bronchus.

Box 5.13 READ MORE
Berdon, W. 2000. Rings, slings, and other things: Vascular compression of the infant trachea updated from the midcentury to the millennium—The legacy of Robert E. Gross, MD, and Edward B. D. Neuhauser, MD. *Radiology* 216:624–632.

PLAIN FILM

- Fluid retention on the right lung in neonatal period or right lung emphysema

WATER SOLUBLE SWALLOW
- Anterior oesophageal impression
- Mass between trachea and oesophagus

ATRIAL SEPTAL DEFECT (ASD)

Most ASDs are found in childhood, although they are usually asymptomatic in early life. Rarely a cause of congestive cardiac failure. See Table 5.1 for a summary of paediatric congenital heart disease.

Three types:

- Ostium secundum (80%–90%)
  - Deficiency of the interatrial septum (patent foramen ovale is a variant)
  - Right axis deviation
- Ostium primum (5%–10%)
  - Low on the atrial septum immediately above the AV valves
  - Left axis deviation
  - Mitral incompetence—may involve the interventricular septum
- Sinus venosus (5%)
  - High in atrial septum near opening of the SVC
  - Associated with anomalous pulmonary venous return

PLAIN FILM

- Right-sided cardiac enlargement rotates the heart, resulting in straightening of the left heart border (also left ventricle and left atrium are small).
- Enlarged right atrium and right ventricle.
- Pulmonary plethora due to increased blood flow and enlarged central veins.
- SVC overlies the spine, small aortic arch due to cardiac rotation.

COARCTATION

In total, 80% is seen in males. It can present at any age with a murmur, hypertensive headache and claudication. Hypertension leads to left ventricular hypertrophy or congestive cardiac failure if there is a critical stenosis. Commonly associated with a biscuspid aortic valve (and aortic stenosis), Turner syndrome and intracerebral haemorrhage.

PLAIN FILM

- 'Figure 3' appearance of aorta—two bulges (dilated subclavian artery above and post-stenotic aortic dilatation below) around a constriction (narrow point at coarctation)
- Bilateral, symmetrical posterior rib notching, seen by 6–8 years of age mostly in ribs 3–8 due to engorged intercostal collaterals
- Prominent left heart border (due to hypertension and aortic stenosis if the valve is bicuspid).

Table 5.2 Cyanotic congenital heart disease

Plethoric	Oligaemic
Total anomalous pulmonary venous return	Tricuspid atresia
Transposition of the great arteries	Tetralogy of Fallot
Tricuspid atresia (only if ventricular septal defect and no pulmonary stenosis)	Ebstein anomaly
Truncus arteriosus	Pulmonary atresia
Single ventricle	

Note: Think of cyanotic heart disease in terms of increased (plethoric) or decreased (oligaemic) pulmonary vascularity.

Box 5.14 READ MORE

Ferguson, E., Krishnamurthy, R., Oldham, S. 2007. Classic imaging signs of congenital cardiovascular abnormalities. *Radiographics* 27:1323–1334.

DOUBLE ARCH

Accounts for up to 60% of vascular rings. Usually an isolated anomaly presenting early in life with stridor, wheezing and dysphagia. The aorta splits in two, each part passing either side of the trachea and oesophagus before reuniting inferiorly. The common carotid and subclavian arteries arise separately from right and left arches.

PLAIN FILM

- Right-sided arch, increased paratracheal soft tissue

WATER SOLUBLE SWALLOW

- Reverse S indentation on AP view
- Posterior indentation on the oesophagus on lateral view

EBSTEIN ANOMALY

Rare congenital heart disease. It presents in the neonatal period when severe. The problem is with malposition of the tricuspid valve leaflets leading to a functional obstruction or 'atrialised' portion of the right ventricle. The right atrium becomes grossly enlarged and the right ventricle small. There is an ASD in up to 50%, which may give rise to a right-to-left shunt and cause cyanosis. Associated with numerous other cardiac defects.

PLAIN FILM

- Cardiomegaly/right atrial enlargement (may be extreme)
- Hypoplastic aorta/pulmonary trunk—unique to Ebstein anomaly
- Oligaemic lungs (if functional right-to-left shunt)

HYPOPLASTIC LEFT HEART SYNDROME

Also known as aortic atresia. This is the most common neonatal cause of congestive cardiac failure. It is two-times more common in males. The left heart is underdeveloped: hypoplastic aortic valve, mitral valves, left ventricle and ascending aorta.

PLAIN FILM
- Interstitial oedema (i.e. cardiac failure)
- Prominent right atrial border
- Absent left ventricular silhouette

INTERRUPTION OF THE AORTIC ARCH

Very rare discontinuity between the ascending and descending aorta, may be complete or partial due to a fibrous band. In total, >95% have another cardiac anomaly, mostly a patent ductus arteriosus (PDA) or ventricular septal defect (VSD).

PLAIN FILM
- Absent aortic knuckle
- Cardiomegaly

PATENT DUCTUS ARTERIOSUS

The ductus arteriosus normally closes within 48 hours of birth. There may be a normal examination at birth, followed by cyanotic episodes and failure to thrive at about 6 months. It is more common in females. It may present after respiratory distress syndrome (RDS)—pulmonary surfactant decreases atelectasis and so pulmonary vascular resistance encourages a shunt to develop. Left-to-right shunts occur as high-pressure blood passes from the aorta to the pulmonary circulation via the patent ductus. The left atrium and ventricle are enlarged and the aorta dilated while the right heart is unaffected. Eisenmenger syndrome may develop in adults. See Table 5.3.

Table 5.3 Abnormalities associated with left-to-right cardiac shunts

	RA	RV	LA	LV	AO	PV
ASD	↑	↑	Normal	Normal	↓	↑
VSD	Normal	↑	↑	↑	↓	↑
PDA	Normal	Normal	↑	↑	↑	↑

Note: ASD: atrial septal defect; VSD: ventricular septal defect; PDA: persistent ductus arteriosus; RA: right atrium; RV: right ventricle; LA: left atrium; LV: left ventricle; AO: aorta; PV: pulmonary vasculature.

PLAIN FILM
- 'Shunt vascularity' (i.e. pulmonary plethora with enlarged pulmonary arteries)
- Cardiomegaly—left atrium and ventricle enlargement
- Enlarged aorta differentiates from VSD

PERICARDIAL AGENESIS

Rare—due to premature atrophy of the common cardinal cardiac vein, which fails to nourish the pericardium. It can be partial or complete. In partial cases, absence of the left-sided pericardium is more common and is managed surgically due to a risk of cardiac herniation. Associated with bronchogenic cysts in 30%, VSD, PDA and mitral stenosis.

PLAIN FILM
- Heart displaced to the left
- Air seen between the base of the heart and the diaphragm

CT
- Preferred modality for diagnosis

PERSISTENT TRUNCUS ARTERIOSUS

Due to a failure of the normal division of the primitive truncus into aorta and pulmonary artery. A single vessel leaves the base of the heart, which gives rise to the pulmonary arteries, coronaries and systemic arteries. There is congestive cardiac failure.

PLAIN FILM
- Cardiomegaly at birth
- Pulmonary plethora
- Right-sided arch (in a third of cases)
- Forked ribs

MRI
- Very useful for depicting anatomy without contrast or radiation

RIGHT-SIDED ARCH

If you see a right-sided arch, then:

- 90% TOF (due to the prevalence of TOF)
- 5% truncus arteriosus
- 5% tricuspid atresia

However, a right sided arch occurs in:

- 33% of patients with truncus arteriosus have a right-sided arch.
- 25% of TOF.
- 5% of tricuspid atresia.

SCIMITAR SYNDROME

Also known as hypogenetic lung syndrome, this is a rare form of partial anomalous pulmonary venous return. It is characterised by an anomalous vein that drains all/part of a sequestered right lung segment. Most commonly, the anomalous vein drains into the inferior vena cava (IVC); it may also drain into the right atrium, portal vein, hepatic veins, azygous vein or coronary sinus. Commonly associated with an ASD.

PLAIN FILM

- Small right lung with mediastinal shift to the right (dextroposition)
- Curvilinear tubular opacity (the anomalous vein) adjacent to the right heart border—looks like a curved Turkish sword (scimitar)

SITUS

'Situs' refers to the position of the cardiac atria and viscera—situs solitus is the name given to the normal configuration.

SITUS INVERSUS

Rare—mirror image of solitus (i.e. right atrium is on the left, left atrium on the right and abdominal organs and lungs also swapped). There is a 3%–5% incidence of congenital heart disease. There may be levocardia or dextrocardia (Table 5.4).

Table 5.4 The frequency of congenital heart disease (CHD) with situs anomalies

Situs	Frequency of CHD
Situs solitus/levocardia	<1%
Situs inversus/dextrocardia	4%
Situs solitus/dextrocardia	95%
Situs inversus/levocardia	95%
Situs ambiguous	50%–100%

SITUS AMBIGUOUS

Also known as 'heterotaxy', there is no clear sidedness. The bowel is malrotated.
  It is classified as either:

- Right-sided isomerism/'asplenia': there is bilateral 'right-sidedness' with no spleen, complex cyanotic congenital heart disease, and centralised liver and lungs, which both have three lobes.

PLAIN FILM

- Bronchial configuration of the right lung on both sides
- Congenital heart disease
- Midline liver

- Left-sided isomerism/'polysplenia': less complex cyanotic congenital heart disease, multiple spleens, bilateral SVC, absent gallbladder, azygous continuation of the IVC common

PLAIN FILM

- Bi-lobed lungs
- Midline liver
- Increased pulmonary arterial flow (Table 5.5)

Table 5.5 Characteristics of polysplenia and asplenia

Polysplenia	Asplenia
50%–60% mortality in the first year	80% mortality in the first year
Females > males	Males > females
Left isomerism	Right isomerism
Semi-annular pancreas	Annular pancreas
Partial APVR	Total anomalous pulmonary
Bilateral SVC	venous return (APVR)
Malrotation 80%	Midline gallbladder
Absent gallbladder	

TETRALOGY OF FALLOT (TOF)

TOF accounts for 8% of congenital heart disease and is usually diagnosed by 3 months of age. There are four features: VSD; over-riding aorta; right ventricular hypertrophy due to right ventricular outflow obstruction (causes right ventricular hypertrophy).

PLAIN FILM (FIGURE 5.9)

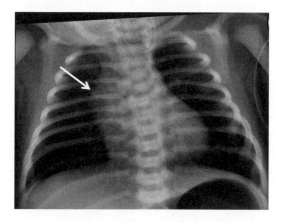

Figure 5.9 Chest radiograph of a young, cyanotic child demonstrating small central pulmonary arteries and a normal-sized heart. Note a right-sided aortic arch (white arrow). The appearance is suggestive of the tetralogy of Fallot.

- Cyanosis, small central pulmonary arteries and a normal-sized heart are strongly suggestive of TOF.
- The most common finding is elevation of the cardiac apex due to right ventricular hypertrophy.
- Heart normal size but 'boot-shaped' (not usually present), arch right-sided.
- Dilated aorta.

TOTAL ANOMALOUS PULMONARY VENOUS RETURN

Due to anomalous drainage of the pulmonary veins into e.g. the SVC, right atrium or portal vein. The end result is complete mixing of pulmonary venous and systemic venous blood, resulting in cyanosis early in life. There are various subtypes; the most common involves the pulmonary veins draining into a common vein connecting to the left brachiocephalic vein. See Table 5.2 for other causes of cyanotic congenital heart disease.

PLAIN FILM

- Snowman appearance—due to a large supracardiac shadow (the anomalous superior mediastinal veins) combined with the cardiac shadow (right atrium dilated). Not useful in infancy due to the presence of the thymus.

CT/MRI

- Both used for depicting anatomy and confirming the diagnosis

TRANSPOSITION OF THE GREAT ARTERIES

This is the most common cyanotic heart disease to present at birth. It is more common in male children of diabetic mothers. Presentation is with cyanosis and heart failure. The aorta is connected to the right ventricle and supplies the systemic circulation; the pulmonary artery arises from the left ventricle. In total, 90% are isolated abnormalities.

PLAIN FILM (FIGURE 5.10)

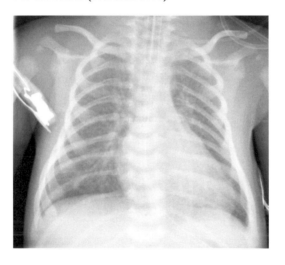

Figure 5.10 Chest radiograph of an unwell young child. There is narrowing of the superior mediastinum, absent aortic knuckle and 'egg-on-side' appearance of the heart. The diagnosis is transposition of the great arteries.

- Shunt vascularity (i.e. pulmonary plethora)—absent if there is a pulmonary stenosis
- Enlarged heart, 'egg-on-side' appearance with narrow superior mediastinum (thymic atrophy)
- Absent aortic knuckle

TRISCUSPID ATRESIA

This is the second most common cause of neonatal cyanosis after transposition. It is characterised by a completely absent tricuspid valve, an ASD and a small VSD. Most occur in the absence of transposition (80%). Treatment with the Fontan procedure is at 3–5 years of age. The pulmonary artery is anastomosed to the right atrium.

PLAIN FILM

- Cardiomegaly, dilated right atrium and left ventricular hypertrophy
- Pulmonary oligaemia
- Chronic pleural effusions may occur post-Fontan procedure

VENTRICULAR SEPTAL DEFECT (VSD)

VSD is the second most common congenital heart defect. It is usually diagnosed in childhood. It is a defect in the interventricular septum that gives rise to a left-to-right shunt. The shunt may be small and insignificant or large, causing increased pulmonary vascular resistance and eventual reversal of the shunt (Eisenmenger syndrome). Most defects are in the membranous segment of the septum. There is an association with Down syndrome.

PLAIN FILM

- Enlarged left atrium and right ventricle (left ventricle is not enlarged as it decompresses into the right ventricle).
- Shunt vascularity after the neonatal period—later on, there is central pulmonary enlargement and peripheral pruning if pulmonary hypertension supervenes.

RESPIRATORY

BRONCHOGENIC CYST

This is the most common foregut malformation in the thorax. It accounts for up to 20% of mediastinal masses. It is an abnormality of the ventral diverticulum of the primitive foregut and is associated with other congenital anomalies, spina bifida, extra-lobar sequestration and congenital lobar emphysema.

PLAIN FILM

- Posterior or middle mediastinal mass, typically subcarinal and more common on the right.
- Can be intrapulmonary—most commonly located in the medial lower lobes.

CT

- Well-circumscribed spherical mass usually with an internal density of 0–25 HU (may be higher).
- May contain an air–fluid level if communicating with an airway.
- Rim-enhancement may be seen, calcification is not typical.

BRONCHOPULMONARY DYSPLASIA

Also referred to as chronic lung disease of prematurity, it is uncommon in children at >30 weeks of gestation. It is defined as oxygen dependency at 28 days of age or 36 corrected weeks of gestation. It is the result of high positive pressure ventilation with high-concentration oxygen. Thought to be the result of a process of scarring and repair. It commonly coexists with pulmonary interstitial emphysema (Table 5.6).

Table 5.6 The four stages of bronchopulmonary dysplasia and the appearance on chest x-ray

Stage	Time	Chest x-ray
I	0–3 days	Identical to respiratory distress syndrome/hyaline membrane disease, bilateral patchy ground-glass opacities with air bronchograms
II	4–10 days	Complete opacification with air bronchograms Bilateral increased density from exudative necrosis
III	10–20 days	Small round lucencies and areas of irregular opacity Honeycombing—air sac distension in dysplastic interstitium
IV	>1 month	Hyperinflation, coarse linear densities and focal areas of emphysema or bubble-like lucencies Fibrosis and cystic emphysema

BRONCHOPULMONARY SEQUESTRATION

This is the second most common pulmonary anomaly diagnosed antenatally. It is composed of a non-functioning lung segment with no communication to the bronchial tree and a systemic arterial supply. More common in males. Hybrid lesions composed partly of a sequestration and congenital pulmonary airway malformation (CPAM) can occur (Table 5.7).

Table 5.7 Characteristics of bronchopulmonary sequestration

Type	Intralobar	Extralobar
Percentage	75% of cases	25% of cases
Presentation	Presents in adulthood with pain, infection and haemoptysis	Presents in infancy with feeding difficulties, respiratory distress, cyanosis and heart failure
Venous drainage	Central drainage to pulmonary venous system	Systemic drainage via inferior vena cava, azygous or hemiazygous
Arterial supply	Systemic feeding vessels from the descending thoracic aorta	Systemic feeding from aorta or from the splenic, gastric or intercostal arteries
Pleural relationship	Enclosed in visceral pleura	Own pleura
Associations	Nil	Diaphragmatic hernia, cardiac anomalies, pulmonary hypoplasia and duplication cyst

CHYLOTHORAX

This is the most common cause of a large pleural effusion in a neonate. It is more common in males and on the right side. Mostly idiopathic, other causes include birth trauma, thoracic duct atresia and lymphangiectasia. Also associated with Turner syndrome, extra-lobar sequestration, CPAM, etc.

PLAIN FILM
- Pleural effusion in a neonate

CONGENITAL PULMONARY AIRWAY MALFORMATION

Previously known as congenital cystic adenomatoid malformation, it is a heterogeneous group of cystic and non-cystic lung lesions arising from airway developmental dysfunction. Most CPAMs have a normal arterial and venous connection. 'Hybrid' lesions may have a systemic supply (cross between a CPAM and sequestration). Typically imaged with chest x-ray and CT (see Figure 5.11).

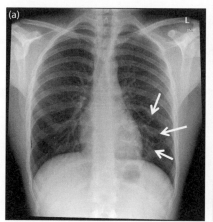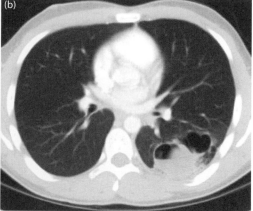

Figure 5.11 (a) Frontal chest radiograph in a young adult showing large cysts in the left lower zone (white arrows). (b) Axial computed tomography image of the thorax shows the cysts lying in the left lower lobe and containing air–fluid levels. The appearance is in keeping with a type-1 congenital pulmonary airway malformation.

Box 5.15 READ MORE
Biyyam, D., Chapman, T., Ferguson, M., Deutsch, G., Dighe, M. 2010. Congenital lung abnormalities: Embryologic features, prenatal diagnosis, and postnatal radiologic-pathologic correlation. *Radiographics* 30:1721–1738.

Three types are demonstrated with imaging:

- Type 1: large cysts (>2 cm), most common, there may be mediastinal shift and air–fluid levels
- Type 2: small cysts, heterogeneous intrapulmonary mass on chest x-ray with small air-filled cavities, CT shows multiple uniform 5–12 mm cysts
- Type 3: microcystic/solid lesions, appear solid on imaging

CONGENITAL LOBAR EMPHYSEMA

Congenital lobar emphysema refers to over-distention of the alveoli of a single lobe of lung, due to maldevelopment of the bronchopulmonary system. Most commonly due to a 'ball valve'-type obstruction from a weak/collapsed airway. Presents in the first 6 months of life with respiratory distress and cyanosis.

PLAIN FILM

- Early neonatal: hazy, mass-like opacity (due to delayed clearing of lung fluid in the emphysematous lobe).
- Later: hyperlucent lung with mass effect and mediastinal shift (once fluid has cleared and the lobe expanded fully) (Figure 5.12a).
- Lobes are affected in the following order: left upper (41%) > right middle (34%) > right upper (21%).

CT

- Hyperlucent and expanded lobe of lung, with attenuated vessels within the affected region (Figure 5.12b)

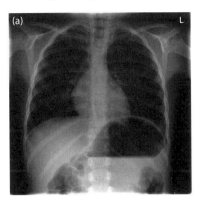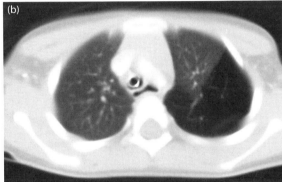

Figure 5.12 (a) Frontal chest radiograph in a child showing increased transradiancy of the left lung, particularly the left upper zone. There is mediastinal shift to the right. (b) Computed tomography image of the thorax in the same patient demonstrating reduced attenuation in an expanded left lower lobe. There is mediastinal shift to the right. The appearance is in keeping with congenital lobar emphysema.

CROUP

Non-specific term, describes acute onset of inspiratory stridor and a characteristic cough seen in children of mean age 1 year. Most commonly due to a viral laryngotracheobronchitis.

PLAIN FILM

- Exclude important differentials (e.g. foreign body, epiglottitis, abscess)
- Tapered upper trachea due to subglottic oedema, 'steeple sign'

CYSTIC FIBROSIS (CF)

Multi-system, autosomal recessive disorder due to abnormal chloride and sodium transporters, which leads to thick secretions. CF is manifested commonly in the lungs and gastrointestinal (GI) tract. It presents in the first year of life with cough and respiratory infection.

PLAIN FILM (MILD DISEASE)

- May be normal at first.
- The first sign is often hyperinflation then bronchial wall thickening.
- Pectus carinatum.

PLAIN FILM (MODERATE/ADVANCED DISEASE)

- Linear streaks and nodules (due to mucous impaction)
- Atelectasis, more common in children, usually right upper lobe
- Cylindrical bronchiectasis (upper lobes most)
- 'Finger in glove' (mucous impaction)
- Cystic spaces (bronchiectasis, may contain fluid levels)
- Enlarged hilum due to pulmonary hypertension or lymph node enlargement
- Pneumothorax

FOREIGN BODY ASPIRATION

Most common in children <3 years of age, it presents with a triad of cough, wheeze and reduced air entry. The paediatric airway diameter increases in inspiration and decreases in expiration—a partial obstruction in inspiration may become complete in expiration, allowing air trapping in expiration. Note: In children, the carina angle is symmetrical, so foreign bodies are as likely to enter either the right or left main bronchus.

PLAIN FILM

- Overinflation
- Atelectasis.
- Infiltrates with or without air trapping, which almost exclusively involves the lower lobes.
- Foreign body seen in only 9% as the majority are radiolucent food material.

KARTAGENER SYNDROME

This is a rare, autosomal recessive syndrome composed of situs inversus, chronic sinusitis and bronchiectasis. Without situs inversus, the disorder is known as primary ciliary dyskinesia. Patients present with respiratory infections beginning in the neonatal period. Associated with chronic middle-ear effusions and infertility due to ciliary dysfunction. Other associations include transposition of the great vessels, pyloric stenosis, post-cricoid web and epispadias.

PLAIN FILM

- Situs inversus
- Hyperinflation
- Bronchial wall thickening
- Lower lobe bronchiectasis (unlike CF)

HIGH-RESOLUTION CT (HRCT)

- Most sensitive to early changes

LANGERHANS CELL HISTIOCYTOSIS (LCH)

Rare—diagnosis peaks at 1–3 years of age. The bones are most commonly affected. There is pulmonary involvement in up to 50% if there is multi-system disease. In children <10 years of age, it may regress spontaneously. In children >10 years of age, the features are as for adults. Hand–Schüller–Christian disease describes a common constellation of LCH symptoms consisting of exophthalmos, diabetes insipidus and lytic skull lesions.

PLAIN FILM

- Diffuse, bilateral symmetrical reticulonodular opacification
- Pleural effusion rarely
- Pneumothorax

HRCT

- Small, multiple bilateral nodules that progress to cysts and honeycombing
- Upper/midzone cysts with spared costophrenic angles

Table 5.8 Causes of lung metastases in children ordered by decreasing frequency

Lung metastases	Peak age of onset
Rhabdomyosarcoma (more common)	1–5 years then 15–19 years
Osteosarcoma	<15 years
Wilms tumour	Females <5 years
	More common in African–Americans
Ewing sarcoma (less common)	1–11 years (peak 3–4 years)

LYMPHOMA

> **Box 5.16 THE ST. JUDE CLASSIFICATION SYSTEM FOR NON-HODGKIN LYMPHOMA**
>
> **I.** Single extranodal tumour/single anatomical area
> **II.** Single extranodal tumour + regional nodes; ≥2 nodal areas on same side of the diaphragm; 2 extranodal tumours with or without nodes on same side of the diaphragm; primary GI tumour with or without nodes
> **III.** 2 extranodal tumours on opposite sides of diaphragm; ≥2 nodal areas on both sides of diaphragm; primary intrathoracic tumours; extensive primary intra-abdominal disease; paraspinal/epidural tumour
> **IV.** Any of the above + central nervous system/bone marrow involvement

This is the third most common paediatric malignancy (behind leukaemia and brain tumours). It is by far the most common cause of an anterior mediastinal mass. In total, 95% of cases are non-Hodgkin lymphomas, although Hodgkin lymphoma is the most common type to affect the mediastinum.

HODGKIN DISEASE

Most commonly affects cervical lymph nodes, mediastinum, abdominal nodes and the spleen. Staging is with the Ann Arbor classification.

NON-HODGKIN LYMPHOMA

Most commonly affects the mandible, mediastinum, abdominal nodes and bone marrow. Staging is with the St. Jude classification.

MACLEOD SYNDROME

Also known as Swyer–James syndrome. It is often an incidental finding in an adult and follows previous childhood infectious bronchiolitis.

PLAIN FILM

- Hyperlucent lung with a paucity of vascular markings
- Normal or small-volume lung and hilum on the affected side

HRCT

- Hyperlucent lung with a reduced number of vessels.
- Bronchiectasis and bronchial wall thickening are common.

NUCLEAR MEDICINE

- Expect a matched ventilation/perfusion defect (non-specific)

MECONIUM ASPIRATION

This is a problem of full-term/post-term neonates, where it is the most common cause of respiratory distress. Meconium inhalation causes medium and small airway obstruction and a chemical pneumonitis.

PLAIN FILM (FIGURE 5.13)

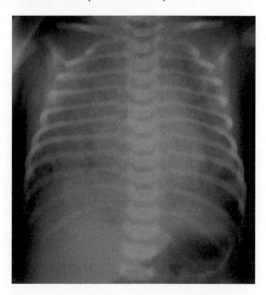

Figure 5.13 Frontal chest radiograph performed in a term neonate showing bilateral, patchy pulmonary opacities and hyperexpansion. No evidence of pneumothorax or pneumomediastinum. The appearance is in keeping with meconium aspiration.

- Most commonly there is widespread asymmetric patchy atelectasis and hyperinflation.
- Pneumothorax, pneumomediastinum and pneumopericardium are common.
- May progress to pulmonary interstitial emphysema.
- Pleural effusions.
- Changes may resolve in 48 hours.

PNEUMONIA

Box 5.17 THE MOST COMMON PATHOGENS IN CHILDHOOD PNEUMONIA ORGANISED BY AGE

Premature infants
Group B *Streptococcus*
Escherichia coli
Listeria
Cytomegalovirus

Infants
Respiratory syncytial virus (RSV)
Chlamydia
Streptococcus pneumoniae
Haemophilus type B

School age
Mycoplasma
Influenza A
Streptococcus pneumoniae

BACTERIAL PNEUMONIA

Various patterns exist, some typical to certain pathogens. Premature infants are most at risk of group B *Streptococcus* pneumonia, especially with a prolonged rupture of membranes or maternal fever during labour.

Plain film

- Lobar consolidation—typically affects one lobe, may cavitate, no volume loss.
- Bronchopneumonia—patchy airspace change, may enlarge and coalesce, volume loss may occur with mucous plugging.
- Round pneumonia—occurs in children <8 years of age, more commonly seen with *Streptococcus* pneumonia, tends to be pleural and in the lower lobes, responds well to treatment and may contain air bronchograms (unlike metastases).
- Pleural effusion—in up to two-thirds of group B *Streptococcus* cases.

VIRAL PNEUMONIA

RSV is the most common culprit in patients aged <2 years (75% of bronchiolitis), otherwise adenovirus.

Plain film (Figure 5.14)

- Parahilar peribronchial infiltrates
- Airspace opacification in up to 50%, otherwise interstitial pattern
- Hyperexpansion
- Effusions common (20%)
- With or without hilar lymph node enlargement

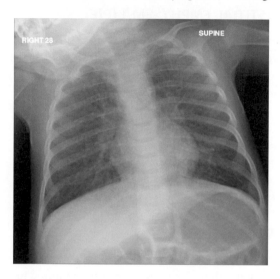

Figure 5.14 Frontal chest radiograph in a child showing hyperexpansion of the lungs and bulky hila bilaterally. There is subtle airspace opacification at the lung bases. The diagnosis in this case was viral infection (RSV).

MYCOPLASMA PNEUMONIA

This is the most common cause of pneumonia in children of school age.

Plain film

- Peribronchial/perivascular infiltrates
- Patchy consolidation
- Ground-glass opacification
- Lower lobes most commonly affected
- Hilar lymph node enlargement
- Small effusions in 20%

BORDETELLA PERTUSSIS

Affects those who have been incompletely immunised/young infants.

Plain film

- Shaggy heart caused by patchy central infiltrates

PULMONARY ARTERIOVENOUS MALFORMATION

Patients can present with orthodeoxia (postural hypoxaemia accompanied by breathlessness) or stroke due to paradoxical emboli. Up to 15% have hereditary haemorrhagic telangiectasia (Osler–Weber–Rendu disease).

PLAIN FILM/CT

- Well-defined, lobulated nodules with a feeding artery and draining vein
- Most unilateral
- Two-thirds in a lower lobe
- May contain small foci of calcification/phleboliths

PULMONARY INTERSTITIAL EMPHYSEMA (PIE)

Due to positive pressure ventilation leading to air leaks from the bronchi to the interstitium in immature lungs (although it can also occur in adults). The lungs become stiff and more difficult to ventilate; this leads to overinflated lungs and higher risk of pneumothorax or pneumomediastinum.

PLAIN FILM

- Overinflated lungs
- Oval, spherical or streak-shaped lucencies
- Subpleural cysts
- Commonly coexists with bronchopulmonary dysplasia

REACTIVE AIRWAYS DISEASE

This condition is precipitated by RSV and *Aspergillus*. Most children who wheeze at <2 years of age do not develop asthma. Imaging often is not required for investigation. Severity of reactive airways disease on chest x-ray does not correlate with clinical severity.

PLAIN FILM

- Peribronchial thickening
- Hyperinflation
- Small parenchymal opacities/atelectasis

RESPIRATORY DISTRESS SYNDROME

Previously known as hyaline membrane disease. It is the most common cause of death in live newborns and respiratory distress in premature neonates—it affects up to 50% of premature babies. It is due to the relative immaturity of type II pneumocytes, leading to a lack of surfactant. This leads to alveolar collapse, non-compliant lungs and decreased lung volumes. Risk factors include multiple gestation and perinatal asphyxia. It may occur in term infants of diabetic mothers. Onset is within hours of birth. See Table 5.9 for differentiating characteristics.

PLAIN FILM

- A normal chest x-ray 6 hours after birth excludes RDS.
- Chest x-ray abnormalities peak at 12–24 hours after birth.
- Reduced lung expansion.
- Bilateral reticulogranular opacities that represent collapsed alveoli.
- Prominent air bronchograms because the larger bronchi do not collapse.
- Generalised atelectasis/white-out if severe.
- Resolves over days.

THYMUS

The thymus peaks in size at 2–3 years of age. It plays a key role in the maturation of the immune system. Thymic lymphoma is the most common thymic malignancy in children.

PLAIN FILM

- Normal thymus appears as a large triangular density in infants and young children, so-called 'sail sign' (present in 5%).

CT

- Normal appearance changes with age—quadrilateral shape in young children, triangular in teenagers with concave borders. It narrows/elongates with respiration.
- Heterogeneous density, calcification or displacement of adjacent structures is concerning.
- Thymic hyperplasia may occur following stress (recovery from illness, post-chemotherapy or radiotherapy, following treatment for Cushing disease, etc.)—the thymus is enlarged and oval-shaped.
- Hypoplasia is also seen in times of stress (also DiGeorge syndrome, steroid use)—it recovers its size and may develop rebound hyperplasia.

Table 5.9 Factors differentiating neonatal chest disease

	Respiratory distress syndrome	Transient tachypnoea of the newborn (TTN)	Meconium aspiration	Neonatal pneumonia
Typical patient	Premature	Term/caesarean section	Post-term stained below cords	Premature rupture of membranes
Time course	<6 hours	24–48 hours	12–24 hours	<6 hours
Lung volume	Decreased	Increased	Increased	Increased
Imaging	Ground glass	Interstitial oedema	Coarse, nodular, asymmetric	Perihilar streaking

TRACHEAL BRONCHUS

Also known as a 'pig' bronchus, the right upper lobe apical segmental bronchus originates from the trachea rather than the right upper lobe bronchus. It is associated with tracheal stenosis.

- Rarely, there may be a duplicated bronchus with a normally located right upper lobe apical segmental bronchus present as well.

TRANSIENT TACHYPNOEA OF THE NEWBORN (TTN)

This is the most common cause of respiratory distress in the newborn. It affects term babies. It arises due to inadequate clearance of lung fluid before the first breath (Note: A third of the fluid is squeezed out through vaginal delivery, a third is resorbed by lymphatics and a third is resorbed by capillaries). There may be a history of caesarean section, precipitous delivery, breech presentation, maternal diabetes or foetal sedation. Symptoms develop within 6 hours of birth, peak at 1 day and are resolved by 2–3 days.

PLAIN FILM
- Hyperinflated lungs with an increase in pulmonary interstitial markings in a term baby
- Linear densities radiating from the hila
- Fluid in the fissures and small pleural effusions
- Clinical and radiographic resolution within 48–72 hours

WILLIAMS–CAMPBELL SYNDROME

A rare congenital deficiency of cartilage in the third- to sixth-generation bronchi.

PLAIN FILM
- Hyperinflated lungs
- Multiple rounded lucencies in the mid-lower zones
- Cystic bronchiectasis beyond the third-generation bronchi

WILSON–MIKITY SYNDROME

Chronic lung disease in premature infants considered part of the spectrum of bronchopulmonary dysplasia. Affects about 2% of those born early with low birth weight.

PLAIN FILM
- Similar to bronchopulmonary dysplasia, but normal in the first week of life.

MISCELLANEOUS

CEPHALOHAEMATOMA

Located beneath the outer layer of periosteum; therefore, it does not cross suture lines. Caput succedaneum is oedema/haemorrhage within the skin and therefore does cross sutures. They are seen in the setting of a traumatic delivery.

CT
- Crescent-shaped lesion adjacent to the outer table of the skull
- May calcify if chronic

NON-ACCIDENTAL INJURY (NAI)

Box 5.18 READ MORE

Lonergan, G., Baker, A., Morey, M., Boos, S. 2003. Child abuse: Radiologic–pathologic correlation. *Radiographics* 23:811–845.

Box 5.19 THE SKELETAL SURVEY

Skull
- AP, lateral, with or without Townes view.
- Skull x-rays should be taken even if a head computed tomography is planned.

Chest
- AP including the clavicles.
- Right and left obliques to show ribs

Abdomen
- Must include pelvis and hips

Spine
- Lateral: This may require separate exposures of the cervical, thoracic and thoraco-lumbar regions.
- If the whole of the spine is not seen in the AP projection on the chest and abdominal radiographs, then additional views will be required.
- AP views of the cervical spine are rarely diagnostic at this age and should only be performed at the discretion of the radiologist.

Limbs
- AP of both upper arms
- AP both forearms
- AP both femurs
- AP both lower legs
- Posterior–anterior (PA) of hands
- Dorsoplantar (DP) of feet

Note: A full survey must always be performed in suspected NAI in those aged <2 years and be guided by clinical findings in those aged >2 years. It must be performed by two radiographers.

Source: Royal College of Radiologists & Royal College of Paediatrics and Child Health. 2008. *Standards for Radiological Investigations of Suspected Non-accidental Injury*. Royal college of Radiologists, UK.

In total, 7% of children experience serious physical abuse at the hands of their parents or carers during childhood. Up to 55% of physically abused children receive injury sufficient to cause a fracture. Injuries may manifest in any pattern; however, injuries in a non-ambulant child or fractures of different ages at different sites are particularly concerning.

PLAIN FILM

- Skeletal injury is the most common form of NAI.
- Transverse diaphyseal fractures are most common (76%).
- Metaphyseal corner ('bucket handle') fractures are most specific—from shearing forces, usually in children <2 years of age.
- Posterior rib fractures (due to squeezing injury).
- Skull fracture in 20% (depressed fractures of the occiput).
- Others: outer third of the clavicle, scapula, spinous processes, spiral long bone, vertebral body.

CT

- Subdural and subarachnoid haemorrhage associated with NAI.
- Parafalcine haematoma is most common due to an interhemispheric injury, shallow posterior fossa subdural haematomas are also seen.
- Also bilateral subdural haematomas, haematomas of different ages and haematoma without fracture suggest shaking.
- Communicating hydrocephalus (due to repetitive subarachnoid haemorrhage).
- Visceral injury—less common, duodenum most affected.

NUCLEAR MEDICINE

- Bone scan is sensitive to injuries within 6 hours of insult.
- Foci of tracer uptake are non-specific, always requires correlation with x-ray.

TUBES AND LINES

UMBILICAL ARTERY CATHETER

Note: There are normally two arteries and a single vein ('Ava'). The catheter follows the course of the vessel to the anterior division of the internal iliac artery, to the common iliac artery and then aorta. The tip is positioned either at T8–10 or inferior to the renal arteries at L3.

UMBILICAL VENOUS CATHETER

Passes from the umbilical vein to the left portal vein, then ductus venosus and hepatic vein and IVC. The tip should be positioned at the junction of the right atrium and IVC at T8–9.

ENDOTRACHEAL TUBE

The tip should lie 1–1.5 cm above the carina.

VACTERL

Refers to a collection of congenital abnormalities arising due to an insult during the fourth gestational week. Finding one feature prompts a search for others. More commonly seen in children of diabetic mothers.

VERTEBRAL

Segmentation anomalies, sacral agenesis, scoliosis and rib anomalies.

ANORECTAL MALFORMATION

Any such malformations.

CARDIAC

Most commonly a septal defect, also arch anomalies, total anomalous pulmonary venous return and TOF.

TRACHEO-OESOPHAGEAL FISTULA

Any such fistulae.

RENAL

Abnormal position or fusion, cystic dysplasia and agenesis.

LIMB ANOMALIES

Radial aplasia/dysplasia, triphalangeal thumb, syndactyly and radioulnar synostosis.

WILLIAMS SYNDROME

Rare, sporadic genetic disorder associated with idiopathic hypercalcaemia in infancy. Associated with elfin-like facies, learning disability, short stature, cardiac anomalies and aortic stenosis, osteosclerosis and metastatic calcification.

US
- Structural renal abnormalities, medullary nephrocalcinosis and stones
- Bladder diverticula

GASTROINTESTINAL

ANNULAR PANCREAS

This is a relatively common congenital abnormality. A ring of pancreatic tissue encircles the duodenum (due to abnormal migration of the ventral pancreas). It is usually asymptomatic, but may present with abdominal pain, vomiting or pancreatitis. It is a cause of duodenal obstruction in the neonate (transition point at D2 in 85%). Commonly associated with other congenital anomalies, including duodenal atresia and Down syndrome.

PLAIN FILM
- Double bubble sign (i.e. dilated duodenum and stomach).
- Obstruction is incomplete, gas is seen in the distal bowel.

CONTRAST MEAL
- Narrowed D2 segment

Box 5.20 THE DOUBLE BUBBLE SIGN
<ul><li>Mostly duodenal atresia (30%)</li><li>Annular pancreas second most common</li><li>Others: duodenal web, midgut volvulus, etc.</li></ul>

ANORECTAL MALFORMATION

This is a complex group of anomalies associated with other congenital abnormalities in up to 70% (most commonly genitourinary). In most cases, the anus is not perforated and the distal bowel is either blind-ending or fistulates. The classification depends on the relationship to the levator sling. Classified as low (most common), intermediate and high. High malformations are most strongly associated with fistula and genitourinary (50%) and VACTERL spectrum anomalies.

PLAIN FILM

- Vertebral segmental/sacral anomalies

MRI

- Performed routinely (also has a role in foetal investigation)
- Spinal dysraphism (e.g. tethered cord)

US

- Identify distal rectal pouch and direction of fistulation
- Screen for spinal dysraphism/tethered cord

MICTURATING CYSTOURETHROGRAM (MCUG)

- Assess genitourinary fistulation

BECKWITH–WIEDEMANN SYNDROME

This is a rare, mostly sporadic overgrowth disorder characterised by omphalocele (exomphalos), gigantism and macroglossia (see Table 5.10 for characteristics of omphaloceles). There is also hemihypertrophy, neonatal hypoglycaemia, pancreatic islet cell hyperplasia and ear abnormalities. There is an increased risk of benign and malignant tumours (particularly Wilms tumours).

US

- Short-interval abdominal US to monitor for malignancy
- Visceromegaly affecting liver, spleen, kidney and adrenal glands
- Wilms tumour (in up to 20%), hepatoblastoma and adrenocortical carcinoma especially high risk

BILIARY ATRESIA

Rare disorder presenting in the neonatal period with jaundice and hepatomegaly. It may be due to a congenital absence of the bile ducts (presents in the first 2 weeks of life) or progressive biliary inflammation, which eventually obliterates the ducts (presents at 2–8 weeks of age). Managed surgically with/without liver transplant.

US

- Echogenic triangular structure at the porta hepatis, 'triangular cord sign' (this is pathognomonic and represents an atretic biliary plate)
- Small or non-visualised gallbladder, absent common bile duct (CBD)
- Periportal oedema
- With or without intrahepatic duct dilatation

NUCLEAR MEDICINE—HEPATIC IMINODIACETIC ACID (HIDA) SCAN

- Phenobarbital is given for 5 days prior to imaging to stimulate biliary secretion.
- Tracers used: technetium-99m, diosgenin or mebrofenin.
- Biliary excretion by 60 minutes is normal.
- Biliary atresia diagnosed if no tracer is seen in the bowel at 24 hours (hepatic uptake is normal).

- Also demonstrates delayed clearance from the cardiac pool and increased renal excretion and bladder activity.
- Neonatal hepatitis is indicated by a delayed/reduced hepatic uptake.

BUDD–CHIARI SYNDROME

Rare (especially in children) syndrome due to hepatic vein occlusion. Associated with congenital membranes, parenteral nutrition, chemotherapy and toxins. It presents with abdominal pain, jaundice, tender hepatomegaly and ascites.

US

- Dilated hepatic veins/flow reversal/collaterals on colour Doppler
- Hepatomegaly
- Ascites

CT

- Enlarged liver with increased enhancement of the caudate lobe
- Patchy enhancement of the other hepatic segments
- Thrombus in the hepatic veins
- Ascites and gallbladder wall oedema

CHOLEDOCHAL CYSTS

Rare (however, they are the most common congenital lesions of the gallbladder), usually present in childhood. They are characterised by aneurysmal dilatation of the CBD, which is thought to be due to reflux of pancreatic enzymes across an anomalous duct junction.

There are five subtypes, with type 1 being the most common (cystic, fusiform dilatation of the CBD below the cystic duct). See Table 3.8.

US

- Fusiform cystic structure at the porta hepatis, separate from the gallbladder
- May be seen to communicate with normal intrahepatic ducts
- Multiple low-reflective areas (bile duct lakes) with a central focus of high reflectivity in the liver (portal vein)

NUCLEAR MEDICINE—HIDA SCAN

- Cystic structure connected to the biliary system

CONGENITAL DIAPHRAGMATIC HERNIA

Relatively common, major surgical emergency in newborns. Mortality is up to 60% due to associated complications including pulmonary hypoplasia, persistent foetal circulation, gastric/midgut volvulus and cardiac and renal abnormalities. Bochdalek hernia is the most common (90%)—it presents in neonates with RDS and is usually associated with a left posterolateral defect. A Morgagni hernia defect is anteromedial parasternal—it rarely presents at birth and is less common (5%).

PLAIN FILM (FIGURE 5.15)

- Classic appearance: loops of bowel in the left hemithorax (CPAM is a differential).
- Mediastinal shift to the right.
- Paucity of bowel gas below the diaphragm.
- Right-sided hernias may contain the liver.
- A mediastinal, basal mass is likely to represent a Morgagni hernia.

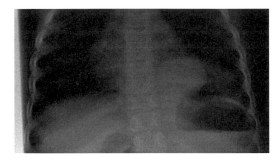

Figure 5.15 There is an opacity projected over the left lung base and the gastric air bubble extends superior to the left hemidiaphragm. The appearance is in keeping with a diaphragmatic hernia—a Bochdalek hernia is most likely.

DISTAL INTESTINAL OBSTRUCTION SYNDROME

This is a common abdominal manifestation of CF. It is a similar pathological entity to meconium ileus and meconium plug syndrome, but occurs in older children. Inspissated stool becomes impacted in the distal ileum and proximal colon, causing an obstruction.

PLAIN FILM

- Small bowel obstruction
- Right lower quadrant 'bubbly' mass

CONTRAST ENEMA

- Water-soluble contrast enema may be therapeutic

DUODENAL ATRESIA

Complete, congenital obstruction of the duodenal lumen. Strongly associated with an annular pancreas (nearly always), Down syndrome (30%), polyhydramnios (40%) and other anomalies (50%). It presents in neonates with bilious vomiting.

PLAIN FILM (FIGURE 5.16)

- Double bubble sign
- No distal gas

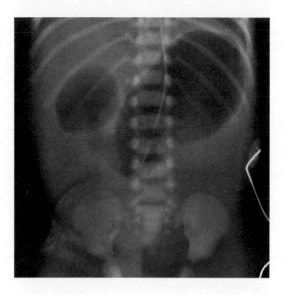

Figure 5.16 Note the presence of an NG tube. This abdominal radiograph shows marked gaseous distension of the stomach and proximal duodenum—the so-called double bubble sign. There is no convincing distal small bowel or large bowel gas, in keeping with complete obstruction. The most common cause is duodenal atresia.

GALLSTONES

Rare in children. Most are pigment stones formed in the setting of a haemolytic disorder, parenteral nutrition, diuretic treatment, an obstructed biliary system, dehydration or short gut syndrome.

US

- Multiple shadow-casting foci within the gallbladder lumen
- Gallbladder wall thickening
- Pericholecystic fluid

GASTROINTESTINAL DUPLICATION CYSTS

GI duplication cysts account for 15% of paediatric abdominal masses. They typically arise from the small bowel and colon. They are usually asymptomatic, but occasionally bleed due to foci of ectopic gastric or pancreatic tissue. Oesophageal duplication cysts present with dysphagia. In total, 4% occur in the rectum, where they are associated with perianal fistulae.

US

- Simple cyst with characteristic two-layered wall (i.e. inner echogenic mucosa and outer hypoechoic muscle)
- 35% found in the distal ileum on the mesenteric side of the bowel

WATER SOLUBLE SWALLOW

- Oesophageal duplication cysts may displace the oesophagus.

Table 5.10 Gastroschisis versus omphalocele

	Gastroschisis	Omphalocele
Position of defect	Right paramedian	Midline
Cord insertion	Normal	At apex of defect
Peritoneal covering	No	Yes
Ascites	No	Common
Liver herniated	Infrequently	Common
Bowel complications	Common	No
Associated abnormalities	Intestinal atresia or stenosis (only 5% of gastroschisis is associated with congenital anomalies)	50% of cases associated with congenital anomalies—chromosomal, intrauterine growth retardation, Beckwith–Wiedemann syndrome, cardiac (ventricular septal defect), neural tube, genitourinary (GU)

HENOCH–SCHÖNLEIN PURPURA

An upper respiratory tract infection that is often a precipitating factor of this acute systemic vasculitis involving the skin, GI tract, joints and kidneys. Children aged 3–10 years are affected. It presents with a purpuric rash on the extensor surfaces, arthralgia and crampy abdominal pain with bloody stool. Severe chronic renal disease may result from a proliferative IgA glomerulonephritis.

US

- Enlarged, slightly hyperechoic kidneys
- Thickening of the terminal ileum
- Intussusception

CT

- Multifocal areas of bowel wall thickening due to intramural haemorrhage and oedema.
- Other GI complications include perforation, bowel infarction and intussusceptions.

HEPATOBLASTOMA

This is the most common primary malignant liver tumour in children. A total of 90% of cases occur in those aged <5 years. It presents with an enlarging abdomen, anorexia and weight loss. Tumours are large (average 10–12 cm) at presentation and lung metastases are common. AFP is abnormally raised. Overall survival is up to 70% with surgery and chemotherapy.

PLAIN FILM

- Right upper quadrant mass.
- 50% demonstrate calcification on plain abdominal x-ray.

US

- Variable appearance, usually hyperechoic to adjacent normal liver.
- Mixed-type hepatoblastomas have a heterogeneous appearance.
- Calcification, haemorrhage and necrosis.

CT

- Slightly hypodense compared to liver on pre- and post-contrast.
- Centripetal and heterogeneous enhancement following contrast.
- Tends not to be multifocal (this would favour hepatocellular carcinoma [HCC]).
- Stippled or coarse calcification are common.

MRI

- Non-specific low T1 and high T2.
- Septations are low on T1 and T2 and enhance.
- Foci of T1 hyperintensity indicate haemorrhage.

HEPATOCELLULAR CARCINOMA (HCC)

Second most common malignant liver tumour of children, but rare unless there is coexisting hepatitis B or C infection or other liver disease. More common in children aged 10–14 years. Growth patterns of HCC are solitary, multinodular and diffuse. AFP is elevated. Poor prognosis overall.

US

- Variable appearance, predominantly hypoechoic.
- Large lesions are heterogeneous due to a mixture of necrosis, fat, haemorrhage, etc.

CT

- Poorly defined, low-density mass(es)
- Enhances most avidly in the hepatic arterial phase (due to the blood supply), may have washed out by the portal venous phase.
- Check the portal and hepatic veins for vascular invasion.

MRI

- Mild T2 hyperintensity, variable T1 signal due to tumour contents
- Arterial enhancement with rapid washout as for CT

Fibrolamellar HCC

Variant of HCC found in older children and adolescents without underlying liver disease. AFP is not elevated.

PLAIN FILM

- Right upper quadrant mass
- Stellate calcification

US

- Heterogeneous mass with or without hyperechoic central scar

CT

- Well-defined, lobulated mass.
- Enhances in the hepatic arterial phase.
- Variable attenuation in the portal phase.
- Central scar does not enhance, so relatively low density.

MRI

- Mildly low T1 and high T2 signal
- Scar is low on T1 and T2 and does not enhance

HIRSCHSPRUNG DISEASE

Functional colonic obstruction characterised by an aganglionic distal segment of colon and proximal dilatation. It accounts for 20% of all neonatal bowel obstructions, and 80% present by <6 months of age. Symptoms include failure to pass meconium at 48 hours, vomiting, abdominal distension and necrotising enterocolitis (NEC). The rectosigmoid colon is most commonly affected (80%), as well as the long segment (15%) and total colonic agangliosis (5%). A biopsy is required for diagnosis.

CONTRAST ENEMA

- Transition zone between the dilated proximal ganglionic bowel and distal aganglionic bowel
- Inversion of the rectosigmoid index (normal neonate rectal diameter > sigmoid diameter)
- Tortuosity and corrugation of the narrowed aganglionic segment
- Difficulty in obtaining good rectal distension

HYPOPERFUSION COMPLEX

Seen in children with hypovolaemic shock who maintain blood pressure by marked vasoconstriction. Poor prognosis.

CT

- Small-calibre aorta due to vasoconstriction
- Flattening of the IVC due to decreased venous return
- Dilated bowel loops with mucosal hyperaemia due to vasoconstriction of mesenteric vessels
- Increased enhancement of the adrenal glands
- Decreased splenic enhancement
- Dense nephrograms due to lack of contrast excretion by the kidneys

INFANTILE HAEMANGIOENDOTHELIOMA

This is the most common benign hepatic tumour occurring in the first 6 months of life; 85% are diagnosed by 6 months. It consists of multiple sinusoidal vascular channels with surrounding connective tissue stroma. Patients present with an abdominal mass, high-output cardiac failure from AV shunting (15%) and red blood cell consumption. The natural history is of regression within 12–18 months.

US

- Ill-defined, complex, heterogeneous mass in the right lobe of the liver containing multiple vascular channels on Doppler US
- Hyperechoic lesions with peritumoural flow on colour Doppler

PLAIN FILM

- Right upper quadrant mass
- Stellate calcification

CT

- Heterogeneous mass with central areas of low density
- Early peripheral nodular enhancement
- Variable delayed central enhancement
- Complete central opacification on delayed images (like an adult haemangioma)

INTUSSUSCEPTION

Typically presents between 6 months to 2 years. It is a common cause of an acute abdomen in infancy. The presentation is with pain, 'red currant jelly' stools and a palpable abdominal mass. The vast majority are idiopathic (95%); otherwise, mucosal oedema and lymphoid hyperplasia post-viral gastroenteritis may be the cause. Most are ileocolic (up to 95%) or ileo-ileocolic (10%).

US (FIGURE 5.17)

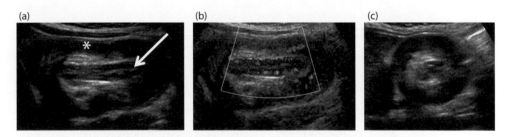

Figure 5.17 These three images depict the classic US appearances of intussusception. (a) Longitudinal view showing the 'pseudo-kidney'. The intussusceptum (white arrow) is surrounded by fatty mesentery (echogenic). The isoechoic rim is the intussuscipiens (asterisk, often colon). (b) Doppler ultrasound showing preserved vascularity of the intussusceptum, a good prognostic indicator for successful pneumatic reduction. (c) Axial ultrasound showing a doughnut appearance of central intussusceptum surrounded by fatty mesentery and outer isoechoic intussuscipiens.

- Large structure (usually greater than 5 cm) displacing bowel loops most commonly found in the subhepatic region
- Pseudo-kidney appearance or 'donut' on axial scanning

Box 5.21 PNEUMATIC REDUCTION

Factors predicting success at reduction
Blood flow within the intussusceptum on ultrasound scan
Onset of <24 hours
Age <12 months
No fluid trapped in the intussusception
No evidence of small bowel obstruction

Risks
Perforation
Failure or recurrence

Contraindications
Hypovolaemic shock
Sick infant
Pneumoperitoneum
Peritonitis

Techniques
Max pressure 120 mmHg
No more than three attempts with up to 3 minutes/attempt
3 minutes between attempts

JUVENILE POLYPOSIS

Rare disorder with autosomal dominant inheritance. It is the most common cause of colonic polyps in children. Polyps in this polyposis syndrome are hamartomatous. Polyps may occur anywhere in the GI tract. Polyps are less numerous than in familial adenomatous polyposis syndrome. Poor prognosis—many patients die before 2 years of age and 15% convert to malignancy by 35 years of age.

KAWASAKI SYNDROME

Idiopathic, acute, febrile, multisystem vasculitis involving large, medium and small arteries with a predilection for the coronary arteries. It affects children primarily (<5 years of age) and is more common in Japan. Classically, it presents with a strawberry tongue, injected fissured lips and bilateral purulent conjunctivitis. There are also skin and joint manifestations. Coronary artery aneurysms are present in up to 20%.

US

- Cardiac echo at diagnosis and for follow-up
- Dilated ('hydrops'), thin-walled gallbladder
- Positive Murphy sign
- Enlarged lymph nodes

CT

- May be useful in selected high-risk patients to demonstrate coronary aneurysms and calcification.

Box 5.22 LIVER LESIONS IN CHILDREN ARE MORE COMMON IN CERTAIN AGE GROUPS (NOTE THE TYPICAL AGE OF PRESENTATION OF THE LESIONS IS CONVENIENTLY IN ALPHABETICAL ORDER!)

Haemangioendothelioma: neonates
Hamartoma: 15–22 months
Hepatoblastoma: <3 years
Hepatocellular carcinoma: >3 years

MALROTATION

Box 5.23 READ MORE

Applegate, K., Anderson, J., Klatte, E. 2006. Intestinal malrotation in children: A problem-solving approach to the upper gastro-intestinal series. *Radiographics* 26:1485–1500.

Common congenital abnormal positioning of the duodenojejunal flexure; 90% present within the first year of life with bilious vomiting (75% in newborns, but can present much later). The mesenteric attachment of the midgut to the caecum is commonly too short, and the gut is prone to anticlockwise rotation around an axis of the superior mesenteric artery (SMA) and superior mesenteric vein (SMV). This is termed 'midgut volvulus' and causes abdominal pain and, ultimately, bowel necrosis. It is a surgical emergency.

US

- 'Whirlpool' sign of twisted mesenteric vessels.
- SMV curled around SMA in clockwise pattern.
- SMV lies on the left of the SMA (i.e. reversed).

CONTRAST STUDY (FIGURE 5.18)

- Paediatric surgical team should attend.
- Small, water-soluble contrast bolus (5 mL often adequate) via nasogastric tube, observe emptying of the stomach and position of the duodenal–jejunal (DJ) flexure, preferably with the patient supine.
- DJ flexure normally lies to the left of a left vertebral body pedicle, at the level of d1.
- Spiral corkscrew appearance of the duodenum/proximal jejunum indicates volvulus.
- Cephalad positioning of the caecum is seen in up to 80%.

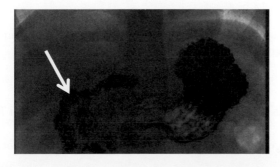

Figure 5.18 Upper gastrointestinal contrast study in an infant showing an abnormal position of the DJ flexure (white arrow) to the right of the midline, in keeping with midgut malrotation.

MECKEL DIVERTICULUM

Box 5.24 RULE OF 2S FOR MECKEL DIVERTICULUM
Found in 2% and 2% become symptomatic 2 inches long, found 2 ft from the iliocaecal (IC) valve Two-thirds have ectopic gastric mucosa

The most common congenital abnormality of the GI tract. This condition arises from persistence of the vitelline duct (connects the midgut to the embryonic sac during early development), which can manifest as a sinus, cyst or diverticulum. It is usually asymptomatic; however, symptomatic diverticula are more often found in children (<10 years of age). The most common presentation in children is bleeding, usually from heterotopic gastric mucosa.

NUCLEAR MEDICINE
- Technetium-99m pertechnetate scan is the best test for evaluating children with acute symptoms; it is 85% sensitive and 95% specific.
- Cimetidine, pentagastrin and glucagon increase sensitivity; perchlorate blocks tracer uptake by gastric mucosa and decreases sensitivity.
- False positives: urinary obstruction, inflammatory bowel disease, appendicitis, intussusception and recent barium enema.
- False negatives: malrotation of the terminal ileum, no gastric mucosa in the diverticulum.

MESENCHYMAL HAMARTOMA

This is a rare, benign liver tumour, typically arising in children aged <2 years. It may be diagnosed antenatally; however, the typical presentation is with painless distension of the abdomen. AFP is normal (unlike hepatoblastoma). Complete surgical excision is the treatment of choice.

US
- Range of appearances, from multiple anechoic cysts with thin septa to solid echogenic portions
- Vascularity on colour Doppler in the solid components and septa

CT
- Complex cystic mass, solid components and septa enhance post-contrast.
- Haemorrhage is atypical.

MRI
- Solid components contain fibrous material and so are low signal on T1 and T2 (but enhance).
- Cysts are high signal on T2, variable signal on T1 depending on protein content.

MECONIUM ILEUS

Small bowel obstruction due to impacted meconium in the distal small bowel. It presents at about 24 hours of age with abdominal distension, bilious vomiting and failure to pass meconium. Water-soluble contrast enema is an effective treatment in 60% (5% perforate).

PLAIN FILM

- 'Soap bubble' appearance in the right lower quadrant
- Small bowel obstruction

CONTRAST ENEMA

- Water-soluble contrast enema (diluted contrast with or without rehydration to counter fluid shift)
- Microcolon (due to under use)
- Pellets of meconium seen as contrast refluxes into the terminal ileum

MECONIUM PERITONITIS

This is a chemical peritonitis that has occurred *in utero* following a bowel perforation due to obstruction or ischaemia. Often an incidental finding, may present with obstruction due to post-inflammatory adhesions.

PLAIN FILM

- Dense calcification/calcified plaques/curvilinear calcification (calcified cyst)
- 'Soap bubble' appearance in the right lower quadrant
- Ascites
- Can rarely involve the thorax or scrotum

US

- Ascites
- Echogenic material between bowel loops with a 'snowstorm' appearance (free-floating meconium)
- Well-circumscribed peritoneal cysts

MECONIUM PLUG SYNDROME

Also known as small left colon syndrome and functional immaturity of the colon. It is a functional obstruction, usually transient and self-limiting. It usually affects term infants, often large babies or babies of diabetic mothers. Believed to be due to relative immaturity of bowel innervation. Water-soluble enema is typically curative (unlike in Hirschsprung disease).

PLAIN FILM

- Dilated proximal colon with a transition point at the splenic flexure.
- Empty descending colon.
- Contrast outlines a column of impacted meconium in the descending colon.
- Patients with Hirschsprung disease have similar findings, but typically return with symptom recurrence.

NECROTISING ENTEROCOLITIS

This is a common cause of an acute abdomen in neonates. The common final pathology is intestinal ischaemia, necrosis and perforation. Multiple factors are involved. Prematurity and congenital heart disease are major risk factors. In total, 10% of neonates weighing <1.5 kg are affected. Typically manifests in the first 2 weeks of life. Clinical features are non-specific but include sepsis, intolerance to feed, vomiting, diarrhoea and bloodstained stool.

PLAIN FILM (FIGURE 5.19)

- Generalised gas-distended bowel—if focal, suggests a deterioration or impending perforation.
- Intramural gas (i.e. pneumatosis intestinalis up to 98%)—almost pathognomic of NEC, most common in the right lower quadrant, curvilinear (subserosal) or bubbly (submucosal) pattern.
- Portal venous gas (up to 30%)—also seen with gas entrained via an umbilical vein catheter.
- Pneumoperitoneum from perforation, horizontal beam or left side down decubitus is optimal. Look for the football sign, Rigler sign and gas outlining the falciform ligament.

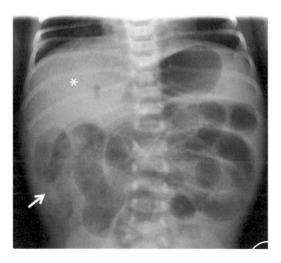

Figure 5.19 Plain abdominal radiograph of a premature neonate. The bowel is gas-filled and dilated. There is a bubbly gas pattern in the right lower quadrant (white arrow) in keeping with intramural gas and further gas is seen within the portal vein and its branches (asterisk). There is no evidence of perforation. The appearance is in keeping with necrotising enterocolitis.

OESOPHAGEAL ATRESIA AND TRACHEO-OESOPHAGEAL FISTULA

There is a spectrum of abnormalities concerning maldevelopment of the oesophagus. It is associated with anomalies including intestinal atresia, annular pancreas, pyloric stenosis, Down syndrome, VACTERL, etc. Atresia presents with excessive drooling while tracheo-oesophageal fistula may present with aspiration during feeding. A failure to pass a nasogastric tube to the stomach is diagnostic.

TYPES

1. Atresia with distal tracheo-oesophageal fistula (85%)
2. Atresia with no fistula (10%)

3. Tracheo-oesophageal fistula only (no oesophageal atresia), 'H-type' (rare)
4. Atresia with proximal and distal fistula (rare)
5. Atresia with proximal fistula only (rare)

WATER SOLUBLE SWALLOW

- Lateral view most useful to demonstrate fistula
- Most useful to demonstrate an H-type fistula

PLAIN FILM

- Atresia: gas-distended proximal oesophagus, feeding tube coiled in the pouch.
- Absence of abdominal gas suggests atresia alone or a proximal fistula.
- Abdominal gas suggests a distal tracheo-oesophageal fistula or H-type fistula.

PYLORIC STENOSIS

Box 5.25 READ MORE
Dias, S. et al. 2012. Hypertrophic pyloric stenosis: Tips and tricks for ultrasound diagnosis. *Insights into Imaging* 3:247–250.

Most common surgical cause of vomiting in the first 2–6 weeks of life. It is more common in first-born males and there may be a family history. The problem is an elongated and thickened pyloric mucosa that fails to relax in order to allow the stomach to empty.

US (FIGURE 5.20)

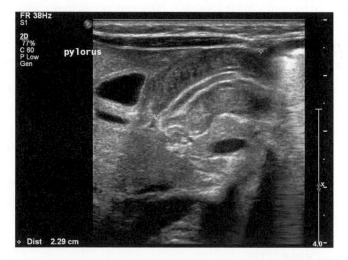

Figure 5.20 Ultrasound scan of the upper abdomen of a young infant. The image shows a view of the gastric pylorus in the longitudinal plane. There is marked thickening of the pylorus and the pyloric canal is abnormally long (normal <12 mm). The appearance supports a diagnosis of hypertrophic pyloric stenosis.

- Perform after feeding, use a high-frequency probe with or without right side down to exclude gas.
- Look for a muscle wall thickness of >3 mm.
- Look for canal length >12 mm.
- Check for passage of fluid through the pylorus—if the pyloric canal opens well, stenosis is excluded.
- 'Cervix sign'—thickened pylorus projects into the gastric lumen.
- Increased gastric peristalsis.

RHABDOMYOSARCOMA OF THE BILIARY TRACT

Rhabdomyosarcoma is a rare, aggressive, soft tissue tumour that may occur anywhere. The biliary variant occurs almost exclusively in children. The presenting features are commonly weight loss, malaise and intermittent jaundice. It is more common in males; 30% have metastases at presentation. See Table 5.8 for other causes of lung metastases in children.

US

- Intra- and extra-hepatic duct dilatation.
- Heterogeneous, hypoechoic soft tissue mass with high Doppler flow at the porta hepatis (most commonly arises from the extra-hepatic duct).
- Check for adjacent organ invasion.

SICKLE CELL DISEASE

This is an autosomal recessive disorder arising from the presence of a mutated form of haemoglobin that is less soluble and more viscous (due to polymer formation in deoxygenated conditions). The end result is a multi-system disease manifest by haemolytic anaemia, painful vaso-occlusive crises and ischaemia-induced damage to the heart, skeleton, spleen and CNS. Symptoms do not usually develop before age 6–12 months due to persistence of foetal haemoglobin.

US

- Enlarged spleen (intrasplenic veins obstruct and trap a large volume of blood within the spleen) with multiple peripheral hypoechoic lesions (splenic sequestration syndrome).
- Over time, the spleen infarcts and becomes small and calcified (autosplenectomy).
- Enlarged kidneys in 50%, thought to be due to increased vascularity.
- Gallstones.

TYPHILITIS

This is an acute inflammation of the caecum, appendix and occasionally terminal ileum. It was initially described in neutropenic children with leukaemia and other forms of immunosuppression, including AIDS and lymphoma. Patients present with abdominal pain and diarrhoea and, on examination, may have a palpable mass in the right iliac fossa.

CT

- Circumferential thickening of the caecum
- Inflammatory fat stranding
- Pericolonic fluid and intramural pneumatosis may be seen

WORMS

Radiographic findings are non-specific. Worms may present as filling defects on lower GI contrast studies or mucosal oedema.

ASCARIASIS

Most common and largest roundworm parasite in humans. It may cause respiratory symptoms, known as Loeffler syndrome. More common in children aged 1–10 years. Presents with abdominal pain, appendicitis, haematemesis and occasionally small bowel obstruction.

PLAIN FILM

- Linear or coiled filling defects of 15–35 cm in length
- Worm intestine may be opacified by contrast material

STRONGYLOIDIASIS

Symptoms are non-specific, as are imaging appearances. May cause respiratory symptoms (Loeffler syndrome).

PLAIN FILM

- Bowel mucosal oedema and fold thickening

GENITOURINARY

ADRENAL HAEMORRHAGE

Rare, but more common in neonates than in children or adults. Causes include trauma, neonatal stress (e.g. asphyxia at birth), sepsis, bleeding disorders and extracorporeal membrane oxygenation. May also occur antenatally or with a difficult delivery, especially with a diabetic mother. Adrenal glands are disproportionately large in young children.

US

- More common on the right (70%)—due to the proximity of the liver.
- Mass of mixed echogenicity, may displace the adjacent kidney.
- Check for patency of the renal vein (may clot with adrenal haemorrhage in children).
- Chronically haematoma becomes cystic ('adrenal pseudocyst') then calcified.
- Haematoma decreases in size on follow-up (unlike neuroblastoma).

ALPORT SYNDROME

Heterogeneous group of inherited disease affecting basement membranes, particularly in the kidney, eye and cochlea. Presents with anaemia, polyuria and haematuria, which progress to renal failure. Ocular abnormalities include congenital cataracts, nystagmus, myopia and spherophakia (rounded lens).

US

- Normal kidneys initially
- Progressive atrophy and increased echogenicity as chronic kidney disease ensues

CT

- Oesophageal leiomyomatosis (late childhood)

AUTOSOMAL RECESSIVE POLYCYSTIC KIDNEY DISEASE (ARPKD)

ARPKD is the most common neonatal polycystic renal disease and is strongly associated with hepatic fibrosis. It arises from a common mutation causing an abnormality of the epithelium of the collecting ducts. This results in ductal proliferation and dilatation. It may be diagnosed antenatally. Large abdominal masses can cause delivery to be difficult. Older children may also present with abdominal distension from renal masses or hepatosplenomegaly. Hepatic fibrosis is progressive, but usually not clinically important to children surviving the perinatal period.

ANTENATAL US

- Oligohydramnios (due to renal failure, leads to pulmonary hypoplasia—this causes neonatal death in up to 50%).
- Small/empty bladder.
- Enlarged, hyperechoic kidneys bilaterally.

US

- Grossly enlarged, hyperechoic kidneys with poor corticomedullary differentiation.
- Microcysts of 1–2 mm, macrocysts imply deterioration (more common in older children).
- Enlarged, echogenic liver with or without cysts in the liver and pancreas.
- Reversal of flow in the hepatic veins (implies portal hypertension).
- Splenomegaly.

CYSTIC PARTIALLY DIFFERENTIATED NEPHROBLASTOMA

Rare—more common in boys aged 3 months to 2 years. These are neoplasms that commonly present with a painless abdominal mass.

PLAIN FILM

- Mass-displacing bowel

US

- Multilocular cystic renal tumour, multiple septa and no solid components
- Beak/claw of normal renal tissue around the mass

CT

- Well-defined renal mass, splays/displaces collecting system.
- May appear solid due to close apposition of septa.
- Enhancing septa.
- Claw-shaped normal parenchyma adjacent to the mass.
- Cystic spaces do not fill with contrast.

ECTOPIC URETER

Box 5.26 WEIGERT–MEYER RULE
1. Upper pole moiety ureter inserts inferior and medial to the lower pole moiety ureter.
2. The upper pole moiety ureter frequently ends in a ureterocele and is prone to obstruction.
3. There is frequently reflux into the distal lower pole moiety ureter.

Due to abnormal ureteral bud migration, which results in distal ectopia. In females, the distal ectopia is most commonly in the lower bladder, urethra, vestibule or vagina; in males, it is most commonly in the lower bladder, posterior urethra, seminal vesicle, vas deferens or the ejaculatory duct. In 50% of affected females, the ectopic ureter therefore bypasses continence mechanisms and causes characteristic continuous dribbling incontinence with a normal voiding pattern.

US

- Obstructed upper pole
- Dilated ureter may be traced to the bladder
- Low ureteral insertion to the bladder

INTRAVENOUS UROGRAM (IVU)

- Less commonly performed (upper pole may not be demonstrated due to poor function)
- 'Drooping lily' sign—inferior displacement of the lower pole collecting system by an unopacified, dilated upper moiety

MCUG

- Demonstrates ureter insertion and reflux

NUCLEAR MEDICINE

- Tc-99m MAG3 (mercaptoacetyltriglycine) is used to assess split renal function.

HAEMOLYTIC URAEMIC SYNDROME

Caused most commonly by *Escherichia coli* infection. It is the most common cause of end-stage renal failure in children. A clinical triad of microangiopathic haemolytic anaemia, thrombocytopaenia and acute oliguric renal failure leading to uraemia.

US

- Mildly enlarged kidneys with hyperechoic cortices

HORSESHOE KIDNEY

This is the most common renal fusion abnormality (affects about 1 in 400). In 90% of cases, the lower renal poles are joined by a parenchymal or fibrous isthmus at L4–5 (just below the inferior mesenteric artery). The renal pelves and ureters are anterior and more prone to pelvi-ureteric junction (PUJ) obstruction. There are commonly accessory renal arteries and a 50% association with genitourinary anomalies including hypospadias, undescended testes, bicornuate uterus and ureteral duplication. Associated non-GU anamolies include trisomy 18, Turner syndrome, GI, cardiac and skeletal anomalies. The risk of transitional cell carcinoma is slightly increased.

US

- Isthmus of soft tissue/band connecting the lower renal poles
- Medially orientated renal long axis

MEDULLARY NEPHROCALCINOSIS

Box 5.27 TOP THREE CAUSES OF MEDULLARY NEPHROCALCINOSIS
Hyperparathyroidism **A**cidosis (renal tubular type 1) **M**edullary sponge kidney

Common—mostly affects the renal pyramids (i.e. 'medullary'), but can also affect the cortex. The most common causes are hyperparathyroidism, distal renal tubular acidosis (most common in children) and medullary sponge kidney. May be seen in preterm neonates with e.g. furosemide treatment.

US

- Punctate/linear foci of increased echogenicity located in the pyramids
- No acoustic shadowing

MESOBLASTIC NEPHROMA

Rare—however, it is the most common renal tumour to occur in patients aged ≤1 year (90% occur within first 3 months). It is a benign fibromyomatoid lesion arising from renal connective tissue. It is associated with prematurity, polyhydramnios, neuroblastoma and malformations of the GI/genitourinary tracts.

US

- Can be seen on antenatal scan.
- Mixed solid/cystic mass with areas of increased echogenicity.

CT

- Large, soft tissue mass, more enhancement peripherally and areas of low attenuation.
- Replaces 60%–90% of renal parenchyma and typically involves the renal sinus.

MULTICYSTIC DYSPLASTIC KIDNEY (MCDK)

Congenital absence of the calyceal system and cystic replacement of the renal cortex. It is unilateral—there must be a functioning kidney on the other side, otherwise it is fatal. There is contralateral reflux or PUJ obstruction in 30%. Associated with other genitourinary anomalies (e.g. hemiuterus, absent uterus, absent testis, seminal vesicle agenesis, etc.).

US

- Numerous cysts of varying sizes with rim calcification
- No/little renal parenchyma

NUCLEAR MEDICINE

- MAG3 is useful for differentiating MCDK from hydronephrosis (no uptake in MCDK).

NEPHROBLASTOMATOSIS

Embryonic renal parenchyma normally disappears by 36 weeks of gestation; if this does not occur, it is known as nephroblastomatosis. This residual tissue is usually occult unless it transforms into a Wilms tumour. If diffuse, it may present a renal mass(es), usually within the first year of life.

US

- Small nodules of varying echogenicity
- Enlarged kidneys with diffuse disease, loss of corticomedullary differentiation
- Cysts in diffuse nephroblastomatosis

CT

- Focal disease causes peripheral parenchymal nodules that enhance less than adjacent cortex—may give kidney a lobulated appearance.
- Diffuse nephroblastomatosis forms a thick rind at the periphery of the kidney with or without striated enhancement.

MRI

- Nodules are low T1 compared to adjacent kidney.
- Reduced enhancement compared to kidney.

MEGAURETER

Enlarged ureter with or without dilatation of the upper tracts. There are various subtypes, including primary (e.g. due to an aperistaltic ureter) or secondary (e.g. downstream obstruction).

US

● Dilated ureter >7 mm
● With or without hydronephrosis and ureteral dilatation above a distal aperistaltic segment
● With or without waves of peristalsis above the abnormal segment

MCUG

● Used to evaluate for reflux

NUCLEAR MEDICINE

● MAG3 demonstrates the effect of the obstruction on function (guides treatment; i.e. is urine draining in spite of the hydronephrosis and megaureter?).

NEUROBLASTOMA

This is the most common paediatric malignancy after leukaemia and CNS tumours. The peak age is 22 months. Tumours arise from anywhere along the sympathetic chain. Two-thirds are abdominal and two-thirds are from the adrenal medulla. They are the most common posterior mediastinal masses in childhood. They commonly present with bone pain due to metastases (in up to 50% at presentation). See Figure 5.21; See Table 5.11 for a summary.

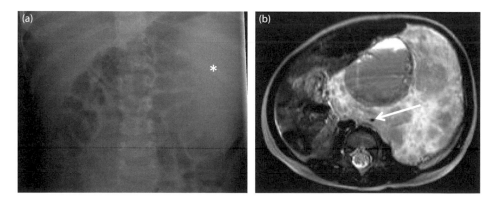

Figure 5.21 (a) Plain abdominal radiograph showing displacement of bowel loops by a soft tissue-density lesion in the left upper quadrant (asterisk). (b) Axial T2-weighted magnetic resonance imaging scan showing a large, mixed-signal mass predominantly on the left, but crossing the midline. Note encasement of the mesenteric vasculature (arrow), which is typical of neuroblastoma.

Box 5.28 STAGING NEUROBLASTOMA

I—limited to organ of origin
II—regional spread, does not cross the midline
III—extends across midline or unilateral tumour with contralateral nodes
IV—tumour involving distant nodes, bone, liver, skin or other organs
IVs—subset in infants <1 year old only, good prognosis

PLAIN FILM

- Posterior mediastinal mass with stippled calcification
- Rib splaying
- Rib erosion
- Permeative bone lesion typically in the metaphysis/submetaphysis of a long bone

US

- Heterogeneous echogenic abdominal mass
- With or without foci of reflectivity (calcification)
- Liver metastases

CT

- Preferred for diagnosis and staging
- Mass with stippled calcification (90%) with or without crossing the midline, encasing (not invading) mesenteric vessels
- Areas of low attenuation
- With or without invading neural foramina
- Bone, nodal or liver metastases (brain and lung also)

NUCLEAR MEDICINE

- About 75% of neuroblastomas take up technetium-99m, bone scan is useful for assessing bones, liver and lungs.
- PET/CT is better than MIBG for detecting metastases.

Table 5.11 The characteristics of neuroblastoma versus Wilms tumours

	Neuroblastoma	Wilms tumour
Age	Younger age (2 years)	3–4 years
Calcification	85%–95%	10%
Mass effect	Suprarenal and displaces ipsilateral kidney and crosses the midline	Displaces vessels and other structures
Inferior vena cava and vessel involvement	Encases vessels	Invasion of inferior vena cava
Metastases	Bone and lymph nodes	Lung primarily, also liver and lymph nodes
Metastases at presentation	70%	10%

POSTERIOR URETHRAL VALVE

This affects males only. It is a congenital membrane extending from the verumontanum to the distal prostatic urethra. It is the most common cause of bilateral hydronephrosis in an infant. Congenital obstruction can give rise to oligohydramnios and therefore pulmonary hypoplasia.

ANTENATAL US

- Diagnosis most commonly made antenatally
- Hydronephrosis
- Oligohydramnios
- Foetal ascites

POSTNATAL US

- Dilated prostatic urethra on perineal US
- Thickened bladder wall
- Urinoma

MCUG

- Dilatation of the posterior urethra with or without radiolucent band (the valve)
- Vesicoureteric reflux (up to 50%)
- Thickened bladder wall

PRUNE BELLY SYNDROME

Absence of the rectus abdominis muscles gives the abdomen a wrinkled, prune-like appearance (also known as Eagle–Barrett syndrome). It almost exclusively affects males and is also associated with abnormalities of the GI, musculoskeletal, respiratory and cardiovascular systems.

US

- Bilateral hydronephrosis and hydroureter
- Renal dysplasia with or without cystic change
- Cryptorchidism (bladder interferes with descent of the testicles)

MCUG

- Vesicoureteral reflux present in 85%
- Elongated and enlarged bladder
- Urachal diverticulum
- With or without posterior urethral valves

PYELECTASIS

US

- Persistent AP measurement of the renal pelvis of >10 mm at birth
- Followed up at 6 weeks

MCUG

- Used to assess cause (e.g. reflux)

NUCLEAR MEDICINE

- Dimercaptosuccinic acid (DMSA) is used to assess for scarring if MCUG shows reflux.
- MAG3 to assess obstruction if no reflux on MCUG.

RENAL LYMPHANGIECTASIA

Rare and benign, caused by a failure of the lymphatics of the developing kidney to connect with the extrarenal lymphatics. Abnormal lymphatic channels dilate, resulting in cystic lesions in the parapelvic, perinephric and, less commonly, retroperitoneal regions.

US

- Large, echo-free, septated cystic collections around both kidneys
- Scalloping of the renal outline

Box 5.29 RENAL ULTRASOUND IN NEONATES
1. Foetal lobulation is prominent.
2. Cortex is more echogenic and renal sinus fat less marked than later.
3. Medullary pyramids are larger and more hypoechoic.
4. Echogenic septa at the anterosuperior and posteroinferior margins of the kidney; these represent the sites of fusion of metanephric elements.
5. Adult pattern by 6 months of age.

RENAL VEIN THROMBOSIS

Risk factors in neonates include nephrotic syndrome, renal transplantation, dehydration, sepsis, birth trauma, adrenal haemorrhage, etc. It is more common on the left due to a slightly longer renal vein. It presents with a palpable mass, elevated urea and creatinine and haematuria.

US

- Enlarged, echogenic kidney
- Reversal of end-diastolic arterial flow
- Loss of corticomedullary differentiation, medullary pyramids prominent and hypoechoic

TESTICULAR TORSION

An acute scrotum in a child is more likely due to epididymitis or torsion of the appendix testis. Testicular torsion is due to twisting of the testis around the spermatic cord, resulting in ischaemia and necrosis if not corrected promptly (100% salvage at 6 hours, 20% at 12 hours).

US

- Normal in the first few hours
- Enlarged, heterogeneous testis with increased peritesticular flow and absent parenchymal flow (testicle may not be salvageable at this point)
- Coarse echotexture
- Hydrocele

TESTICULAR TUMOUR

Rare in boys; however, >95% of intratesticular masses are malignant (mostly non-seminomatous germ cell tumours; e.g. yolk sac tumour [80%], teratoma, embryonal carcinoma and choriocarcinoma). Yolk sac tumours peak at 2 years of age. Treatment is with orchidectomy.

US

- Yolk sac tumour commonly presents as a heterogeneous solid mass replacing the entire testis.
- Teratoma has solid and cystic components.

URINARY TRACT INFECTION (UTI)

Vesicoureteric reflux is diagnosed in up to 30% of children with their first UTI. No imaging is advised for children aged >6 months, with a simple UTI responding to antibiotics within 48 hours.

AGE <6 MONTHS

- Urgent US if atypical infection or recurrent
- US at 6 weeks if responds to treatment in 48 hours
- DMSA and MCUG if it is an atypical or recurrent UTI

AGE 6 MONTHS TO 3 YEARS

- No imaging acutely or follow-up if responds to treatment in 48 hours
- Urgent US and DMSA follow-up if atypical
- Follow-up US and DMSA if recurrent infection

AGE >3 YEARS

- No imaging acutely or follow-up if responds to treatment in 48 hours
- Urgent US only if atypical infection
- Follow-up US and DMSA if recurrent infection

Box 5.30 THE INTERNATIONAL GRADING SYSTEM FOR VESICOURETERIC REFLUX
I. Reflux into the ureter only
II. Reflux into the pelvi-calyceal system, no dilatation
III. Pelvi-calyceal reflux with mild dilatation and hydroureter
IV. Reflux into a tortuous ureter with clubbed calyces
V. Reflux into a markedly dilated and tortuous ureter and marked pelvi-calyceal dilatation.

WILMS TUMOUR

Box 5.31 WILMS TUMOUR RULE OF 10s
10% unfavourable histology 10% bilateral 10% vascular invasion 10% calcify 10% have lung metastases at diagnosis

Box 5.32 STAGING WILMS TUMOUR	
I.	Tumour limited to the kidney
II.	Extension into the perinephric space with or without vessel invasion
III.	Abdominal or pelvic nodes affected or peritoneal invasion
IV.	Haematogenous spread to lung/liver/brain/bone; nodes outside the abdomen or pelvis
V.	Bilateral renal tumours at diagnosis

Also known as nephroblastoma, it is the most common renal tumour of childhood. The peak age is 3–4 years and 80% occur at <5 years of age. It is bilateral in nearly 15%. It is associated with Beckwith–Wiedemann syndrome and hemihypertrophy. In total, 90% present with a painless abdominal mass. Treatment is with nephrectomy and chemotherapy. The cure rate is up to 90%. See Table 5.11 for a summary.

PLAIN FILM

- Calcification seen in 20%

US

- Heterogeneous mass of average size 12 cm at presentation.
- Check the IVC for tumour extension.

CT

- Well-defined, heterogeneous, partially cystic mass that contains foci of calcification and fat.
- Check for extension to the IVC and liver metastases.
- Spreads by direct extension with displacement of adjacent structures.

MRI

- Non-specific low signal on T1 and high T2 signal
- Most sensitive for demonstrating caval patency or tumour

Central Nervous System, Head and Neck

TRAUMA

Box 6.1 NATIONAL INSTITUTE FOR HEALTH AND CARE EXCELLENCE (NICE) GUIDELINES FOR IMAGING ACUTE HEAD INJURY

Immediate scan—Glasgow Coma Scale (GCS) <13 in first 2 hours post-injury, or GCS <15 at 2 hours after injury, possible fracture, post-traumatic seizure, focal neurology and amnesia, loss of consciousness (LOC) and coagulopathy

Within 8 hours—>0.5 hours of amnesia before trauma, amnesia/LOC and aged >65 years/high-energy trauma.

CONTUSIONS

These usually involve the cortex and are haemorrhagic. Contusions that start out non-haemorrhagic are typically haemorrhagic after 72 hours. The bases of the frontal lobes are more commonly affected as they impact on cribriform plate, orbits and frontal bones; the temporal lobes collide with the greater sphenoid wing.

CT (FIGURE 6.1)

- Hyperdensity (i.e. haemorrhage) at frontal and temporal lobe tips, undersurface of frontal lobes, dorsolateral midbrain

DIFFUSE AXONAL INJURY

This is a shearing injury due to deceleration and rotation. It is the most common cause of a persistent vegetative state, with a mortality rate of 50%.

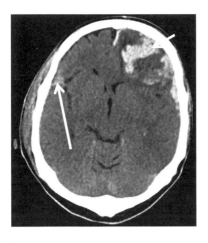

Figure 6.1 Unenhanced computed tomography (CT) scan of the brain showing extensive left frontal lobe contusion (short arrow) with subarachnoid haemorrhage (long arrow). There is marked mass effect and midline shift to the right.

CT

- Initially normal in up to 85%.
- Small haemorrhagic foci in the frontotemporal, grey–white junction, basal ganglia, corpus callosum and dorsal midbrain regions.
- Diffuse axonal injury in the brainstem is most often seen at the superior cerebellar peduncles/medial leminisci.
- Relative sparing of the cortex.

HAEMATOMA—EXTRADURAL

In total, 85% of extradural haematomas are associated with a skull fracture. They cause the dura to strip from the inner skull table and therefore cross dural attachments (but not sutures).

CT (FIGURE 6.2)

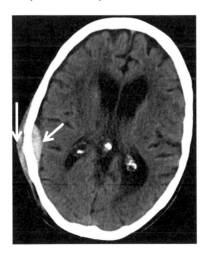

Figure 6.2 Unenhanced CT scan of the brain showing a lenticular hyperdense collection overlying the right occipital lobe (short arrow). Note the swelling of the overlying soft tissues (long arrow). This is an acute extradural haemorrhage. There is likely to be an underlying skull fracture.

- Lenticular-shaped hyperdense collection.
- Look for the skull fracture.
- Check for midline shift.

HAEMATOMA—SUBDURAL

Subdural haematomas cross sutures but not dural attachments.

CT (FIGURES 6.3 AND 6.4)

- Irregularly shaped collection that may overlie a whole hemisphere.
- Non-clotted hypodense (fresh) blood mixed with clotted hyperdense blood denotes active bleeding, the 'swirl sign'.

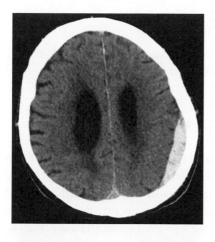

Figure 6.3 Unenhanced computed tomography scan of the brain showing a hyperdense collection overlying the left parietal lobe with associated mild mass effect (note the slightly effaced sulci and left lateral ventricle). This is an acute subdural haemorrhage.

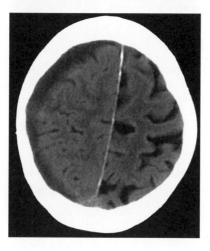

Figure 6.4 Unenhanced computed tomography scan of the brain showing a low-density collection overlying the right cerebral convexity. There is mass effect (effacement of the sulci and probable movement of the falx to the left). The appearance is in keeping with a chronic subdural haemorrhage.

MANDIBLE FRACTURE

Mostly following an assault. Assess with PA, lateral, Towne and oblique views and orthopantomogram.

PLAIN FILM

- Expect multiple and bilateral fractures.
- Condylar process/angle of mandible fractures is most common following assault.
- Open fracture where there is external communication via tooth socket/skin laceration.

CT

- Regularly used to characterise fractures prior to surgery

> **Box 6.2 FRONTAL SINUS FRACTURE**
>
> If the posterior wall is fractured, it is considered an open fracture and likely to result in pneumocephalus. The superior or medial orbital wall is also likely to be involved with a frontal sinus fracture.

MIDFACE—LE FORT FRACTURE

All involve the pterygoid plates. It follows severe facial trauma. A strict definition needs bilateral fractures; otherwise, technically it is a hemi-Le Fort fracture.

CT

- I—'Floating palate', transverse fracture above the hard palate and through the maxilla. Involves **nasal septum**, all walls of maxillary sinuses and pterygoid plates.
- II—'Floating maxilla', pyramidal fracture involving the nasoethmoid region and the orbital floor, including the **inferior orbital rim**. Facial bones may displace posteriorly, known as 'dish face'. Infra-orbital nerve often affected.
- III—'Craniofacial disjunction', horizontal fracture through the orbits and **zygomatic arches** separating the face from the skull base. Orbits appear elongated on Water and Caldwell views.

NASOETHMOIDAL FRACTURES

Nasoethmoidal complex injury. Follows blow between the eyes.

PLAIN FILM

- Expect an orbital fracture.

CT

- Look for a skull base fracture (if the anterior cranial fossa is injured → CSF leak, dural tear, injury to nerve I), clivus fracture or pneumocephalus.

ORBITAL FRACTURE

Blowout fracture is due to a sudden increase in intra-orbital pressure.

CT

- Orbital floor fracture—comminuted fractures may cause orbital contents to herniate inferiorly, resulting in entrapment of the inferior rectus.
- Medial orbital wall fracture (less common).
- Check for injury to soft tissues (e.g. optic nerve, extra-ocular muscles, globe rupture).

> **Box 6.3 OCULAR TRAUMA**
>
> Wrinkling of the posterior sclera is seen with globe rupture and collapse ('flat tyre' sign). The lens may be displaced posteriorly.

TEMPORAL BONE FRACTURE—LONGITUDINAL

Longitudinal fractures account for up to 80% of temporal bone fractures. Due to a temporoparietal impact. Complications include dislocation of the ossicular chain and conductive hearing loss, the tympanic membrane is often ruptured. There may be a delayed VII palsy due to nerve oedema.

CT

- Fracture line extending along the axis of the temporal bone.
- Air in the temporomandibular joint is indicative.

TEMPORAL BONE FRACTURE—TRANSVERSE

This tends to follow a frontal–occipital impact and may lead to transection of VIII and sensorineural hearing loss. VII is also more likely to be transected, resulting in a permanent palsy.

CT

- Fracture line crosses the temporal bone transversely and crosses the VII nerve canal.
- A medial fracture may cross the VIII nerve canal, leading to nerve transection.

ZYGOMA FRACTURES

Fractures tend to be complex and involve all three of McGrigor's lines (e.g. 'tripod' or 'quadripod'). The 'jug handle' view is preferred for zygoma evaluation on plain film.

PLAIN FILM/CT

- Zygomaticofrontal suture diastasis.
- Posterior zygomatic arch fracture.
- Inferior orbital rim fracture and lateral maxillary wall fracture. Note: The infraorbital nerve is at risk with a fracture of the infraorbital rim.

CEREBROVASCULAR DISEASE

AMYLOID ANGIOPATHY

Deposition of β–amyloid protein in small vessel walls in the cortical, subcortical and leptomeningeal regions. Tends to lead to lobar haemorrhage/multifocal haemorrhage, more common in the elderly, rare in those aged <55 years. Linked to progressive senile dementia in 30%. Consider in elderly normotensive patients with spontaneous bleed.

CT

- Frontal and parietal lobe haemorrhage with sparing of the grey matter
- Extensive small vessel disease

MAGNETIC RESONANCE IMAGING (MRI)

- Extensive background small vessel disease
- Superficial cortical siderosis (black dots on gradient echo [GE])

ARTERIOVENOUS MALFORMATION (AVM)

This accounts for about 5% of intracranial haemorrhage. AVMs have a 2%–3% annual risk of bleed with a cumulative risk of 70%. They are associated with seizures. There is no increased risk of bleeding in pregnancy. AVMs are the most common cause of brain haemorrhage in a newborn. See Figure 6.5.

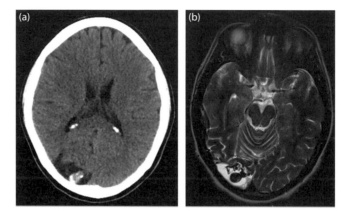

Figure 6.5 (a) Unenhanced axial CT scan of the brain showing a well-defined, hyperdense lesion with calcification in the right occipital lobe that replaces brain parenchyma. (b) Axial T2 magnetic resonance image at the same level showing a vascular lesion and T2 hyperintensity (CSF) replacing brain tissue peripherally. There is no oedema. The appearance is in keeping with an arteriovenous malformation.

MRI

- May be difficult to visualise AVMs after a bleed.
- No mass effect, replaces brain tissue.
- Only oedema if there has been a haemorrhage.
- Commonly, there is atrophy of adjacent brain tissue, due to vascular steal.
- Most AVMs are supplied by the internal carotid artery (ICA).

INTERVENTION

- Angiography is performed to plan treatment or embolise.

BASILAR INFARCTION

Basilar infarction is often fatal, as respiratory and cardiac regulatory centres are disabled. Pontine infarcts can lead to 'locked in' syndrome. The thrombolysis window for basilar infarction is up to 24 hours.

CT (FIGURE 6.6)

- Hyperdense basilar artery in an obtunded (i.e. GCS 3) patient
- 'Tip of basilar' syndrome = infarction in the thalami, posterior limb of internal capsule and midbrain

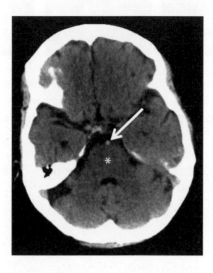

Figure 6.6 Unenhanced axial CT scan of the brain of an obtunded patient showing a hyperdense basilar artery (white arrow) and low-density brainstem (asterisk), in keeping with basilar artery thrombosis.

CADASIL

Cerebral autosomal dominant arteriopathy with subcortical infarctions and leukoencephalopathy. Think of this when a young patient presents with strokes or transient ischaemic attacks (TIAs). No link to vascular risk factors.

MRI

- Similar appearance to small vessel disease—high signal white matter dots on T2.
- Involvement of the anterior temporal lobe white matter is characteristic.

CAROTID ARTERY STENOSIS

ULTRASOUND (US)

- Peak systolic velocity of >230 cm/second in the ICA and end-diastolic velocity of >100 cm/second.
- Ratio of peak systolic velocities between the internal and common carotid arteries of >4 suggests a stenosis of >70%.

CAVERNOUS MALFORMATIONS (CAVERNOMA)

These are low-pressure, slow-flow anomalies with a low risk of haemorrhage (<1%/year). Seizures are the most common presentation. See Figure 6.7.

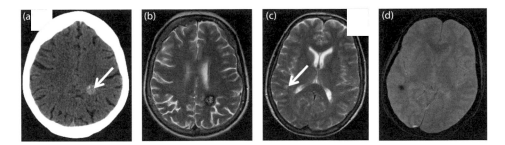

Figure 6.7 (a) Unenhanced axial CT scan of the brain showing a small, solitary hyperdense lesion in the subcortical white matter of the left parietal lobe (white arrow). (b) On T2 MRI, the lesion is high signal with a low signal rim. The appearance is in keeping with acute central haemorrhage (methaemoglobin) surrounded by old blood products (haemosiderin), typical of a cavernoma. In a different patient, (c) a small focus of high signal is demonstrated on the T2 magnetic resonance image in the right occipital lobe (white arrow); this is of marked low signal (susceptibility artefact) on the gradient echo sequence (d).

CT

- 80% supratentorial, 75% solitary
- Hyperdense lesion with patchy enhancement
- Speckled calcification

MRI

- Single best sequence is GE, which shows marked 'blooming' or susceptibility artefact (Figure 6.7d).
- Popcorn or mulberry appearance, area of central enhancement with a rim of chronic blood products.
- Central high T2 signal (methaemoglobin) with outer low signal intensity rim (haemosiderin) (Figure 6.7b).

Box 6.4 DIFFERENTIATING OLD HAEMORRHAGE FROM CAVERNOMA

- Haemorrhage is slit-like, cavernoma is round
- Haemorrhage leads to volume loss and gliosis, cavernoma does not

---

DEVELOPMENTAL VENOUS ANOMALY (VENOUS ANGIOMA)

This is an anomalous vein draining the normal brain, a large stellate venous complex extending to the cortical or ventricular surface. They do not haemorrhage themselves, but are associated with a cavernous malformation in 30%—these can bleed.

MRI

- Haemorrhage best demonstrated on GE
- Medusa's head appearance of vessels

CAPILLARY TELANGIECTASIA

These are nests of dilated capillaries that coexist with cavernous malformations. No other clinical significance.

MRI

- Area of brain showing slow, abnormal contrast enhancement
- May develop in children after whole-brain radiotherapy

DISSECTION

This tends to affect the internal carotid arteries (ICA) or the vertebral arteries. It presents with sudden neck pain, stroke and Horner syndrome and may follow insignificant-seeming trauma.

CT

- Subtle narrowing of the vessel (rarely dissection flap seen) on the affected side.
- The ICA is often affected at the bifurcation, skull base or supraclinoid segment.
- The vertebral artery is more commonly affected at C6 (entry to the foramen transversarium) and C1 (entry to the foramen magnum).

FIBROMUSCULAR DYSPLASIA (FMD)

A total of 90% of cases occur in women aged 40–60 year; 95% involves the high ICA with or without vertebral arteries. It is bilateral in up to 70%. It is generally asymptomatic and may occur in the context of rheumatoid arthritis. Smooth muscle proliferation is the underlying pathology.

CT

- Short stenoses with aneurysmal dilatation between—'string of beads' appearance

MRI

- Best for detection of a stroke arising as a complication

FISTULAE—DURAL ARTERIOVENOUS

Probably arises from sinus thrombosis. Most are supplied by dural branches of the external carotid artery.

CT/MRI

- Rarely seen
- Most diagnosed on angiography

FISTULAE—CAROTICOCAVENOUS

There are high-flow and low-flow subtypes:

1. High = direct: usually young men due to trauma, ruptured aneurysm or FMD. Drains via ophthalmic vein, which is therefore enlarged on CT.

2. Low = indirect: middle-aged men, often asymptomatic, arise from aberrant communication between the internal and external carotid arteries via the cavernous sinus.

Signs include pulsatile exophthalmos, chemosis, reduced visual acuity and cranial nerve palsies (commonly III and VI).

MRI

- Enlarged, oedematous extraocular muscles
- Dilated superior ophthalmic vein with flow void (think high flow)
- Enlargement of the cavernous sinus
- Enlargement of the superior orbital fissure and sellar erosion when chronic

---

Box 6.5 A DIFFERENTIAL FOR SUPERIOR OPHTHALMIC VEIN DISTENSION

Caroticocavernous fistula
Cavernous sinus thrombosis
Superior ophthalmic vein thrombosis
Pseudotumour
Grave disease
Obstructive orbital mass

GENERALISED CEREBRAL ANOXIA

In adults this is more often due to trauma, severe hypotension/hypertension, radiation and venous sinus occlusion. In children, suspect dehydration, anoxia or child abuse.

CT (FIGURE 6.8)

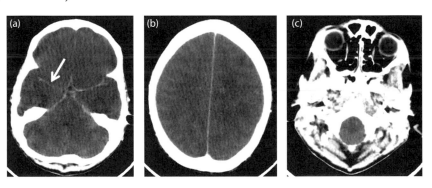

Figure 6.8 (a, b) Unenhanced CT scan of the brain shows marked cerebral oedema with generalised effacement of the CSF spaces (sulci and ventricles). The overall density of the brain parenchyma is reduced, giving vessels and reflections a hyperdense appearance, the pseudosubarachnoid haemorrhage sign (white arrow). (c) There is soft tissue seen in the foramen magnum, a pre-terminal sign of raised intracranial pressure known as coning.

- Loss of grey–white matter differentiation and generalised low-density cortex
- Sulcal effacement.
- Pseudosubarachnoid haemorrhage (widespread reduction in brain density make normal vessels and reflections appear more conspicuous; note basal cisterns are normal CSF density).

- Cerebellum is more resistant to hypoxia and therefore may be of high density compared to the low-density cortex, known as the 'reversal sign'.

MRI

- Diffuse signal abnormalities on diffusion-weighted imaging (DWI), watershed infarcts
- Laminar necrosis (bright coating of the cortex on T1, thought to be lipid laden macrophages)

HAEMORRHAGIC NEOPLASM

Due to tumour necrosis, vascular invasion, neovascularity and coagulopathy. Glioblastoma is highest risk for haemorrhage, but metastases also tend to bleed. If there is doubt about the presence of tumour, follow up with CT in 3–6 weeks.

CT/MRI

- An enhancing component post-contrast suggests either vascular malformation or tumour (Note: Old haemorrhage also shows rim enhancement).
- There is more prominent and persistent oedema with tumour.
- If it is a benign haemorrhage, the oedema resolves in about 1 week (Tables 6.1 and 6.2).

Table 6.1 The characteristics of haemorrhage on computed tomography (CT)

CT	Timescale	Density
Acute	<3 days	80–100 HU Note: With a low haemoglobin (Hb) (<8 g/dL), haemorrhage is not hyperdense!
Sub-acute	3–14 days	Range from hyperdense → hypodense, with or without rim enhancement
Chronic	>2 weeks	Hypodense

Note: CT is the mainstay for the detection of haemorrhage in the acute setting.

Table 6.2 The appearance of haemorrhage on magnetic resonance imaging (MRI) depends on the binding of iron to haemoglobin

Stage	T1	T2
Hyperacute up to 6 hours	Isodense	Bright Oxyhaemoglobin is bright as it contains bound Fe
Acute 8–72 hours	Isodense	Dark Deoxyhaemoglobin is paramagnetic and so dark on T2-weighted imaging
Early subacute 3–7 days	Bright	Dark Intracellular methaemoglobin
Late subacute 1 week to months	Bright	Bright Extracellular methaemoglobin, erythrocyte has lysed
Chronic Months to years	Dark No T1 signal	Dark T2 shortening, so dark—haemosiderin

ISCHAEMIC STROKE (ACUTE)

The middle cerebral artery (MCA) is involved in 75% of infarcts (posterior cerebral artery in 15%), mostly due to atheroma in the internal or common carotid arteries. Key small branches include lateral lenticulostriates (basal ganglia) and hemispheric branches (lateral cerebral surface). In young patients with a stroke, consider trauma, drug abuse, coagulopathy, vasculitis, oral contraceptive pill, steroids and CADASIL.

CT (FIGURE 6.9)

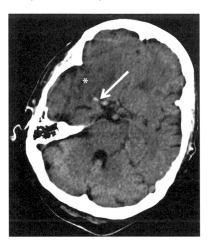

Figure 6.9 Unenhanced axial computed tomography scan of the brain shows a hyperdense right middle cerebral artery (white arrow) and adjacent hypodensity (cytotoxic oedema; asterisk) in keeping with middle cerebral artery thrombosis and infarction.

- 60% have an abnormal CT at 3–4 hours, 100% at 24 hours.
- Low density conforming to a vascular territory with loss of differentiation between grey and white matter (insula and putamen especially; i.e. oedema).
- Hyperdense MCA.

MRI (FIGURE 6.10; TABLE 6.3)

- DWI is most sensitive for the detection of cytotoxic oedema, positive within minutes of infarction.

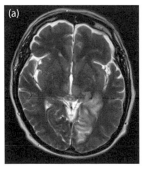
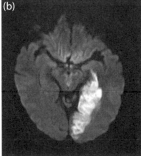
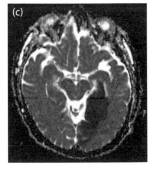

Figure 6.10 (a) T2-weighted axial brain MRI showing an area of signal intensity in the left occipital lobe, conforming to the distribution of the posterior cerebral artery. (b) On this diffusion-weighted image, there is a well-defined area of high signal in the same territory. (c) There is a matching area of low signal on the apparent diffusion coefficient (ADC) map, in keeping with true restriction of diffusion. The appearance is in keeping with acute infarct.

- First 30 minutes—high signal in vascular territory on DWI with corresponding low signal on the ADC.
- Normal T2 signal when hyperacute.
- Check for absence of MCA flow void.

Box 6.6 CAUSES OF RESTRICTED DIFFUSION ON BRAIN MAGNETIC RESONANCE IMAGING

Abscess
Seizure
Hypoglycaemia
Infarct
Trauma

CT/MR ANGIOGRAPHY

- May be used to demonstrate a clot in the M1 segment, which might be amenable to thrombectomy.

Box 6.7 ALBERTA STROKE PROGRAM EARLY CT SCORE (ASPECTS) SCORING

This is a reproducible grading system of early ischaemic changes on pre-treatment computed tomography for patients with suspected MCA-territory infarcts.

- Scoring is done on axial cuts at the level of the basal ganglia and at the supraganglionic level (i.e. including corona radiata/centrum semiovale).
- 1 point is deducted for evidence of ischaemia in the caudate head, insula ribbon, internal capsule, lentiform nucleus and six divisions of the MCA.
  - ASPECTS 10 = normal
  - ASPECTS 0 = total MCA territory infarct
  - ASPECTS ≤ 7 = bad prognosis

Table 6.3 The magnetic resonance imaging characteristics of acute infarct

Time	T1	T2	Diffusion-weighted imaging	ADC
0–6 hours	Iso	Iso	High	Low
6 hours–4 days	Iso	High	High	Low
4–14 days	Low	High	T2 shine-through	Pseudo-normalisation
>14 days	Low	High	T2 shine-through	High

Note that areas of infarction maintain the characteristic high signal on diffusion-weighted imaging and low signal on the ADC map for approximately 4 days.

ISCHAEMIC STROKE (SUBACUTE)

Peak oedema is at 3–7 days. Oedema lasting >1 month suggests a tumour.

CT

- Haemorrhagic transformation in up to 75% as reperfusion occurs (peak at 1–4 days).
- 'Fogging effect'—as oedema settles, the abnormality may be masked.

- After 3–7 days, there may be some gyral enhancement with contrast (good prognostic indicator).
- Long term the infarcted area is filled with CSF as macrophages remove dead tissue—expect *ex vacuo* dilatation of the adjacent ventricle.

MRI

- Look for blood products lying on the gyri (GE most sensitive)—haemorrhagic transformation.
- First week—DWI increases due to restricted diffusion and may remain bright due to T2 shine through.
- Weeks 1–4—ADC returns to normal.
- >4 weeks—DWI dark/ADC bright due to unrestricted diffusion of water within gliosis.
- Chronically, there is atrophy of the corresponding part of the corticospinal tract, giving the cerebral peduncle a shrunken appearance, 'Wallerian degeneration'.

Box 6.8 PERFUSION IMAGING IN STROKE

- Mean transit time—how long it takes blood to reach a bit of tissue, not a good predictor of later events.
- Cerebral blood volume—total blood volume circulating in a given volume of tissue, low volume correlates with later infarct.
- Cerebral blood flow—flow of blood within a voxel, used experimentally to predict likelihood of infarction.

MELAS

Mitochondrial myopathy, encephalopathy, lactic acidosis and stroke-like episodes. This is an inherited genetic mitochondrial mutation with onset in childhood/early adulthood.

CT

- Symmetrical basal ganglia calcification

MRI

- Stroke-like lesions crossing vascular territories with 'shifting spread' (appear, disappear and reappear somewhere else)

Box 6.9 CAUSES OF BASAL GANGLIA CALCIFICATION

- Idiopathic (most common)
- Infections (toxoplasmosis, cytomegalovirus [CMV])
- Inherited (Cockayne syndrome, MELAS)
- Poisoning (carbon monoxide, lead)
- Radiation therapy
- Hypo/hyper (hypoparathyroidism, pseudohypoparathyroidism, hyperparathyroidism, hypoxia at birth)

MOYAMOYA DISEASE

This is an idiopathic angiopathy that translates as 'puff of smoke' from Japanese. The puff of smoke describes the appearance of a collateral network that arises within the brain from congenital, bilateral occlusion of the intracranial ICAs. It commonly presents with intraventricular haemorrhage. Moyamoya syndrome gives the same appearance on angiography, but is not the result of a congenital ICA occlusion (it is associated with NF1, sickle cell, radiation, chronic infection, tuberculosis [TB], atherosclerosis, etc.).

MRI

- 'Ivy sign' = high signal seen in the sulci (engorged pial collaterals)
- Multiple small flow voids in basal ganglia
- Watershed infarcts

ANGIOGRAPHY

- Prominent lenticulostriate/thalamostriate collaterals appearing like a puff of smoke

PERIVASCULAR SPACES

Also known as a Virchow–Robin space, they represent CSF bathing perforating vessels and are a normal finding in all ages. The frequency and size increase with age.

CT

- Well-defined foci of CSF density, typically bilateral and in the inferior basal ganglia/medial temporal lobes

SMALL VESSEL DISEASE

Patients may be completely asymptomatic or have a focal neurological deficit or dementia. The typical patients are elderly with cerebrovascular risk factors.

CT

- Scattered, small foci of low density, typically in the periventricular and deep white matter, basal ganglia and pons.

MRI

- Foci of T2/FLAIR hyperintensity, no restriction on DWI
- Black dots on GE (similar appearance to chronic hypertension and amyloid)

SMALL VESSEL ISCHAEMIA—LACUNAR INFARCTS

These account for up to 20% of all infarcts. Syndromes include pure motor, pure sensory, hemiparetic ataxia, dysarthria and hand deficits.

CT/MRI

- Focal area of infarction in the deep grey or deep white matter (i.e. basal ganglia, pons, internal capsule/corona radiata, brain stem, deep cerebellum, corpus callosum and parasagittal white matter)

SUBARACHNOID HAEMORRHAGE (SAH) AND ANEURYSMS

In total, 90% of SAHs are due to a ruptured aneurysm—the rest are due to e.g. trauma, AVM, etc. There is a 2% annual risk of rupture with a known aneurysm if no previous rupture. 50% die within 1 month of first rupture. The first 2 weeks are critical. Vasospasm occurs in up to 40% post-SAH, with peak at 7–10 days. It may cause infarction. See Figure 6.11.

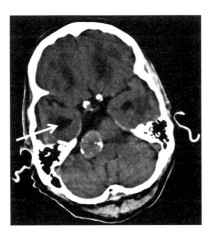

Figure 6.11 Unenhanced axial CT scan of the brain showing a large, dense lesion in the posterior fossa abutting the right cerebellar hemisphere and displacing the brainstem. There is also dilatation of the temporal horns of the lateral ventricles (arrow) and low-density white matter (small vessel disease). This is an unusual finding of a giant basilar artery aneurysm.

Box 6.10 INTRACRANIAL ANEURYSM ASSOCIATIONS

Syndromes caused by aneurysms
1. Cavernous sinus syndrome secondary internal carotid artery aneurysm
2. Optic chiasmal syndrome secondary anterior communicating artery (ACOM) aneurysm (30%–35% of all)

Conditions associated with aneurysms
1. Adult polycystic kidney disease
2. Ehlers–Danlos syndrome
3. Aortic coarctation
4. Fibromuscular dysplasia

Box 6.11 THE CONTENTS OF THE CAVERNOUS SINUS

Internal carotid artery
Ophthalmic vein
Cranial nerves III, IV, V$^{1-ophthalmic}$, V$^{2-maxillary}$ (not V$^{3-mandibular}$) and VI

CT (FIGURE 6.12)

- Overall CT sensitivity is about 90% for acute SAH, but after 3 days, it drops to 66% due to absorption of blood products. After 1 week, it is inconspicuous.
- Hyperdense fluid in basal cisterns, Sylvian fissure and subarachnoid space.
- Check vessels for aneurysm, sensitive to about 1 mm (at <5 mm, the risk of rupture is small).

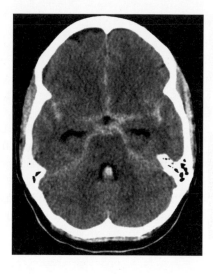

Figure 6.12 Unenhanced axial CT scan of the brain showing extensive hyperdense material (blood) in keeping with acute subarachnoid haemorrhage. Haemorrhage is seen within the suprasellar cistern, fourth ventricle and within the tissues, Fisher grade IV. There is dilatation of the temporal horns in keeping with hydrocephalus.

- Blood in the Sylvian fissure suggests a MCA aneurysm.
- Communicating hydrocephalus at 1 week is common.

Box 6.12 THE FISHER SCALE FOR GRADING SUBARACHNOID HAEMORRHAGE
1. No haemorrhage apparent
2. <1 mm depth
3. >1 mm depth
4. Intraventricular/parenchymal extension

MRI

- FLAIR is best for detecting acute SAH and is more sensitive than CT for subacute SAH.
- Chronic SAH best detected on GE due to susceptibility artefact.
- MRI is useful for screening for aneurysms >3 mm.
- Look for T2 and FLAIR hypointensity along the pial surface/subarachnoid space of the brain and cerebellar vermis in chronic SAH (haemosiderosis).

INTERVENTION

- Cerebral angiography is best performed within 48 hours.
- Overall, coiling has better morbidity and mortality than neurosurgery.

PARENCHYMAL HAEMORRHAGE

Initial mortality exceeds infarct, but if recovering, morbidity is less than for an infarct of a similar size. The causes include AVM, drug effects, amyloid angiopathy (if >60 years of age), tumour, trauma, anticoagulation and collagen vascular disorder (Table 6.4).

CT (FIGURE 6.13)

- Up to 85% of hypertensive haemorrhages occur in the basal ganglia/putamen or subcortical white matter (where the penetrating arteries are).

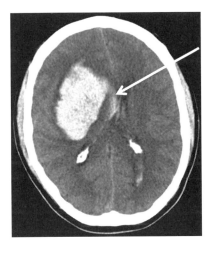

Figure 6.13 Unenhanced axial CT scan of the brain showing a large, solitary, intra-axial hyperdensity arising from the deep white matter of the right parietal lobe, in keeping with acute haemorrhage. There is a marked midline shift and extension into the subarachnoid space (white arrow). The diagnosis was hypertensive haemorrhage.

Table 6.4 Causes of solitary versus multiple haemorrhage

Large solitary	Multiple
Amyloid	Amyloid
Infarct	Multiple cavernous malformations
Venous infarct	Multiple hypertensive haemorrhages
Cocaine	Previous trauma/diffuse axonal injury
Arteriovenous malformation	Multiple haemorrhage telangiectases
Tumour	Haemorrhagic metastases
Hypertension	

- 'Spot sign' = spot of contrast within subacute haematoma, predicts haemorrhage enlargement.
- A residual cavity is left chronically.

Box 6.13 PRIMARY HAEMORRHAGE OR HAEMORRHAGIC INFARCT?
1. Haemorrhagic infarct should correspond to a vascular territory, minimal mass effect.
2. Haemorrhagic infarcts do not result in intraventricular blood.

VASCULITIC INFARCTION

Causes include infection, systemic inflammation and drugs. Inflammation/necrosis of the intima and media vessel layers causes occlusion and then infarction/aneurysm/ haemorrhage. There is a 50% mortality rate for haemorrhage secondary to vasculitis. Treatment is with steroids/cytotoxic agents.

CT/MRI

- Infarcts scattered across multiple arterial territories
- May be small or large vessel infarctions

ANGIOGRAPHY

- Look for characteristic vessel beading.

VEIN OF GALEN MALFORMATION

This is a group of vascular anomalies comprising a central AVM and dilated vein of Galen. It presents in neonates or later with heart failure due to high-output shunt (type 1 malformation).

MRI

- Dilated midline venous structure

INTERVENTION

- Conventional angiography for diagnosis and treatment with embolisation

VENOUS THROMBOSIS/INFARCTION

The typical presentation is seizures in a young patient. Causes include thrombophilia, pregnancy, infection (e.g. direct invasion from sinuses), dehydration, meningitis and tumour (compressing a vein causing stasis). The parasagittal sinus is most susceptible to thrombosis.

CT (FIGURE 6.14)

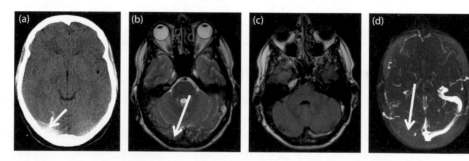

Figure 6.14 Unenhanced axial CT scan of the brain (a) showing an area of hyperdensity in the posterior fossa abutting the right occipital lobe (arrow). On a T2-weighted magnetic resonance image of the same patient (b), absent signal is seen in the right sigmoid sinus (long arrow), which is confirmed post-contrast administration (c, d). The appearance is in keeping with sinus thrombosis of the right sigmoid sinus.

- Haemorrhagic infarction in deep cortical/subcortical regions (not conforming to a vascular territory), rounded and spares the cortex.
- May cause symmetrical infarction of the basal ganglia, thalami and midbrain.
- Presence of haemorrhage does not preclude anticoagulation in a patient with venous sinus thrombosis.

CT VENOGRAM

- Look for a filling defect in the contrast-filled posterior sagittal sinus (deep veins more commonly in children), the 'empty delta' sign, appears 1–4 weeks after sinus occlusion.

MRI

- Loss of the normal flow void indicates thrombus.
- Acute thrombus is isointense to grey matter on T1, therefore easily missed.
- High signal on FLAIR in the parasagittal cortex.
- Subcortical signal change is typical.
- Gyral enhancement in periphery of infarction (Tables 6.5 and 6.6).

Table 6.5 Typical patterns of venous infarction

Site of thrombosis	Infarct location
Sagittal sinus	Bilateral parasagittal
Transverse/sigmoid sinus	Temporal lobe
Deep veins/straight sinus or vein of Galen	Bilateral basal ganglia

Table 6.6 Ageing venous sinus thrombosis on magnetic resonance imaging—there is a distinctive pattern to the appearance of the thrombus

	T1	T2
Acute (<5 days)	Isointense	Hypointense
Sub-acute	Hyperintense	Hyperintense
Chronic	Isointense	Hyperintense

WATERSHED INFARCTION

The watershed zones are border zones lying between the major arterial territories. They are most vulnerable to ischaemia. Transient global hypoperfusion may give rise to bilateral infarcts here (e.g. post-arrest, haemorrhage, anaphylaxis, surgery, etc.). The main border zones are between the anterior cerebral artery/MCA, posterior cerebral artery/MCA and lenticulostriate branches/MCA.

CT

- Small, deep white matter hypodensities in the watershed territories (i.e. occipitoparietal and mid-frontal regions)

MRI

- Corresponding signal abnormalities on DWI and ADC map (i.e. restriction of diffusion)

MISCELLANEOUS CENTRAL NERVOUS SYSTEM (CNS) DISEASE

CARBON MONOXIDE AND METHANOL POISONING

Carbon monoxide causes necrosis in the globi pallidi and diffuse cerebral oedema.

CT

- Symmetrical hypodensity in the globus pallidus

MRI

- Low T1 signal, high T2 signal and FLAIR in the medial portions of the globus pallidus.
- Caudate, putamen and thalamus occasionally involved.
- Methanol poisoning causes retinal and optic disc necrosis, cerebral oedema and necrosis of the lateral putamen and frontal lobes (grey and white matter).

Box 6.14   CAUSES OF BILATERAL HYPODENSITY IN THE GLOBUS PALLIDUS
• Carbon monoxide poisoning • Cyanide poisoning • Manganese poisoning

CREUTZFELDT–JAKOB DISEASE (CJD)

Spongiform encephalopathy leading to a rapidly progressive dementia. It is a triad of progressive dementia, myoclonic jerks and sharp wave electroencephalogram activity. There are four types—sporadic (most common 85%), variant, familial and iatrogenic.

CT

- Cerebral atrophy most common

MRI

- Foci of high T2 signal in the basal ganglia, especially the caudate and putamen and also the thalami—bilateral. Classic type seen in older age group and genetically linked.
- Symmetrical hyperintensity of the pulvinar nuclei of the posterior thalami on T2—pulvinar sign is seen in the variant type.
- Hyperintensity in the cerebral cortex on DWI and T2 (most common early manifestation).
- Restricted diffusion on DWI (considered most sensitive sign).

NEUROFIBROMATOSIS TYPE 1 (NF1, VON RECKLINGHAUSEN DISEASE)

Autosomal dominant inheritance, with 50% spontaneous (long arm mutation on chromosome 17). Fifteen-times more common than NF2. It is a dynamic, slow-growing disease with features that peak at about 10 years of age before regressing. CNS, spine, MSK and renal systems most commonly affected.

MRI

- Optic nerve glioma (astrocytoma) is the most common intracranial abnormality (30%). Look for a diffusely thickened optic nerve with avid enhancement (may extend into the subarachnoid space) and enlargement of the optic nerve foramina.

- Foci of abnormal signal intensity (or unidentified bright objects) on T2/FLAIR, typically in the basal ganglia and thalami, deep white matter and cerebellum.
- No mass effect or enhancement and no restriction on DWI.
- Check for flow voids—Moyamoya syndrome—due to bilateral ICA stenosis.

SPINE MRI

- Affected in 60%, neurofibroma cause bony abnormalities: kyphosis, scoliosis, posterior vertebral scalloping, enlargement of the neural foramina.
- Also lateral thoracic meningoceles and dural ectasia.

NEUROFIBROMATOSIS TYPE 2 (NF2)

Tends to present with hearing loss with or without vertigo aged between 20 and 40 years. Accounts for about 10% of NF, inherited by autosomal dominance (deletion on chromosome 22).

MRI

- Bilateral acoustic schwannoma with or without enlargement of the internal acoustic meatus. May contain foci of calcification, rarely cystic. Diffuse enhancement.
- There are schwannomas on spinal roots in up to 90% and other cranial nerves in up to 50%.
- Associated with cord/brain ependymoma in up to 10%.

NEUROSARCOIDOSIS

May be intramedullary or leptomeningeal. CNS disease affects 5% of those with sarcoidosis. Bilateral facial palsies in young adults is a typical history.

MRI (FIGURE 6.15)

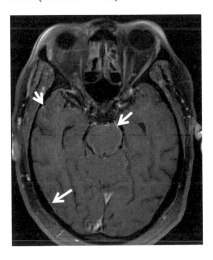

Figure 6.15 Axial T1-weighted MRI of the brain post-contrast showing multiple small leptomeningeal foci of enhancement (arrows). There is a differential for this appearance, including malignancy, tuberculosis, sarcoidosis, etc.

- Diffuse leptomeningeal thickening/nodular thickening.
- Thickening typically shows enhancement with intravenous gadolinium.

- Enhancement of the optic apparatus, floor of the third ventricle and pituitary infundibulum.
- Disease confined to the basal cisterns is usually TB or sarcoid.
- Homogeneous enhancement in active disease and spotty enhancement in end-stage parenchymal disease.
- Enhancing T2 hyperintense deep white matter lesions.
- Multiple or solitary parenchymal masses may also occur—these have a ring-like appearance and mimic malignancy.

Box 6.15 CAUSES OF FOCAL LEPTOMENINGEAL ENHANCEMENT

- Neurosarcoidosis
- Tuberculosis meningitis
- Lymphoma
- Leptomeningeal carcinomatosis (e.g. breast, lung, melanoma, glioblastoma multiforme)

TEMPORAL LOBE EPILEPSY

This is the most common cause of intractable complex partial seizures. The mesial temporal lobe is most commonly affected. Two-thirds of cases have mesial temporal sclerosis.

Mesial temporal sclerosis is associated with hippocampal volume loss (in 80%), which is bilateral in 10%–15%. Temporal lobe resection is helpful/curative in up to 90%.

MRI

- Coronal FLAIR, T2 and T1
- Hippocampal volume loss with *ex vacuo* dilatation of the adjacent temporal horn

NUCLEAR MEDICINE

- SPECT and FDG positron emission tomography (PET) can be used to identify the ictal nidus.

TUBEROUS SCLEROSIS

Autosomal dominant disease presenting with myoclonic seizures in infancy or early childhood. Seizures, mental retardation and adenoma sebaceum are the classical triad seen in about a third of cases. The CNS is affected by subependymal hamartomas, cortical tubers, heterotopic grey matter islands and subependymal giant cell astrocytomas.

CT (FIGURE 6.16)

- Subependymal hamartomas are the most common neurological abnormality (up to 85%) and are readily identified by calcification.
- 50% of cortical tubers are calcified, most commonly found in the frontal lobes, multiple and may show rim calcification.
- Look for hypodense, focal islands of tissue within the cerebral white matter (i.e. heterotopic grey matter).

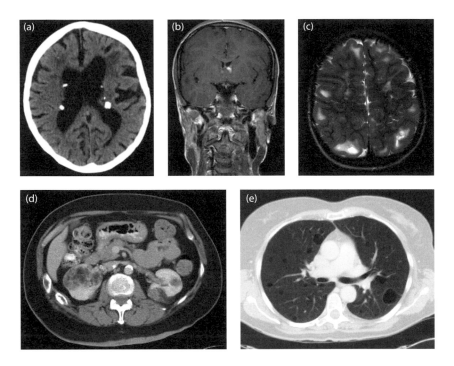

Figure 6.16 The imaging characteristics of tuberous sclerosis. (a) Unenhanced axial CT scan of the brain showing multiple calcified subependymal lesions in keeping with subependymal hamartoma. (b) Coronal T1 post-contrast MRI showing a well-defined enhancing lesion lying near the foramen of Monro in keeping with subependymal giant cell astrocytoma. (c) Axial T2-weighted MRI of the brain shows multiple hyperintense lesions in the frontal and parietal lobes, in keeping with cortical tubers. (d) Post-contrast axial CT scan of the abdomen showing fatty masses arising from both kidneys in keeping with angiomyolipomas (AMLs). (e) CT scan of the thorax showing multiple thin-walled lung cysts (i.e. lymphangioleiomyomatosis).

- Subependymal giant cell astrocytoma is found at the foramen of Munro. It is a well-defined mass with calcification that enhances uniformly (unlike hamartoma and tubers).
- Expect hydrocephalus with giant cell astrocytoma.

MRI (FIGURE 6.16)

- Subependymal hamartomas are high signal on T1, low on T2.
- Cortical tubers are hyperintense on T2, no enhancement with gadolinium.

Box 6.16 CAUSES OF INTRACRANIAL CALCIFICATION

5Ts + O
- **T**reated metastases or lymphoma
- **T**reated toxoplasmosis
- **T**uberculosis
- **T**umour (multifocal glioblastoma multiforme)
- **T**uberous sclerosis
- **O**ld haematoma

WERNICKE AND KORSAKOFF SYNDROMES

Both are due to thiamine depletion. Korsakoff syndrome is the long-term result of thiamine deficiency. It presents with ataxia, oculomotor palsies and confusion.

MRI

- Bilateral and symmetrical high signal on T2 and FLAIR and enhancement with intravenous contrast in the mammillary bodies, basal ganglia, paraventricular/medial thalamic regions, brain stem and periaqueductal grey matter.
- Korsakoff syndrome is associated with mammillary body atrophy and dilatation of the third ventricle.

BASICS OF BRAIN TUMOURS

Box 6.17 PATTERNS OF MENINGEAL CONTRAST ENHANCEMENT

The leptomeningeal pattern of enhancement ('thin'—pia/arachnoid light up).
The pachymeningeal pattern ('thick'—dural surfaces light up).
Smirniotopoulos, J., Murphy, F., Rushing, E., Rees, J., Schroeder, J. 2007. Patterns of contrast enhancement in the brain and meninges. *Radiographics* 27:525–551.

The brain is mostly composed of neuroepithelial cells, so most tumours are neuroepithelial in origin, i.e.

- Astrocytoma (glial)
- Oligodendroglioma (glial)
- Ependymoma (glial)
- Choroid plexus tumour (glial)

Mature neurons *do not* divide, so generally they cannot become neoplastic.

- Intracerebral tumours mostly affect adults and are mostly metastases.
- At <15 years of age, 70% of tumours arise in the posterior fossa.

FOUR QUESTIONS TO ASK YOURSELF

1. IS IT A MASS?

There must be mass effect. Note: Early infarct looks like a mass on CT, so either DWI or a follow-up CT after 3–6 weeks is used for differentiation.

2. IS IT EXTRA-AXIAL OR INTRA-AXIAL?

This is crucial to formulating a differential diagnosis. See Table 6.7.

3. ZONE OF TRANSITION

Intra-axial tumours lack a capsule, so there is no distinct margin, unlike in extra-axial masses.

4. LOCATION

E.g. posterior fossa versus supra-tentorial, and determine which lobe is affected.

Table 6.7 Imaging characteristics of extra-axial and intra-axial lesions

Extra-axial

- Buckling of the grey–white matter interface.
- Expansion of the subarachnoid space.
- CSF cleft sign or pseudocapsule.
- Thin rim of CSF between the tumour and brain parenchyma.
- Medial displacement of the vessels in the subarachnoid space.
- Thinned fronds of white matter (it looks crowded).
- Normal differentiation of grey and white matter.
- May involve bone.
- External blood supply (e.g. dural branches).

Intra-axial

- Expansion of white matter and cortex.
- Thickened white matter fronds and blurring of the grey–white interface.
- Bone is rarely involved.
- CSF spaces may be effaced and the vascular supply is internal.
- Pial vessels peripheral to the mass.

Table 6.8 The differentiation of tumour recurrence versus radiotherapy damage

	Radiation injury	Tumour recurrence
MRI spectroscopy	↓choline	↓NAA
		↑choline
CT perfusion	↓rCBV	↑rCBV
Thallium SPECT	↓	↑

Abbreviations: CT: computed tomography; MRI: magnetic resonance imaging; NAA: N-acetylaspartate; rCBV: regional cerebral blood volume

WORLD HEALTH ORGANISATION (WHO) GRADING

This is the most commonly used grading system for CNS tumours and is useful for treatment planning. Grades III/IV are considered high grade.

- *Grade I*: Low proliferative potential, possibility of cure with surgery alone (e.g. pilocytic astrocytoma).
- *Grade II*: Infiltrative in nature, low-level proliferation but often recur. Some tend to progress to higher grades (e.g. oligodendroglioma).
- *Grade III*: Malignant histology (nuclear atypia, increased mitotic activity). Most treated with adjuvant radiation/chemotherapy (e.g. anaplastic astrocytoma).
- *Grade IV*: Cytologically malignant, prone to necrosis, rapid pre- and post-treatment growth/infiltration of surrounding tissue and fatal outcome (e.g. glioblastoma).

COMMON TUMOUR CHARACTERISTICS

CT

- Typically hypodense surrounded by white matter oedema.
- If the lesion is hyperdense, think of lymphoma (medulloblastoma if a child) and metastases from melanoma, breast, renal, thyroid, lung and choriocarcinoma.

MRI

- Typically low signal on T1, high on T2 with surrounding oedema
- Tumoural haemorrhage—tends to be intermittent, so you get blood products of differing ages in the same lesion—it may cause blood–fluid levels.

Box 6.18 ENHANCEMENT AND BRAIN TUMOURS

1. For enhancement to occur, there must be a breakdown in the blood–brain barrier (e.g. tumour, radiation necrosis, abscess, etc.).
2. The pituitary and pineal are exceptions, as they do not have a blood–brain barrier! These can be useful to help you determine whether a scan is pre- or post-contrast.
3. Granulation tissue appears within 72 hours of surgery, and this also enhances.
4. Differentiating tumour recurrence from radiotherapy damage can be challenging (see Table 6.8).

Box 6.19 MAGNETIC RESONANCE IMAGING SPECTROSCOPY

A high-grade tumour is typically:

- Low in N-acetylaspartate (viable neurons are high in N-acetylaspartate)
- High in choline (very cellular)
- High in lactate (indicates metabolism outstripping blood supply)

HERNIATION

SUB-FALCINE

The cingulate gyrus herniates under the falx, hence it is also known as cingulate herniation. The anterior cerebral artery may be compressed with herniation, which may cause ischaemia/infarction.

UNCAL

The uncus (i.e. medial temporal lobe), when pushed down through the tentorial incisura, squashes the brainstem and its cranial nerves, especially III—so it presents with a 'blown pupil'. The blown pupil is ipsilateral to the herniated uncus. Look for an effaced ambient/suprasellar cistern and contralateral ventricular dilatation.

CENTRAL

There is upward (ascending) or downward (descending) displacement of the brainstem through the tentorial incisura, often due to bilateral supratentorial masses.

TONSILLAR

The cerebellar tonsils are displaced downward through the foramen magnum (i.e. coning).

HYDROCEPHALUS

Hydrocephalus can be non-communicating (obstruction to CSF flow) or communicating (CSF not reabsorbed in the usual way by the arachnoid villi, the fourth ventricle often appears normal).

CT/MRI

- Superior bowing of the lateral ventricles
- Inferior bowing of III (see sagittal)
- Enlarged temporal horns
- Corpus callosum stretched (see sagittal)
- Sulcal effacement
- Interstitial oedema ('transependymal CSF flow')—periventricular hypodensity on CT/high signal on T2 due to CSF being forced into the interstitium

Normal-pressure hydrocephalus

Classical clinical picture of dementia (wacky), gait disturbance (wobbly) and incontinence (wet). Symptoms improve with a shunt.

CT

- Diffuse ventriculomegaly, upward bowing of the corpus callosum

MRI

- Pronounced aqueductal flow void

Intracranial hypotension

More common in women aged 30–40 years. From previous lumbar puncture, surgery or spontaneous. It is associated with postural headaches.

MRI

- Dural thickening with uniform enhancement (due to dural venous dilatation that occurs with reduced CSF volume)
- Sagging midbrain with low-volume basal cisterns

Box 6.20 A DIFFERENTIAL DIAGNOSIS FOR LESIONS CAUSING NON-COMMUNICATING HYDROCEPHALUS

Foramen of Monro
Colloid cyst, subependymal nodule

Third ventricle
Pituitary mass, craniopharyngioma

Cerebral aqueduct
Pineal mass
Stenosis
Tectal nodule

Fourth ventricle
Tumour
Congenital anomaly (e.g. Chiari and Dandy–Walker malformations)

- Depression of the optic chiasm
- Small bilateral subdural hygromas
- Increased enhancement of the pituitary
- Tonsillar/insular herniation
- Increased risk of venous thrombosis/infarct, especially in the medulla or brainstem

INTRA-AXIAL TUMOURS

ASTROCYTOMA

This is a family of tumours accounting for 70% of gliomas, mostly in adults. They show a range of malignancy. Subtypes include:

- Pilocytic astrocytoma (WHO grade I)
- Fibrillary astrocytoma (WHO grade II)
- Anaplastic astrocytoma (WHO grade III)
- Glioblastoma multiforme (GBM; WHO grade IV)

ATYPICAL TERATOID/RHABDOID TUMOUR (ATRT)

Patients are usually <5 years of age. This is a rare tumour of childhood (consider as a differential for medulloblastoma). It is aggressive (WHO grade IV).

CT

- Posterior fossa mass (50%), often lying at the cerebellopontine (CP) angle (medulloblastoma tends to arise from the midline)
- Hyperdense, heterogeneous enhancement

MRI
- Heterogeneous with haemorrhagic foci
- May restrict on DWI

Box 6.21 TOP DIFFERENTIALS FOR CYSTIC POSTERIOR FOSSA TUMOURS

Children
Atypical medulloblastoma
Pilocytic astrocytoma

Adults
Haemangioblastoma
Metastases

BRAINSTEM GLIOMA

Peak at 3–10 years of age. Mostly astrocytoma and tends to be high grade in children. It presents with VI and VII palsy (due to expansion of the brainstem), hydrocephalus and long tract signs (e.g. clonus, muscle spasticity and bladder dysfunction).

CT

- Iso- or hypo-dense mass with patchy and variable enhancement.
- The mass typically enlarges the pons and encases the basilar artery.
- The medulla or cervical cord may also be involved.
- They may calcify (suggests lower WHO grade).
- Cystic change (rarely) or haemorrhage in about 25%.
- Expect effacement of the usual contour of the fourth ventricle, exophytic growth into the basal cisterns.
- A tectal glioma is a low-grade subtype that is centred on the tectum—it has a good prognosis, requiring imaging follow-up only.

MRI

- High signal on T1- and T2-weighted sequences

DESMOPLASTIC INFANTILE GANGLIOGLIOMA (DIG)

This is rare and generally presents at <1 year of age. It is more common in boys (WHO grade I) and presents with a rapidly enlarging head.

MRI

- Mixed solid/cystic mass, shows contrast enhancement

DYSEMBRYOPLASTIC NEUROEPITHELIAL TUMOUR

The tumour most commonly associated with refractory complex partial seizures. It tends to affect young patients between 10 and 30 years of age. It is low grade (WHO grade I) with good prognosis.

MRI

- Cortically based mass (often temporal lobe), may be exophytic
- Minimal mass effect and no contrast enhancement
- Soap bubble multicystic lesion ± calvarial erosion/remodelling
- Usually no oedema

DYSPLASTIC CEREBELLAR GANGLIOCYTOMA

Also known as Lhermitte–Duclos disease. Typically presents at about 30 years of age with ataxia. Associated with Cowden syndrome (colonic polyposis). This is a benign hamartomatous tumour (WHO grade I).

MRI

- Characteristic hyperintense, striated 'corduroy' mass on FLAIR
- No enhancement and minimal oedema
- Bright on DWI
- Low choline on magnetic resonance spectroscopy

GANGLIOGLIOMA

Benign (WHO grade I) with a good prognosis. Children and young adults aged <30 years are more commonly affected. There is an insidious onset of focal seizures. It is the most common tumour seen with chronic temporal lobe epilepsy.

CT

- Partially cystic mass, often calcified (30%) with variable contrast enhancement
- Usually in the temporal lobe
- Minimal mass effect and surrounding oedema
- Occasionally involves the calvarium with remodelling

GLIOBLASTOMA MULTIFORME (GBM)

This is the most common primary brain malignancy in adults (peak from 70–80 years of age). It is very malignant (WHO grade IV) with overall survival of about 15 months.

CT

- Most commonly affects the deep white matter of the centrum semiovale with increased incidence in the frontal and temporal lobes and basal ganglia.
- Heterogeneous, poorly defined, low-density mass.
- Extensive oedema and mass effect.
- Rim contrast enhancement.
- Calcification, cyst formation and necrosis are rare.
- May spread along the white matter tracts and cross the midline to ventricles and leptomeninges.
- 'Butterfly glioma' is GBM that has spread through the corpus callosum to involve both frontal lobes; it looks like oedema (Figure 6.17).
- Other patterns include posterior fossa disease and multifocal distribution.
- Chemotherapy and radiotherapy may cause a transient increase in the lesion size; this denotes a response.

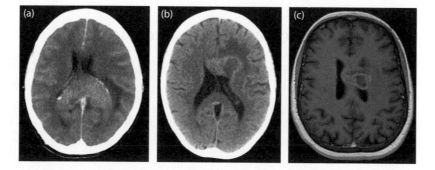

Figure 6.17 Axial computed tomography scan of the brain post-contrast (a), pre-contrast (b) and axial T1 magnetic resonance image post-contrast (c) showing lesions spreading across the midline. The appearance has a differential that includes glioblastoma multiforme, lymphoma and multiple sclerosis.

Box 6.22 DIFFERENTIAL FOR LESIONS CROSSING THE CORPUS CALLOSUM

Glioblastoma multiforme
Lymphoma
Demyelinating disease—multiple sclerosis

GLIOMATOSIS CEREBRI

Diffuse white matter infiltration by neoplastic cells, by definition involving two or more lobes. Often there are mild symptoms. Peak at 30–40 years of age. Rare and poor prognosis, average survival is <1 year.

CT

- Can be normal, no mass lesion or contrast enhancement
- Often bilateral
- Loss of grey–white matter differentiation with minor enlargement of the cortex

MRI

- Diffuse, low T1 signal and high T2 signal, especially in the centrum semiovale, hypothalamus, basal ganglia and thalamus
- Loss of grey–white differentiation
- Typically no areas of necrosis or contrast enhancement
- May look like progressive multifocal leukoencephalopathy (PML), herpes encephalitis or acute demyelinating encephalomyelitis

HAEMANGIOBLASTOMA

This is the most common primary cerebellar lesion in adults. However, metastases are still a more common cause of cerebellar mass overall. In total, 80% are found in those aged between 30 and 60 years. Associated with polycythaemia. Up to two-thirds of patients with Von Hippel–Lindau (VHL) disease are affected: multiple haemangioblastomas are pathognomic for VHL. Overall prognosis is good if there is no underlying VHL. See Table 6.11 for a differential.

CT (FIGURE 6.18)

- 80% affect the cerebellum, rarely spinal cord (usually posterior), medulla, cerebral hemispheres
- Paravermian distribution with hyperdense nodule on non-contrast
- Enhancing solid nodule post-contrast with associated cysts (but 40% are just solid)
- Haemangioblastoma does not calcify
- The nodule is superficial (it gets its blood from the pia) and is the active tumour—the cysts are not malignant
- Surrounding oedema

MRI

- Cystic lesion is low on T1 and high on T2.
- The nodule is hypervascular and may show flow voids.

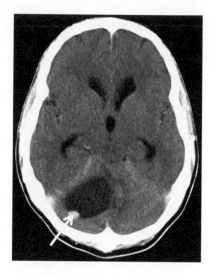

Figure 6.18 Axial CT scan of the brain following intravenous contrast showing a large, predominantly cystic nodule in the right cerebellar hemisphere. There is a small, enhancing mural nodule (arrow), mass effect (midline shift) and hydrocephalus with dilatation of the temporal horns. The appearance and location are typical of haemangioblastoma.

LYMPHOMA

Mostly B-cell non-Hodgkin lymphoma in an immunocompromised host. A solitary lesion in a patient with AIDS is more likely lymphoma than toxoplasmosis. If there is doubt, the lesion is treated as toxoplasmosis and a further scan is performed 3 weeks later. Lymphoma shows a good initial response to steroids and radiotherapy, but may then rebound ('ghost tumour').

CT

- Hyperdense mass with vasogenic oedema and homogeneous contrast enhancement.
- 85% are supratentorial, predominantly periventricular and 50% in basal ganglia.
- Crosses the midline and often involves the corpus callosum—'butterfly' appearance.
- Rarely calcify or haemorrhage (more commonly seen with AIDS).
- Note: If spine is involved, then it is more likely a secondary lymphoma rather than primary CNS lymphoma.

MEDULLOBLASTOMA

Medulloblastoma typically affects children aged <5 years. It is more common in boys and with Gorlin and Turcot syndrome. Treatment is surgery and adjuvant chemoradiotherapy (they are radiosensitive). Survival is 50% at 2 years (WHO grade IV).

CT

- Solid, hyperdense midline lesion arising from the cerebellar vermis (85%).
- 60% show cystic/necrotic change, 20% calcify, rarely haemorrhage.

- Oedema and heterogeneous enhancement.
- There is commonly hydrocephalus due to obstruction of the fourth ventricle.
- Sclerotic bone metastases in 5%.

MRI
- Low on T1, variable T2.
- Restricted diffusion.
- 50% have leptomeningeal metastases—the whole spine must be imaged.

METASTASES

Account for a third of all intracranial masses with average survival of 3–12 months. They typically present with seizures and focal neurology; however, lung cancer and melanoma metastases are often silent. Most are supratentorial, renal cell carcinoma (RCC) has a predilection for the posterior fossa (Table 6.9).

Table 6.9 Common sources and locations of central nervous system metastases

Intra-axial	Extra-axial	Haemorrhagic
Lung	Breast	Melanoma
Breast	Prostate	Renal cell carcinoma
Melanoma	Lung	Thyroid
Colon	Neuroblastoma	Choriocarcinoma

CT
- Multiple low-density lesions, most often at the junction of the grey and white matter.
- Pre-contrast hyperdensity in brain metastases most likely indicates haemorrhage.
- Extensive oedema and dense contrast enhancement (may be solid, nodular or rim).

MRI
- Contrast-enhanced MRI is the most sensitive investigation.
- Lesions are typically low T1/high T2.
- Some metastases are low T2 signal—due to haemorrhage (RCC), mucin production (gastrointestinal) or marked cellularity (e.g. germ cell tumours).
- Equally, some metastases are high on T1 (e.g. melanoma, renal, lung, choriocarcinoma, bowel).

Box 6.23 CAUSES OF RING ENHANCEMENT

Metastases/lymphoma
Abscess
Glioblastoma multiforme
Infarct (sub-acute)
Contusion
Demyelinating disease
Resolving haematoma/radiation necrosis

> **Box 6.24 LEPTOMENINGEAL SPREAD**
>
> Leptomeningeal carcinomatosis/carcinomatous meningitis—either from primary or secondary.
>
> - Breast, lung or melanoma most often.
> - Basal cisterns are often affected → patient presents with a cranial nerve palsy.
> - Post-contrast magnetic resonance imaging with fat suppression or FLAIR are most sensitive.

OLIGODENDROGLIOMA

Rare tumour with peak between 30 and 50 years of age. It is more common in males and 85% are supratentorial. They are slow-growing tumours (WHO grade II) with 10–year survival in up to 60%. Histology may show elements of astrocytoma, known as 'mixed' or 'oligoastrocytoma'. See Table 6.10 for a summary and differential characteristics.

CT

- 70% demonstrate calcification (heavy, in large clumps)
- Large, well-demarcated mass involving the frontal cortex and white matter
- May erode the inner table of the skull (differentiating from a meningioma)
- Little mass effect, variable contrast enhancement (50% enhance)

MRI

- Mixed signal T1, hyperintense T2
- 20% have haemorrhage and cysts

> **Box 6.25 GLIAL TUMOURS THAT CALCIFY ('OL AGE')**
>
> **Ol**igodendroglioma
> **A**strocytoma
> **G**lioblastoma multiforme (rarely)
> **E**pendymoma

PILOCYTIC ASTROCYTOMA

This low-grade (WHO I) tumour commonly presents at <9 years of age. It is the most common intracranial tumour in childhood and is closely related to neurofibromatosis type 1 (20% of these patients suffer from it). See Table 6.11 for a differential.

CT

- Most commonly located in the cerebellar vermis
- Classically unilocular cyst with enhancing solid mural nodule (two-thirds of cases)
- Can also present as a solid lesion with a necrotic centre (a third of cases)
- About 20% calcify, rarely haemorrhage

MRI

- Low on T1 and high on T2
- No restriction of diffusion

SUPRATENTORIAL PRIMITIVE NEUROECTODERMAL TUMOUR

This is a congenital tumour. It develops from embryonic neuroepithelial cells that may originate in the germinal matrix. Peak onset is at 5 years of age (WHO grade IV); 35% are alive at 5 years. Seizures due to raised intracranial pressure are typical at presentation.

MRI

- Well-demarcated, solid/cystic mass often in/around ventricles and causing hydrocephalus.
- Haemorrhage (mixed signal), calcium (low on T2) and necrosis are common (i.e. aggressive tumour).
- Minor oedema but dense contrast enhancement.
- Check for leptomeningeal metastases.

Table 6.10 Intra-axial tumours that calcify

	Incidence	Location	Type of calcification	Character	Enhancement
OLigodendroglioma	Rare	Frontal	Clump	Large mass Slow growth Bony destruction	Variable
Astrocytoma	Common	Cord child	Patchy	Variable depending on grade	Enhances more with higher grade
Glioblastoma multiforme	Common	Deep white matter, frontal and basal ganglia	Rarely	Haemorrhage Necrosis Mass effect Oedema	Avid
Ependymoma	Less common	Fourth ventricle—child Spine—adult	50% do	Hydrocephalus Haemorrhage	Patchy

Note: Try remembering them with the mnemonic 'Ol AGE'.

Table 6.11 Cystic intra-axial tumours characterised by enhancing nodules

	Link	Location	Age	Characteristics
Haemangioblastoma	Von Hippel–Lindau disease	Cerebellum/ spine	Adult	Cyst with solid nodule No calcification Likely haemorrhage Flow voids Polycythaemia
Pilocytic astrocytoma	NF1	Cerebellum	Child	Calcification Rarely haemorrhage Can be solid with necrotic centre

EXTRA-AXIAL TUMOURS

CENTRAL NEUROCYTOMA

Mostly affects those aged 20–40 years (WHO grade II). They arise from the septum pellucidum/wall of the lateral ventricle. The appearance is similar to intraventricular oligodendroglioma. The diagnosis is suggested by the combination of patient age, location, dense calcification and contrast enhancement.

CT

- Well-defined, hyperdense mass with multiple cystic spaces ('bubbly' appearance)
- Calcification is common
- Mild to moderate enhancement
- Ventricular dilatation and intraventricular haemorrhage (Note: Oligodendroglioma do not bleed into the ventricles)

MRI

- Isointense T1, iso-/hyper-intense T2 with cystic regions
- Prominent flow voids
- Mild to moderate enhancement

CRANIOPHARYNGIOMA

Benign, arises from an epithelial remnant, the 'pars tuberalis'. More common in males aged 5–10 years and 50–60 years. Presents with hydrocephalus (obstruction at the foramen of Monro), optic nerve palsy and hypothalamic symptoms. It is the most common suprasellar mass of childhood. A suprasellar mass in a child or adolescent should be considered to be a craniopharyngioma until proven otherwise.

CT

- Mixed solid/cystic lesion
- 90% have foci of calcification (especially in children)
- Enhancing solid/nodular components and cyst wall
- Enlarged J-shaped sella with bone erosion

MRI (FIGURE 6.19)

- Typically high T2 signal
- Enhancement of the solid components with contrast
- Variable signal on T1 due to proteinaceous content

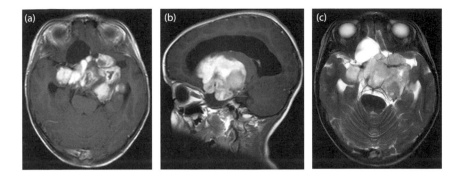

Figure 6.19 Axial and sagittal T1 post-contrast magnetic resonance images of the brain of a child (a, b) showing a large, enhancing, suprasellar lesion. The lesion has areas of low T1 signal/high T2 signal that are cystic (c). There is gross hydrocephalus. The diagnosis is craniopharyngioma.

CHOROID PLEXUS PAPILLOMA/CARCINOMA

These tumours are more common in children <5 years of age and they present when large. Papilloma is benign (WHO grade I), while carcinoma is malignant (WHO grade III)—they cannot be distinguished with imaging alone. There is commonly hydrocephalus due to increased CSF production, reduced CSF reabsorption and obstruction of CSF circulation.

CT

- Tend to affect the lateral ventricle in children, fourth ventricle in adults.
- Iso- to hyper-dense smooth, lobulated mass that enhances brightly post-contrast.
- Calcium in the choroid plexus in those aged <10 years is abnormal—suggests papilloma.

MRI

- Well-defined, multi-lobulated (cauliflower) mass associated with the choroid plexus.
- Invasion of adjacent structures suggests malignancy.
- Avid enhancement, heterogeneous appearance from cysts, haemorrhage, flow voids.
- Drop metastases to the spinal cord.

COLLOID CYST

Benign with adult onset. The characteristic presentation is severe headache, exacerbated by tilting the head forwards: the 'Brun phenomenon'.

CT (FIGURE 6.20)

- Hyperdense or hypodense cyst in the anterosuperior third ventricle, near the foramen of Monro
- 40% show rim contrast enhancement—not solid enhancement
- May have solid central nodule, 'fried egg' appearance

MRI

- Variable appearance depending on cyst contents, low T2 and high T1 is common

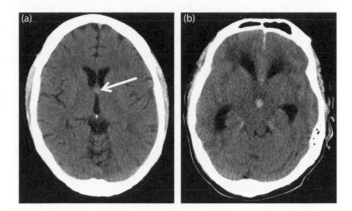

Figure 6.20 (a) Unenhanced axial CT scan of the brain shows a small hyperdense lesion at the anterior margin of the third ventricle (arrow), a characteristic location and appearance of a colloid cyst. (b) Another hyperdense colloid cyst in a different patient, this time presenting with acute hydrocephalus.

DERMOID CYST

Composed of all layers of the ectoderm remnant from the neural tube, including the pilosebaceous unit. It is more common in males, with peak presentation at 20–30 years. Cyst rupture causes a chemical meningitis.

CT (FIGURE 6.21)

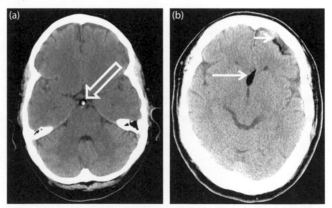

Figure 6.21 Unenhanced axial CT scans of the brain showing (a) a small focus of calcification in the suprasellar cistern with adjacent low density (consistent with fat, open arrow). (b) In a different patient, a focus of fat density is seen (long arrow) centrally, with a smaller focus in the subarachnoid space overlying the left frontal lobe (short arrow). The appearance is in keeping with a dermoid cyst and ruptured dermoid cyst, respectively.

- Low-density (due to fat content) lesion more commonly in the midline, parasellar/sella region.
- A fat–fluid level is pathognomic.
- No enhancement.
- Also appear in the lumbar spine (associated with spinal dysraphism).

MRI

- High signal on T1 and T2 with chemical shift artefact (due to fat)
- Signal voids at points of calcification
- No enhancement

Box 6.26 MASSES IN THE FOURTH VENTRICLE

- Meningioma
- Choroid plexus papilloma
- Ependymoma—most common in children
- Metastasis
- Haemangioma

EPENDYMOMA

Ependymal cells line the ventricular system and central canal of the spinal cord. Patients aged 1–5 years are most commonly affected. They usually present with hydrocephalus. Note: A spinal cord tumour in an adult is most likely to be an ependymoma (most at the conus/filum terminale). Spinal ependymoma is also associated with NF2. The overall 5–year survival rate is 50% (WHO grade II).

CT

- Isodense, heterogeneous mass most commonly found in the fourth ventricle (trigone is most common supratentorial site).
- 50% calcify and 50% have cystic change.
- May haemorrhage.
- Ependymoma in children tend to spread locally via the foramina of Luschka or Magendie to the CP angle and cistern magna, 'plastic ependymoma'.

MRI

- Low T1, high T2 (mixed signal with haemorrhage)
- Mild heterogeneous enhancement post-contrast (Table 6.12)

Table 6.12 Medulloblastoma versus Ependymoma

	Medulloblastoma	Ependymoma
Age	<5 years	Children and adolescents
Location	Vermis	Floor of the fourth ventricle
	Roof of the fourth ventricle	
Unenhanced CT	Hyperdense	Isodense
Contrast enhancement	Moderate	Minimal
Calcification	Uncommon	50%—punctate
Cyst	Rare	Common
Spread	CSF seeding	Local spread through the foramen of Luschka and Magendie

HAEMANGIOPERICYTOMA

Think about this if you see an atypical meningioma (WHO grade II).

CT

- No calcification
- Frank erosion of adjacent bone

MRI

- Vascular flow voids

HYPOTHALAMIC HAMARTOMA

Affects the tuber cinereum (at the base of the infundibulum). More common in boys <2 years of age, it presents with precocious puberty, seizures, developmental delay and hyperactivity. Associated with Pallister–Hall syndrome.

CT

- Well-defined homogeneous mass with no enhancement
- Can be a difficult diagnosis

MRI

- Non-enhancing mass/nodules on the floor of the third ventricle
- Isointense T1, iso-/hyper-intense T2

MENINGIOMA

Meningioma is the second most common primary after glioma. It is the most common extra-axial mass with peak incidence between 50 and 60 years of age (rare in children, unless neurofibromatosis type 2). It is more common in women and hormone sensitive, so may enlarge during pregnancy. In total, 95% are 'typical' and non-aggressive. See Figure 6.22.

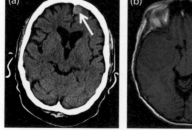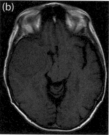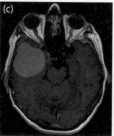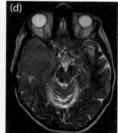

Figure 6.22 (a) Unenhanced axial CT scan of the brain showing a small, extra-axial parafalcine hyperdense lesion abutting the medial left frontal lobe (white arrow). The appearance is typical of a meningioma. (b–d) Axial slices from a brain MRI in a different patient; T1 pre- and post-contrast and T2 showing a large, well-defined, homogeneously enhancing mass. There is crowding of the white matter and mass effect (compression of the brainstem), but no oedema. The appearance is in keeping with an extra-axial lesion. The diagnosis was meningioma.

CT

- Well defined, hyperdense on pre-contrast and enhance avidly.
- 90% are supratentorial, 50% parasagittal—meningioma is the most common tumour to arise from the ventricular trigone in adults.
- Variable oedema, may be absent (they grow slowly).
- Up to 30% calcify.
- Hyperostosis of the adjacent skull.
- Pneumosinus dilatans (i.e. enlarged sinuses).
- Dural tail (tumour extends along the dura) or 'en plaque' (spreads out across skull base).
- Heterogeneous enhancement, haemorrhage, cystic appearance, rapid growth or bone erosion suggest malignancy.

MRI

- Generally non-specific iso-/hypo-intense T1 and iso-/hyper-intense T2
- May be heterogeneous signal due to cysts, vessels and calcium
- May contain flow voids

INTERVENTION

- For pre-operative evaluation, the characteristic appearance is a prolonged arterial blush.
- With or without embolisation of feeding vessels (usually a branch of the middle meningeal artery, so the angiogram includes the external carotid artery).

Box 6.27 PINEAL GLAND MASSES

- 60% are germ cell tumours (e.g. germinoma, teratoma, embryonal cancer, endodermal sinus tumour, choriocarcinoma).
- A calcified pineal at <10 years of age or >1 cm of calcium in an adult suggest tumour.
- Mostly affects neonates/children/young adults.

Box 6.28 PINEAL TUMOUR DIFFERENTIAL BY AGE

Young children
Pineoblastoma
Teratoma

Young adults
Germinoma
Pineocytoma

PINEAL CYST

These are common and benign.

CT/MRI

- CSF density cyst—difficult to distinguish from tumour

PINEAL GERMINOMA

More common in male children and young adults. They typically present with hydrocephalus due to compression of the cerebral aqueduct. 'Parinaud syndrome' is the classic presentation—paralysis of upward gaze due to compression of the tectal plate/superior colliculus.

CT

- Solid, well-circumscribed, hyperdense mass in the posterior aspect of the third ventricle (may be suprasellar)
- Calcification is very common and is central if present
- Enhances avidly post-contrast

MRI

- Isointense signal on T1 and hypointense on T2
- Cystic foci high signal on T2

PINEOBLASTOMA

This affects young children and is pathologically very similar to medulloblastoma. Pineoblastoma spreads via the CSF (WHO grade IV). Pineoblastoma with bilateral retinoblastoma is known as 'trilateral retinoblastoma'.

CT

- Slightly hyperdense mass
- Avid contrast enhancement
- 'Exploded' calcification/peripheral calcification similar to pineocytoma

PINEOCYTOMA

Mostly occurs in young adults.

CT

- Well-demarcated, calcified, slow-growing tumour
- Peripheral calcification

PITUITARY APOPLEXY

Haemorrhagic or non-haemorrhagic necrosis of the pituitary gland. It causes a sudden onset of a headache and commonly presents with cranial nerve palsies (e.g. III, IV and VI). In total, 5% of tumours undergo apoplexy.

CT

- Insensitive for diagnosis
- Pituitary may be hyperdense/heterogeneous

MRI

- May be hyperintense on T1 due to haemorrhage, variable signal on T2
- Enhancement is variable, there may be ring enhancement around a non-enhancing infarcted portion

PITUITARY MACROADENOMA

Box 6.29 GENERAL FEATURES OF THE PITUITARY ADENOMAS
• 90% of sellar masses are pituitary adenomas. • Coronal and sagittal T1 pre- and post-contrast magnetic resonance imaging is the gold standard for imaging the pituitary. • Normal anterior pituitary is isointense on T1 and T2. • Normal posterior pituitary is hyperintense on T1, isointense on T2. • Note that adenoma is indistinguishable from pituitary carcinoma by imaging alone (carcinoma is very rare).

Lesions >10 mm are macroadenomas. They are twice as common as microadenomas. Both can present with hormone imbalance, but macroadenomas can also be symptomatic due to mass effect (e.g. bi-temporal hemianopia, hydrocephalus, hypopituitarism and cranial nerve defects).

MRI

- Look for a sellar mass that may extend to the suprasellar cistern and encase vessels (ICA, cavernous sinus).
- Mass is isointense to brain on T1 and T2.
- Contrast enhancement is heterogeneous due to necrotic/cystic/haemorrhagic foci.
- 'Snowman' configuration due to wasting at the level of the diaphragm sellae on coronal.
- Sellar enlargement in 90%–100%.
- May cause hydrocephalus by obstructing the foramen of Monro.

PITUITARY MICROADENOMA

Microadenoma measure <10 mm. Prolactinoma is the most common (50%) microadenoma. It affects the lateral gland and causes galactorrhoea, amenorrhoea and impotence. May be a mixed picture.

MRI

- Lesion best seen on coronal.
- Low signal on T1, iso- to hyper-intense T2.
- They enhance late (about 30 minutes post-contrast) and more slowly than normal tissue, look for area of low signal.

Box 6.30 A DIFFERENTIAL FOR MASSES IN THE SUPRASELLAR REGION
• Craniopharyngioma • Aneurysm/arachnoid cyst/abscess • Teratoma • Suprasellar extension of adenoma • Sarcoid • Hypothalamic glioma, hamartoma, histiocytosis • Optic nerve tumour • Metastasis • Meningioma

RATHKE CLEFT CYST

Benign cystic lesion. Arises from epithelial remnants of Rathke's pouch in the pituitary gland, the 'pars intermedia'. It is incidental and does not cause symptoms.

CT

- Low-density cyst <2 cm in size and rarely extending beyond the boundaries of the sella
- No calcification
- Peripheral rim enhancement
- Characteristic bean/ovoid shape on axial reconstruction and lies between the anterior and posterior pituitary

MRI

- High signal on T1 and T2 due to proteinaceous/mucoid cyst contents.
- Can also be hypo- or iso-intense depending on contents.
- The cyst does not enhance (sometimes a small rim of peripheral enhancement may be seen due to surrounding compressed pituitary tissue).
- Small, non-enhancing intracystic nodule can be identified in the majority of cases and is pathognomonic (Table 6.13).

Table 6.13 Craniopharyngioma versus macroadenoma versus Rathke cleft cyst

Craniopharyngioma	Macroadenoma	Rathke cleft cyst
Solid/cystic	Predominantly solid	Cystic Intracystic nodule
Enhancement of solid/nodular components	Intense uniform enhancement	Cyst does not enhance Peripheral rim enhancement
Calcification common	Calcification rare	No calcification
Can be a large mass with mass effect symptoms	Suprasellar extension with 'snowman' appearance	Rarely extends beyond boundaries of the sella

SCHWANNOMA

Schwannoma is a nerve sheath tumour. Schwann cells form part of the insulating myelin sheath. It affects the cranial nerves, and 90% affect VIII. They are benign (WHO grade I) tumours and rarely intracerebral. Vestibular schwannoma is the most common cerebellopontine (CP) angle tumour. Bilateral vestibular schwannoma is pathognomic for NF2.

CT

- Isodense.
- Enhances with cystic components.
- 80% emerge from the internal acoustic canal and expand it (i.e. >8 mm).

MRI

- Large lesions look like an ice cream in a cone in the internal acoustic canal (IAC)/ CP angle.
- Iso-intense T1 signal, hyper-intense on T2.

- Homogeneous enhancement.
- Larger tumours (>3 cm) have central areas of necrosis and haemorrhage.
- Look for characteristic thickening of the labyrinthine segment of VII with facial nerve schwannoma (Table 6.14).

Table 6.14 Acoustic neuroma versus meningioma

Acoustic neuroma	Meningioma
Involves the cerebellopontine angle and IAM	Rarely involves the IAM
Acute angle with dura	Obtuse angle with the petrous bone
Expands internal auditory meatus (IAM)	Does not expand
Calcifies rarely	30% calcify
No dural tail	Dural tail of enhancement
Bright on T2	Iso-/hyper-intense T2

Box 6.31 A DIFFERENTIAL FOR CEREBELLOPONTINE ANGLE LESIONS

- Acoustic schwannoma
- Meningioma
- Ependymoma
- Neuroepithelial cyst (arachnoid/epidermoid)

SUBEPENDYMAL GIANT CELL ASTROCYTOMA

Affects 10% of those with tuberous sclerosis; it is very rare otherwise (WHO grade I).

CT

- Mass arising from the foramen of Monro
- Causes hydrocephalus
- Commonly calcifies and enhances avidly

MRI

- Well-defined mass
- High signal on T2
- Uniform enhancement

SUBEPENDYMOMA

Arises from the glial layer underneath the ependymal cells (WHO grade I). It tends to affect elderly males and is often asymptomatic.

CT

- Well-circumscribed, lobulated, intraventricular (usually the lateral ventricles or fourth ventricle)
- Commonly multiple
- A third calcify, a quarter are cystic with variable enhancement
- May bleed into the subarachnoid space

CONGENITAL INTRACEREBRAL LESIONS

ARACHNOID CYST

These arise by secretion of CSF from the lining cells of the cyst. They may cause hydrocephalus by obstructing the CSF flow.

MRI

- 50% are found in the middle cranial fossa (also frontal convexity, suprasellar or quadrigeminal cistern, posterior fossa).
- Same signal as CSF on all sequences—high T2, low T1 and FLAIR.
- Scalloping of adjacent bone (due to CSF pulsation).
- No enhancement.
- Calcification rarely present.
- Note: These lesions show free diffusion on DWI (i.e. they do not restrict).

EPIDERMOID CYST

Contains components of the ectoderm left from closure of the neural tube. They are rare and benign. They present in early adulthood and grow slowly. They are 10-times more common than dermoid cysts and may cause cranial nerve symptoms.

CT

- Well-defined para-midline lesion with calcification (25%).
- 50% at the CP angle.
- With or without rim enhancement.
- If you see one in the posterior fossa, consider Klippel–Feil syndrome.

MRI

- Low signal on T1 and high on T2.
- These lesions restrict on DWI.

Box 6.32 EPIDERMOID CYST VERSUS ARACHNOID CYST

- Both follow CSF signal intensity on T1, T2 and computed tomography
- Epidermoid shows increased signal on proton density, FLAIR and diffusion-weighted imaging.

LIPOMA

Usually an incidental finding.

CT

- Fat-density mass
- Typically at interhemispheric falx (85% midline), tectal plate or suprasellar region
- May contain calcific foci

MRI

- High signal on T1
- Non-enhancing
- Vessels and nerves pass through them
- Definitive diagnosis with demonstration of fat suppression on fat saturated T1 or signal loss on 'out-of-phase' imaging

CNS INFECTION

CONGENITAL CNS INFECTION: TORCH (TABLE 6.15)

Box 6.33 'TORCH', A DIFFERENTIAL FOR CONGENITAL INFECTION. TRANSMISSION IS EITHER TRANSPLACENTAL OR INTRAPARTRUITION

Toxoplasmosis
Other = syphilis
Rubella
Cytomegalovirus
Herpes simplex virus

TOXOPLASMOSIS

This causes a necrotising encephalitis with microcephaly and mental retardation in the long term.

MRI

- Scattered white matter calcification, especially affecting the basal ganglia and cortex
- Dilated ventricles and cortical loss

RUBELLA

Rare thanks to the immunisation programme. Maternal infection in the first trimester gives rise to meningoencephalitis, infarction and then necrosis. Long-term sequelae include microcephaly, ocular abnormalities and deafness.

CT

- Calcified basal ganglia and cortex
- Reduced white matter volume

CYTOMEGALOVIRUS

CMV is the most common cause of congenital CNS infection. It results from maternal infection crossing the placenta in up to 50% and is a congenital disease in 5%. The infection multiplies in the germinal matrix and ependyma and so causes a periventricular pattern of abnormality.

US

- Periventricular hyporeflectivity with or without calcification (not in the basal ganglia or cortex)

MRI

- Loss of periventricular white matter causes microcephaly and ventriculomegaly.
- Note: CMV in the first trimester causes neuronal migration defects (e.g. agyria, heterotopias, cortical dysplasia, deafness). It is less likely to arise with infection later in gestation.

HERPES SIMPLEX VIRUS (HSV)

Most due to transmission of herpes simplex 2 (i.e. genital HSV) being passed to the foetus during parturition. It presents with fever, lethargy, rash and seizures in the first few weeks of life. CNS infection leads to severe/fatal infarction.

US

- Echogenic brain parenchyma

CT

- Diffuse oedema, patchy low attenuation (i.e. infarct)
- Encephalomalacia emerges in the chronic phase

HIV ENCEPHALITIS

Transmission via the placenta, childbirth or breast feeding.

MRI

- Affects the white matter and basal ganglia, causing diffuse volume loss and symmetrical basal ganglia calcification (especially in the globi pallidi).
- With or without vasculopathy, dilation and ectasia of intracranial arteries.

Table 6.15 Congenital central nervous system infection in a nutshell

	Pattern	Abnormality	Chronic sequelae
Cytomegalovirus	Germinal matrix Ependymal Periventricular	Hypoechoic on ultrasound Periventricular calcification	Microcephaly Ventriculomegaly (If in first trimester, neuronal migration defects—agyria, heterotopias, cortical dysplasia)
Toxoplasmosis	White matter Basal ganglia Cortex	Scattered calcification	Necrotising encephalitis → microcephaly, chorioretinitis, mental retardation

continued

Table 6.15 (*Continued*) Congenital central nervous system infection in a nutshell

	Pattern	Abnormality	Chronic sequelae
Herpes simplex virus	Parenchymal	Hyperechoic on ultrasound early on Diffuse oedema on computed tomography with patchy low-density foci (i.e. infarcts)	Necrosis Encephalomalacia
HIV	White matter Basal ganglia (especially globus pallidus)	Symmetrical calcification Vasculopathy—ectatic arteries	
Rubella	Basal ganglia Cortex	Meningoencephalitis Infarction Necrosis	Microcephaly Ocular abnormalities Deafness

EXTRA-AXIAL INFECTION

MENINGITIS—BACTERIAL

Most arise from bacteraemia, so cardiac anomalies, chronic pneumonia, etc., are risk factors.

Box 6.34 PATHOGENS COMMONLY ASSOCIATED WITH MENINGITIS

- Neonates: *Escherichia coli*, group B *Streptococcus*
- Children: *Haemophilus*
- Adults: *Haemophilus influenzae* B, *Neisseria meningitides* or *Streptococcus pneumoniae* in 80%

CT

- Usually normal.
- *H. influenzae* B may be associated with large, bilateral subdural effusions (2% become an empyema).
- May have dense material in the ventricles (exudate), diffuse cerebral oedema or meningeal enhancement.
- Meningitis in infancy may cause cortical atrophy and ventriculomegaly.

MENINGITIS—TB

Complicates TB elsewhere in up to 10%. It is spread by haematogenous dissemination (e.g. from the lungs).

CT

- Thickened, enhancing meninges, characteristically along the basal cisterns ('basilar meningitis'), which may obstruct CSF flow and cause hydrocephalus.
- Look for intra-axial involvement (unusual unless immunocompromised)—abscesses/tuberculomas/miliary appearance and infarcts from arteritis.
- Fungal meningitis also causes basilar meningitis and hydrocephalus.

> **Box 6.35 INDICATIONS FOR AN URGENT HEAD CT SCAN PRIOR TO LUMBAR PUNCTURE WITH SUSPECTED MENINGITIS**
>
> Imaging is reserved for the detection of complications; otherwise, a lumbar puncture is better for prompt diagnosis. The most common complication is hydrocephalus.
>
> 1. Age >60 years
> 2. Immunocompromised
> 3. Seizure <1 week prior to presentation
> 4. Focal neurology
>
> *Source*: Hasbun, R., Abrahams, J., Jekel, J., Quagliarello, V. 2001. Computed tomography of the head before lumbar puncture in adults with suspected meningitis. *New England Journal of Medicine* 345:1727–1733.

SUBDURAL AND EPIDURAL EMPYEMA

Paranasal sinusitis, otomastoiditis, orbital infection, injury/surgery and infection of an existing collection are causes. Pott puffy tumour is a complicated frontal sinusitis leading to osteomyelitis then epidural/subdural empyema. Subdural collections spread freely around the brain surface and require urgent surgery.

CT

- High-density subdural/epidural collection with rim/dural enhancement
- Complications include adjacent cerebritis, venous sinus thrombosis, venous infarction

MRI

- DWI is important in assessing sterile collection versus empyema.
- Empyemas restrict diffusion (i.e. hyperintense DWI and low on ADC), free diffusion for sterile collections/effusions—restricted diffusion is due to the viscosity of the purulent material.
- Collections are often high on T1 and T2.
- Expect rim and dural enhancement.

INTRA-AXIAL INFECTION

ABSCESS AND CEREBRITIS (FIGURE 6.23)

Entry to the CNS is mostly via the haematogenous (intravenous drug user [IVDU], pneumonia, endocarditis and congenital heart disease) route; therefore, the MCA territory is most often involved. Direct invasion may occur due to e.g. surgery, trauma, sinusitis, etc. Features depend on the stage of infection.

CT

- Early cerebritis—normal/mild oedema, mild mass effect, patchy enhancement of lesions typically found at the corticomedullary (i.e. grey–white) junction.
- After 1–2 weeks, there is more pronounced oedema, mass effect, irregular rim enhancement.

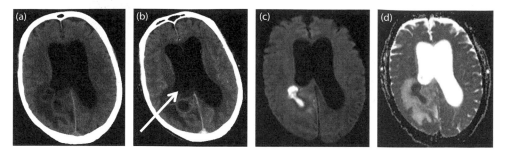

Figure 6.23 (a) Unenhanced axial computed tomography scan of the brain showing multiple rounded lesions in the right occipital lobe with marked perilesional oedema. One lesion abuts the posterior horn of the right lateral ventricle. There is hydrocephalus. (b) Post-intravenous contrast, the lesions show rim enhancement. The appearance is in keeping with abscesses, with possible rupture into the ventricular system (arrow). (c) On diffusion-weighted imaging, there is high signal in several lesions, which is matched with an area of low signal on the ADC map (d), in keeping with diffusion restriction.

- After 2 weeks or more, a capsule begins to form—the abscess has a low-density centre and is surrounded by a smooth, thin rim of contrast enhancement.
- The capsule may persist for up to 8 months, abscess cavity may be multiloculated with thinning of its wall on the side adjacent to the ventricle (due to relative undervascularisation), prone to rupture into the ventricle.

MRI

- Abscess is high signal on T2 and FLAIR with restricted diffusion on DWI.
- Persistent restriction on DWI can indicate failed treatment.
- Ependymal enhancement suggests ventriculitis.

Box 6.36 DIFFERENTIATION BETWEEN ABSCESSES AND METASTASES

- Wall enhancement is thin in abscess (thick enhancement should raise the suspicion of metastasis).
- Restricted diffusion of pus in abscess—opposite in necrotic tumours.

ACUTE DEMYELINATING ENCEPHALOMYELITIS

Acute demyelination that may be triggered by a viral illness, vaccination or occur spontaneously. It is thought to be autoimmune. Mortality is up to 20%; however, a good response to steroids is often seen. Imaging appearances are similar to multiple sclerosis (MS), but the patient and disease course are different. Hurst disease is a hyperacute, haemorrhagic subtype and is usually fatal.

MRI (FIGURE 6.24)

- Multifocal, large, confluent or punctate lesions in the subcortical white matter and cerebellum
- Lesions are hyperintense on T2 and FLAIR

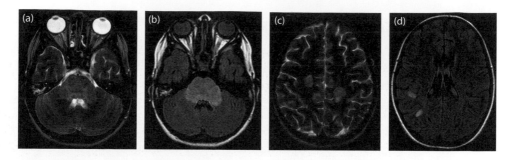

Figure 6.24 Axial T2-weighted magnetic resonance image of the brain showing increased signal intensity in the pons and cerebellar peduncles (a) with a corresponding signal abnormality on FLAIR (b). Further focal white matter lesions are demonstrated on T2 slightly more superiorly (c) and on FLAIR (d). There is a differential for multifocal white matter lesions; this case was acute demyelinating encephalomyelitis.

Box 6.37 A DIFFERENTIAL FOR WHITE MATTER LESIONS ON MAGNETIC RESONANCE IMAGING

- Demyelination
- Acute demyelinating encephalomyelitis
- Vasculitis
- Migraine
- Neurosarcoid
- AIDS
- Progressive multifocal leukoencephalopathy

CYTOMEGALOVIRUS (CMV)

Causes encephalitis and ependymitis, affecting the brainstem and periventricular white matter.

CT

- Multiple hypodensities in the brainstem and periventricular white matter

MRI

- High T2, patchy, diffuse, periventricular white matter change
- Ependymal enhancement

CRYPTOCOCCUS

This is the most common fungal CNS infection in AIDS and the third most common pathogen after *Toxoplasma* and HIV.

MRI

- Widening of the subarachnoid spaces due to mucoid material
- Mild hydrocephalus
- Cryptococcomas: lesions in the basal ganglia and pons, high signal on T2 and low signal on T1
- No oedema or enhancement of cryptococcoma

HERPES SIMPLEX VIRUS (HSV)

HSV accounts for 90% of all viral encephalitis. It is the most common cause of sporadic encephalitis (neonates—HSV-2; adults—HSV-1). There are often no symptoms other than a fever. Mortality is up to 70%.

CT

- Normal for first 3–5 days, then a unilateral abnormality first
- Ill-defined hypodensities, typically affecting the temporal lobes (especially the hippocampus), frontal lobes and insula
- Patchy gyriform enhancement

MRI

- High signal on T2 and FLAIR in temporal lobes, insula, frontal lobes and cingulate gyrus.
- Involvement of the cingulate gyrus is characteristic and bilateral temporal lobe involvement is nearly pathognomic.
- FLAIR and DWI are most sensitive.
- Oedema extends to involve the cortex.
- Leptomeningeal and gyral enhancement.

Box 6.38 DIFFERENTIATING HERPES SIMPLEX VIRUS FROM MIDDLE CEREBRAL ARTERY INFARCT

- Bilateral changes with herpes simplex virus
- Posteromedial temporal lobe affected (supplied by the posterior cerebral artery [PCA])

Box 6.39 CENTRAL NERVOUS SYSTEM INFECTION WITH HIV AND AIDS

Two-thirds have intra-axial central nervous system infection at some point. The most common manifestations are HIV encephalitis, toxoplasmosis, cryptococcosis, cytomegalovirus, herpes simplex virus, mycobacterial tuberculosis, progressive multifocal leukoencephalopathy and neurosyphilis. See Table 6.16 for differentials for CNS lesions in HIV and AIDS.

HIV ENCEPHALITIS

Causes atrophy of the white matter, especially the centrum semiovale. In adults, it causes the 'AIDS dementia complex'; in children, it causes HIV-associated progressive encephalopathy. Appearances improve with treatment.

MRI (FIGURE 6.25)

- Diffuse bilateral symmetrical periventricular white matter lesions with characteristic sparing of the grey matter
- No enhancement post-contrast
- Cerebral atrophy

LYME DISEASE

Transmitted by ticks found on deer (beware hikers and trail runners!). There is CNS involvement in 10%–15%.

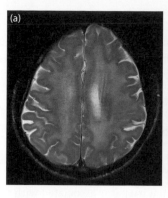 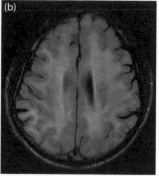

Figure 6.25 Axial T2 (a) and FLAIR (b) images showing diffuse white matter signal intensity with sparing of the grey matter. There is volume loss with prominence of the sulci. The appearance is in keeping with HIV encephalitis.

MRI

- Multiple small white matter lesions with nodular or rim enhancement.
- The appearance is similar to MS, neurosarcoid or vasculitis.

NEUROCYSTICERCOSIS

This parasite originates from a pork tapeworm, *Taenia solium*. The brain is affected in up to 80%. Cysts may rupture and cause a ventriculitis.

CT

- CSF-containing cysts with mural contrast enhancement, most occurring at the corticomedullary junction.
- Old lesions calcify.
- Cysts can occur in the ventricles and cause hydrocephalus.

MRI (FIGURE 6.26)

- 'Pea in a pod' appearance on T1—live larvae in the cysts
- Ring or disc enhancing lesion—dying larvae

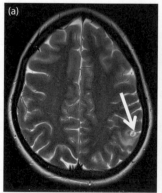 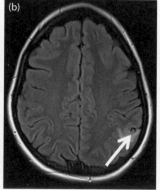 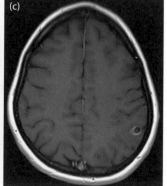

Figure 6.26 (a) Axial T2-weighted image of the brain showing a small hyperintense lesion in the left parietal lobe (arrow). Note the small low-signal focus in the centre of the lesion. (b) On FLAIR, the lesion is mostly low signal and there is surrounding oedema (arrow). (c) Post-contrast T1 shows low signal in the centre of the lesion with peripheral rim enhancement. The appearance is in keeping with neurocysticercosis. Rim enhancement of the lesion suggests dying larvae.

NEUROSYPHILIS

In total, 5% of untreated patients with primary disease get it, often without symptoms. It rarely causes granulomas. It can cause a large to medium vessel arteritis and lead to infarct.

MRI

● Infarcts affecting the brain stem, basal ganglia and MCA territory

PROGRESSIVE MULTIFOCAL LEUKOENCEPHALOPATHY

PML is due to reactivation of the JC polyomavirus. It is associated with severe immunocompromise and CD4 <200 cells/μL. There is multifocal demyelination and necrosis of the white matter.

MRI

● Multifocal, bilateral, asymmetrical high signal in the parieto-occipital lobes with scalloping due to involvement of the subcortical 'U' fibres
● No mass effect and minimal enhancement

Table 6.16 Central nervous system lesions in HIV and AIDS

	Location	Abnormality
HIV encephalitis	Diffuse, bilateral, symmetrical Periventricular white matter lesions	Diffuse atrophy Patchy ↑T2 White matter vacuolation No contrast enhancement
Toxoplasmosis	Basal ganglia Corticomedullary junction Thalamus	Multiple enhancing lesions, ↑T2 and diffusion-weighted imaging Mass effect Vasogenic oedema Haemorrhagic
Primary central nervous system lymphoma	Deep white matter Cortex/periventricular location Corpus callosum	Solid/rim enhancement Crosses midline Lesions iso-/hyper-intense on T2
Fungal encephalitis	Basal ganglia	Pseudocysts of CSF density Minimal oedema
Progressive multifocal leukoencephalopathy	White matter	Multifocal demyelination No oedema
Tuberculosis	Corticomedullary regions	Target lesions Hydrocephalus Dural enhancement

SUB-ACUTE SCLEROSING PANENCEPHALITIS

Affects children and adults with a recent history of measles (<2 years). It is invariably fatal. It causes dementia, paralysis, myoclonus and death.

MRI

- Diffuse T2 hyperintense lesions involving the subcortical and deep white matter
- Cerebral oedema

TOXOPLASMOSIS

This is the most common cause of a mass lesion in patients with AIDS. It occurs in patients with a CD4 count <200 cells/μL. This causes toxoplasmosis reactivation and a necrotising encephalitis.

CT

- Multiple <2–cm rim enhancing lesions typically involving the basal ganglia, corticomedullary junction and thalamus
- Marked vasogenic oedema and mass effect

MRI (FIGURE 6.27)

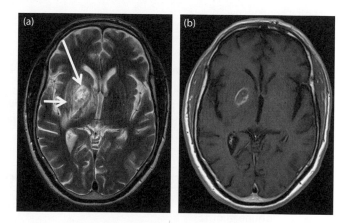

Figure 6.27 (a) Axial T2-weighted magnetic resonance image of the brain in a patient with HIV and severe immunocompromise showing a diffuse area of high signal in the right basal ganglia (long arrow) and adjacent oedema (short arrow) and mild mass effect. (b) Post-intravenous contrast, the lesion shows rim enhancement. The appearance is in keeping with cerebral toxoplasmosis.

- Lesions are typically high signal on T2 and restrict on DWI.
- Lesions may be haemorrhagic (so high signal on T1).

DEMYELINATING DISEASE

CENTRAL PONTINE MYELINOLYSIS

Demyelination of the pons, classically due to rapid correction of hyponatraemia. Occurs in patients with malnutrition, alcoholism, etc. The syndrome involves a generalised encephalopathy (due to hyponatraemia), then a rapidly evolving corticospinal tract syndrome with quadriplegia, altered mental state and then 'locked in' syndrome. The prognosis is poor. See Figure 6.28.

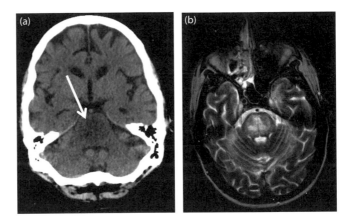

Figure 6.28 (a) Unenhanced axial computed tomography scan of the brain showing focal low attenuation in the central pons (arrow). (b) Axial T2 magnetic resonance image in the same patient shows focal, symmetrical high signal confined to the central pons, in keeping with central pontine myelinolysis.

MRI

- Isolated high signal in the central pons on T2 and FLAIR is characteristic.
- Low signal on T1.
- The abnormality is typically bilateral and symmetrical.
- Other sites affected are the cerebellum, thalamus, globus pallidus, putamen, subcortical white matter and lateral geniculate body.

Box 6.40 DIFFERENTIAL FOR HIGH T2 SIGNAL IN THE PONS

- Central pontine myelinolysis
- Pontine glioma
- Infarction

Box 6.41 CENTRAL NERVOUS SYSTEM DISEASE ASSOCIATED WITH ALCOHOL ABUSE

- Bilateral haemorrhagic necrosis of the putamen (methanol intoxication)
- Atrophy of the cerebellum and particularly the vermis (chronic alcohol abuse)
- Wernicke encephalopathy
- Marchiafava–Bignami disease

MARCHIAFAVA–BIGNAMI DISEASE

This is a form of demyelination seen mostly in alcoholics. There is primary degeneration of the corpus callosum with symmetrical demyelination or necrosis of the central corpus callosum.

CT

- Linear low density in the corpus callosum

MRI

- High signal in the middle layers of the corpus callosum on T2 is nearly pathognomic (FLAIR is sensitive).

MULTIPLE SCLEROSIS

MS is associated with autoimmune destruction of myelin sheaths. It is two-times more common in women. The disease is mostly the 'chronic relapsing' subtype. With known MS, MRI will detect a lesion in 90%. FLAIR is most sensitive, but STIR and proton density sequences are preferred for the posterior fossa and spine due to pulsation artefact. The key characteristic is multiple white matter lesions separated in time and place.

Box 6.42 THE MCDONALD CRITERIA

Diagnosing MS can be done on clinical grounds alone; however, the McDonald criteria allow magnetic resonance to be used instead of some clinical parameters, facilitating earlier diagnosis with a higher degree of specificity and sensitivity. Revised in 2010.

Further reading
Polman, C. et al. 2011. Criteria for multiple sclerosis: 2010 revisions to the McDonald criteria. *Annals of Neurology* 69:292–302.

MRI (FIGURE 6.29)

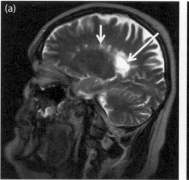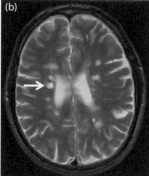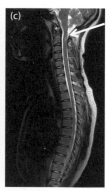

Figure 6.29 Sagittal and axial T2-weighted magnetic resonance images of the brain and upper cord (different patients). There are multiple T2 hyperintense white matter lesions (arrows), most conspicuously in the periventricular white matter and cervical cord. The lesions are oval-shaped and orientated perpendicular to the lateral ventricles (b). A larger, more aggressive-appearing lesion is also demonstrated (long arrow, a). Note expansion of the cord at C2, which suggests acute disease (arrow, c). The appearances are in keeping with multiple sclerosis.

- Typically periventricular (80%) oval lesions with their long axis perpendicular to the lateral ventricles (Dawson's fingers).
- Lesions on the inferior aspect of the corpus callosum are also characteristic.
- Brain lesions are low on T1, cord lesions are high on T1.
- Other sites commonly affected include the internal capsule, centrum semiovale, cerebellar/cerebral peduncles, medulla, cord and optic tract.

- Active lesions show contrast enhancement, adjacent oedema and restricted diffusion.
- Enhancement continues for up to 12 weeks after lesion activity.
- Chronic lesions have a low-signal, target-like appearance.
- Aggressive, 'tumefactive' MS looks like a tumour—a large, deep, white matter mass with a leading edge of contrast enhancement (active demyelination).
- Rings of concentric tumefactive MS are known as 'Balo's concentric sclerosis'.
- In advanced MS, there is white matter loss, with plaques of low T2 signal, ventricular dilatation and thinning of the corpus callosum.

NEUROMYELITIS OPTICA (NMO, DEVIC DISEASE)

This is a relapsing inflammatory/necrotising process associated with optic neuritis and acute myelitis. NMO IgG antibodies are 90% specific.

MRI

- Focal white matter lesions showing contrast enhancement
- Typically affects the parenchyma around the third and fourth ventricles, optic tract and cord

POSTERIOR REVERSIBLE ENCEPHALOPATHY SYNDROME (PRES)

The cause of PRES is uncertain, but it may be due to transient breakdown of auto-regulation in the posterior circulation with hypertension, causing a blood–brain barrier compromise and resultant vasogenic oedema. It is associated with eclampsia, cyclosporine toxicity, renal failure, haemolytic uraemic syndrome, thrombocytopenic purpura, systemic lupus erythematosus, etc.

CT

- Low-density lesions in the occipital lobes

MRI

- High signal on T2 (vasogenic oedema) in the parieto-occipital lobes, posterior frontal, cortical and subcortical white matter/watershed zones.
- Lesions do not enhance or restrict on DWI.
- May be complicated by infarct or haemorrhage.

Box 6.43 EPENDYMITIS GRANULARIS

High signal on T2/FLAIR at the tips of the frontal horns of the lateral ventricles. May extend around the ventricles in old age. It is normal!

RADIATION LEUKOENCEPHALITIS

Associated with doses >40 Gy. Radiotherapy induces a vasculopathy, leading to white matter damage. It is benign and responds to steroids. It tends to occur within 3 months of treatment.

MRI

- Non-specific high signal on T2 (oedema) in diffuse areas of exposed white matter (especially subcortical white matter)

RADIATION NECROSIS

This is a serious complication of radiotherapy. It is dose related and may be progressive and fatal. It tends to occur between 1 and 10 years post-treatment.

CT/MRI

- Lesion with mass effect and rim enhancement at the focus of previous radiotherapy.
- Can look very similar to tumour recurrence—however, it regresses over time, is PET negative and tumour recurrence shows a choline peak on MRI spectroscopy.
- Large vessels included in the radiotherapy field may stricture or there may be telangiectasia mimicking an AVM.

LEUKODYSTROPHY

ADRENOLEUKODYSTROPHY

Typically affects boys aged 5–10 years. Coexists with adrenal insufficiency (neurological symptoms appear first). Death occurs within 2 years.

MRI

- Preferential symmetrical involvement of the optic and auditory pathways, the splenium of the corpus callosum, posterior periventricular white matter.
- Areas of active inflammation enhance with contrast.

ALEXANDER DISEASE

Presents in infancy. Histology shows increased density of Rosenthal fibres.

MRI

- Progressive demyelination beginning with the frontal lobes and eventually involving the entire hemispheres
- Brain enlargement

CANAVAN DISEASE

From build-up of N-acetylaspartate (NAA) from enzyme deficiency. Begins in first year of life. Macrocephaly and brain enlargement.

MRI

- Involvement of all white matter and deep grey matter (especially the basal ganglia and thalami)
- Marked NAA peak on MRI spectroscopy

KRABBE DISEASE

This is typically diagnosed at 3–6 months of age. Expect dysmorphic facies and enlarged ears. It is fatal by 2 years of age.

CT
- Hyperdense thalami and corona radiata

MRI
- Optic nerve hypertrophy

LEIGH DISEASE

A mitochondrial defect of childhood/infancy. May be due to low thiamine (like Wernicke/Korsakoff syndrome).

MRI
- Focal areas of necrosis in the basal ganglia, thalamus and sub-cortical white matter
- Characteristically involves the periacqueductal grey matter (like Wernicke/ Korsakoff syndrome)

METACHROMATIC LEUKODYSTROPHY

This is an autosomal recessive disease presenting at <2 years of age. It is the most common leukodystrophy and is associated with gait disturbance and learning disability. Death occurs within 5 years.

MRI
- Progressive, symmetrical white matter lesions.
- Perivascular white matter is relatively spared, which gives the white matter a stripy 'tigroid' appearance.

PELIZAEUS–MERZBACHER DISEASE

X-linked disease leading to hypomyelination. Typically presents in young males and has a protracted course.

MRI
- Diffuse high T2 signal in the white matter with involvement of the sub-cortical U-fibres in all cases.
- Relative sparing of the perivascular white matter, which produces a 'tigroid' appearance like metachromatic leukodystrophy.

METABOLIC DISORDERS

ACROMEGALY

Caused by excess growth hormone secretion by the anterior lobe of the pituitary gland. Associated with abnormalities of the brain and cranium as described below.

MRI

- Pituitary macroadenoma

CT

- Sellar enlargement and erosion (>15 mm length, height >12 mm)
- Prognathism (elongation of the jaw) and enlargement of the jaw
- Frontal bossing
- Enlargement of the frontal sinus with prominence of the supraorbital ridge
- Thickening of the calvaria

CEREBRAL CALCIFICATION

May occur with hypo- or hyper-parathyroidism, Fahr disease, post-anoxia, neonatal AIDS or Cockayne disease.

CT

- Look for calcification elsewhere, suggesting a systemic problem.

WILSON DISEASE

This is an autosomal recessive disorder related to copper metabolism. Hepatic disease appears first, typically in late adolescence.

MRI

- Variable signal abnormality mostly in the basal ganglia (especially the putamen) and midbrain (tegmentum).
- There may be high signal on T1 from the paramagnetic effects of copper, but mostly high T2.
- Characteristically, the red nuclei and substantia nigra are spared, giving the 'face of the giant panda' sign on T2.

DEGENERATIVE DISORDERS

ALZHEIMER DISEASE

This is the most common degenerative dementia. It affects up to 50% of those aged >85 years.

CT/MRI

- Hippocampal atrophy is the cardinal feature. Perihippocampal fissures are more prominent.
- Focal atrophic change in the medial temporal lobe with subsequent marked enlargement of the temporal horns.
- Suprasellar cisterns and Sylvian fissures are also dilated (not the case with normal ageing).
- Spares the deep white matter, basal ganglia and cerebellum.

FRIEDREICH ATAXIA

Most commonly inherited progressive ataxia.

MRI

- Thinning of the cervical spinal cord and medulla with associated mild cerebral atrophy

HUNTINGTON DISEASE

Autosomal dominant inherited neurodegenerative disease associated with choreoathetosis and dementia. The average age of onset is 40 years.

MRI

- Heart-shaped enlargement of the frontal horns (due to atrophy of the caudate resulting in *ex vacuo* dilatation of the frontal horns).
- There may be iron deposition in the basal ganglia, which is low on T2.
- A juvenile form is associated with high T2 signal in the caudate and the putamen.

LEWY BODY DEMENTIA

Associated with Parkinsonian features. There is fluctuating cognitive impairment and visual hallucinations.

MRI

- Similar to Alzheimer disease, but less sparing of the occipital lobes.
- Affects the parietal and occipital lobes and the cerebellum.

Box 6.44 CAUSES OF CEREBELLAR ATROPHY ('GRAMP PA'S')
• **G**luten insensitivity
• **R**adiation
• **A**taxic telangiectasia
• **M**ultisystem atrophy
• **P**henytoin
• **P**araneoplastic syndrome (e.g. bronchial tumour)
• **A**lcohol
• **S**teroids

MULTISYSTEM ATROPHY

A progressive disease with pyramidal, extrapyramidal and autonomic symptoms (i.e. a combination of Parkinsonian and cerebellar signs).

MRI

- Severe brainstem and cerebellar atrophy and high signal in the pons, the 'hot cross bun' sign
- Low T2 signal in the basal ganglia (iron deposition)

PANTOTHENATE KINASE DEFICIENCY

Also known as Hallervorden–Spatz syndrome, this is a hereditary movement disorder.

MRI

- Low T1 and T2 signal in both pallidum (iron deposition). This gives the 'eye of the tiger' sign.

PICK DISEASE

This is a rare frontotemporal dementia with onset in young adults.

CT/MRI

- Asymmetrical temporal (and sometimes) frontal lobe atrophy
- Similar pattern seen with alcoholism and schizophrenia

PROGRESSIVE SUPRANUCLEAR PALSY (PSP)

This is a combination of Parkinson disease, supranuclear ophthalmoplegia (paralysis of downwards gaze), pseudobulbar palsy and early-onset dementia.

MRI

- Atrophy of the midbrain, globus pallidus and frontal lobes
- Dilatation of the third ventricle, enlargement of the interpeduncular cistern

HEAD AND NECK

Box 6.45 PATHOLOGICAL LYMPH NODES IN THE HEAD AND NECK
- Positron emission tomography (PET)/computed tomography is highly sensitive for diagnosis and follow-up of head and neck cancer. - Standardised uptake value (SUV) is a measure of the relative activity of a lesion on PET, adjusted according to dose given and patient size. SUV >3 is pathological. - In patients with head and neck cancer, a single ipsilateral enlarged node means a reduction of survival by 50%. - Know the lymph node levels of the head and neck and their boundaries (e.g. the hyoid/carotid bifurcation divides II from III; the junction of the hyoid muscle with the sternocleidomastoid muscle divides III from IV).

Read more:
Som, P. et al. 1999. An imaging-based classification for the cervical nodes designed as an adjunct to recent clinically based nodal classifications. *Archives of Otolaryngology—Head and Neck Surgery* 125:388–396.

Box 6.46 CHARACTERISTICS OF MALIGNANT LYMPH NODES

- Peripheral enhancement/central necrosis
- Extracapsular spread
- Conglomerate nodal masses
- Round shape, heterogeneous

Box 6.47 DIFFERENTIAL OF NECK MASSES IN CHILDREN AND ADULTS

- Childhood neck masses are benign in 90%; malignancy in this age group is most likely rhabdomyosarcoma or lymphoma.
- 90% of adult neck masses are malignant. In those aged <40 years, lymphoma is most likely, and in those aged >40 years, metastasis is most likely.

ADENOID CYSTIC CARCINOMA

This is the most common carcinoma of the minor salivary glands.

MRI

- Small lesion with poor encapsulation
- Spreads along the VII nerve

ANTROCHOANAL POLYPS

These are benign, expansile lesions of the maxillary sinus and cause bone remodelling due to the mass effect.

CT

- Homogeneous low-density lesion (due to oedema) filling the antrum with or without extending into the nasal cavity
- Bone remodelling

MRI

- Low signal on T1, high on T2 with peripheral contrast enhancement.
- Lesion fills the antrum and may extend into the ipsilateral nasal cavity.
- Mucoceles do not extend into the nasal cavity.

CHOANAL ATRESIA

This is a paediatric emergency. It is due to congenital failure of perforation of the oronasal membrane. It is associated with malrotation, DiGeorge syndrome and foetal alcohol syndrome.

CT

- Bilateral air–fluid levels in the nasal cavity
- Thickening of the vomer
- Inward bowing of the maxilla
- Narrowing of the posterior choanae to <3 mm in a child <2 years of age

---

Box 6.48 FINESSE YOUR COMPUTED TOMOGRAPHY SINUS REPORTS

Vaid, S. et al. 2011. An imaging checklist for pre-FESS CT: Framing a surgically relevant report. *Clinical Radiology* 66:459–470.

CHRONIC SINUSITIS

Air–fluid levels and mild mucosal thickening is only indicative with a relevant history. Usually a viral aetiology. Complications of sinusitis include polyps, mucous retention cyst and mucocele.

CT

- Opacification of the sinus/mucosal thickening.
- Sinus expands and bone remodels (bony wall may thin due to pressure necrosis).
- Peripheral enhancement.
- Complete absence of air in the sinus represents a mucocele.
- If there is some air in the sinus, it may represent a mucous retention cyst (difficult to distinguish from a polyp).

FUNGAL SINUSITIS

Mostly from aspergillus or mucormycosis.

CT

- Bone erosion is seen with allergic sinusitis—look for polyps.
- Extension outside the sinus without bone erosion is known as invasive sinusitis—this is more common with immunocompromise and diabetes.

JUVENILE NASOPHARYNGEAL ANGIOFIBROMA

This is the most common benign nasopharyngeal tumour. The typical scenario is a teenaged boy with epistaxis. These are highly vascular tumours and can be locally aggressive.

CT

- Densely enhancing mass involving the nasal wall, retromaxillary or pterygopalatine fossa.
- Widening of the pterygopalatine fossa in 90%—pathognomonic.
- Erosion of the medial pterygoid plate is characteristic.
- Homogeneous intense enhancement post-contrast.

INTERVENTION

- Intense tumour blush on angiography.
- Lesions are embolised prior to surgery to reduce bleeding.

LARYNGEAL MALIGNANCY

Associated with smoking and alcohol. In total, 90% are squamous cell carcinomas (SCCs), rarely adenoid cystic carcinomas (these characteristically invade the recurrent laryngeal nerve). Most laryngeal tumours (60%) are glottic—these tend to be small at diagnosis and have a good prognosis. Supraglottic tumours are often large when diagnosed. Subglottic tumours often represent tumour extension from above and have a poor prognosis.

CT

- Most useful for staging
- Asymmetry of the vocal cords with an enhancing mass (may be very small)

MUCOEPIDERMOID CARCINOMA

This is the most common malignant salivary gland primary. It is a high-grade tumour.

CT

- Heterogeneous, enhancing mass with cystic areas
- Spreads along the VII nerve

MRI

- Low signal on T1, heterogeneous on T2
- Early involvement of nodes—jugulodigastric (level II) first

---

Box 6.49 A DIFFERENTIAL FOR TUMOURS AT THE CAROTID BIFURCATION

- Carotid body tumour
- Hypervascular lymph nodes
- Schwannoma

PARAGANGLIONOMA

'Carotid body tumour'. These arise at the carotid bifurcation and splay the internal and external carotid arteries. They typically occur in the fifth decade and present with a slow-growing pulsatile neck mass that may compress an adjacent nerve.

MRI

- 5% are bilateral
- Often multiple masses that enhance densely
- Low T1, high T2 mass with multiple flow voids giving a salt and pepper appearance

PARANASAL SINUS MALIGNANCY

In total, 80%–90% are SCCs. It is often clinically silent or may present with an obstructive sinusitis and bone destruction. Esthesioneuroblastoma is a destructive tumour arising from the olfactory nerve/neurosensory cells of the nasal mucosa and often invades the anterior cranial fossa.

CT
- Soft tissue lesion typically at the fossa of Rosenmüller

PARANASAL SINUS PAPILLOMA

These are rare. In total, >50% arise from the nasal septum. An inverting papilloma is where the lesion arises from the lateral nasal cavity wall and inverts to extend to the ethmoidal air cells/adjacent maxillary sinus. Up to 25% degenerate to SCC, so they are excised.

MRI
- Intermediate signal on T1 and T2
- Avid enhancement differs it from mucocele

PLEOMORPHIC ADENOMA (PAROTID)

The rule of 80%: pleomorphic adenoma accounts for 80% of benign parotid tumours, 80% of pleomorphic adenomas occur in the parotid and 80% occur in the superficial lobe. Up to 20% undergo malignant degeneration.

US
- Hypoechoic multiloculated mass

SIALOGRAM
- Clawed fist appearance

CT
- Well-defined, homogeneous mass that is slightly higher attenuation than muscle

MRI
- Usually bright on T2 (differentiates it from parotid malignancy, which is hypo-intense)
- Iso-intense to muscle on T1 sequences
- Avid enhancement with contrast

RANULA

This is a retention cyst arising from the sublingual gland. The simple type is confined to the sublingual space; the diving type extends to the submandibular space.

MRI
- Best demonstrated on T2 sequences. Look for a fluid signal lesion in the sublingual space (simple) or extending to the submandibular space (diving).
- Thick wall enhancement suggests infection.

TORNWALD CYST

This is a posterior nasopharyngeal cyst. It is common and benign. It is filled with proteinaceous material that will intermittently discharge its contents, causing halitosis and a bad taste. They rarely become infected.

CT
- High-attenuation (due to protein content) nasopharyngeal cyst

MRI
- Thin-walled cyst
- High signal on T1 and T2 (protein content)
- No enhancement

VOCAL CORD PARALYSIS

This may be due to causes including iatrogenic (postoperative/intubation), trauma, thyroid/parathyroid neoplasm, lymphadenopathy and tumour.

CT
- Look for medialisation of the arytenoid and adduction of the vocal cord with resulting enlargement of the ipsilateral piriform sinus.
- Atrophy of the cricothyroid muscle.
- Absent thyroid (e.g. post-thyroidectomy).

WARTHIN TUMOUR

This is the most common benign tumour of the parotid tail. Patients are typically aged 50–70 years.

US
- Well-defined heterogeneous mass.
- 10% are bilateral.

MRI
- Well-defined mass
- Low T1 relative to the parotid, heterogeneous high T2 signal

NUCLEAR MEDICINE
- This is the only parotid tumour demonstrating uptake on technetium-99m pertechnetate.

WEGENER GRANULOMATOSIS

Think of this when there is involvement of the nasal cavities, paranasal sinuses and the orbits. Carcinoma is the principal differential.

CT

- Nasal septal perforation
- Bony erosion
- Soft tissue mass

EAR

CHOLESTEATOMA

Can be congenital or acquired. It is an epidermoid cyst in the temporal bone. The vast majority are acquired and may be complicated by erosion of the ossicles/tegmen tympani/lateral semicircular canal. The tympanic membrane is grossly abnormal and recurrence is common. Congenital cholesteatomas have an intact tympanic membrane and mass lateral to the ossicular chain.

CT

- Bone erosion—typically the scutum is affected (acquired cholesteatoma).
- Mass either lateral (acquired) or medial to the ossicular chain.
- Check for intracerebral abscess.

MRI

- Non-enhancing mass that is low signal on T1 and high signal on T2.
- Unlike other middle ear masses, cholesteatomas restrict on DWI.

CHOLESTEROL GRANULOMA

This is a complication of chronic middle ear infection/mastoiditis.

MRI

- High signal on T1 and T2 in the air cells of the petrous apex (due to cholesterol content)
- With or without low-signal haemosiderin rim
- Thinning of the adjacent bone

GLOMUS TYMPANICUM PARAGANGLIONOMA

This is the most common primary middle ear tumour in adults. It presents with pulsatile tinnitus and hearing loss and 30% have a VII palsy. Examination demonstrates a pulsating cherry-red mass behind the tympanic membrane. Differentials include an aberrant carotid artery, persistent stapedial artery (look for an absent foramen spinosum) and jugular bulb variants.

CT

- Densely enhancing mass at the cochlear promonitory.
- Arises from the wall of the middle ear.
- Does not erode the ossicles—it engulfs them.

INTERVENTION

- Most have a vascular supply from the ascending pharyngeal branch of the external carotid artery, which may be amenable to pre-operative embolisation.

LABYRINTHITIS OBLITERANS

An inflammatory process (due to e.g. infection, trauma or surgery) that may give rise to hearing loss and vertigo.

CT

- Bony proliferation and effacement of the cochlear

Box 6.50 SKULL BASE MALIGNANCY
• The vast majority of skull base malignancies are due to metastatic disease, most commonly from breast cancer.   • Primary sources include chordoma (clivus), chondrosarcoma, sarcoma, paraganglionoma etc.

MALIGNANT OTITIS EXTERNA (NECROTISING EXTERNAL OTITIS)

This is a serious infection of the external ear canal, almost always due to *pseudomonas*. It is more common in the immunocompromised, especially diabetics. It erodes the skull base, causing cranial nerve palsies and sigmoid sinus thrombosis.

CT

- Soft tissue mass in external auditory canal, with bone erosion
- Fluid-filled opacification of mastoid air cells

MRI

- Best for early detection of osteomyelitis, granulation tissue is low on T1 and T2.
- Check for sinus thrombosis.

OTOSCLEROSIS

Also known as otospongiosis, this is the most frequent cause of hearing loss in young adults. Vascular/fibrotic bone changes are the cause of the sclerosis. Subtypes are fenestral (affects the oval window and stapes) and retrofenestral (affects the otic capsule around the cochlear).

CT

- Small bone lucencies either anterior to the oval window (fenestral) or around the cochlear (retrofenestral).
- Findings are subtle and often symmetrical.

THYROID, PARATHYROID AND SALIVARY GLANDS

GRAVE DISEASE

This is an autoimmune disease associated with human leukocyte antigen (HLA) antibodies. Typically, it presents with thyrotoxicosis, goitre and eye disease (bilateral enlargement of the extraocular muscles).

US

- Enlarged gland, heterogeneous echotexture with spotty hypoechoic appearance
- Marked hyperaemia—'thyroid inferno'

CT/MRI

- Useful for establishing a diagnosis of thyroid associated ophthalmopathy.
- Enlargement of the extraocular muscles with sparing of the tendon insertions: muscles most commonly affected are **i**nferior > **m**edial > **s**uperior > **l**ateral > **o**blique (mnemonic = 'I'M SLO').
- May only involve the retrobulbar fat.

NUCLEAR MEDICINE

- Uniform increased uptake
- Elevated iodine uptake in up to 80%

HASHIMOTO THYROIDITIS

The typical patient is a 40–year-old woman with gradual enlargement of the thyroid. Patients are usually euthyroid; however, 20% present with hypothyroidism. There is an increased risk of malignancy, mostly non-Hodgkin lymphoma. Rapid enlargement of the gland suggests malignancy. There is a low threshold for nodule biopsy (e.g. focal bulge, adenopathy, etc.).

US

- Diffusely hypoechoic gland, avascular when acute
- Chronic phase causes an enlarged hypoechoic/heterogeneous gland, fibrous septae separating hypoechoic areas
- Hyperaemic in chronic phase due to effect of increased thyroid stimulating hormone (TSH)

NUCLEAR MEDICINE

- Generalised reduced uptake of technetium-99m

PARATHYROID ADENOMA

This is the most common cause of primary hyperparathyroidism and is benign.

US

- Normal glands up to about four in number, 3–4 mm in width, hypoechoic nodules posterior to the thyroid gland (outside of the thyroid capsule).
- Adenomas cause parathyroid gland enlargement and hyperaemia.

NUCLEAR MEDICINE

- Technetium-99m sestamibi concentrates in parathyroid adenomas.
- The test is also useful for detecting ectopic parathyroid adenomas.

SIALOLITHIASIS

Up to 90% of stones are found in Wharton's ducts in the submandibular gland. Stones are typically solitary and radiopaque. Sialolithiasis may be complicated by abscess or sialadenitis.

US

- Echo-casting calculus with duct dilatation

SIALOGRAM

- Obstructing filling defect/opacity

THYROID CANCER

Thyroid cancer is three-times more common in women. It usually presents with a palpable solitary nodule without thyroid dysfunction. Fine needle aspiration (FNA) is used for diagnosis. See Table 6.17.

US

- Non-specific features

NUCLEAR MEDICINE

- Typically, a cold nodule on radio-iodide scan, may be warm/hot on pertechnetate scan.
- Radioactive iodine can be used for detecting metastases—however, this is no good for anaplastic or medullary types.

CT

- Bone metastases are typically lytic.

Table 6.17 Features of thyroid malignancy

Type	Age group	% of tumours	Characteristics	Prognosis
Papillary	35–40 years	80%	Metastasises to cervical nodes	90% at 10 years
Follicular	40–70 years	10%	Hürthle cell is a slightly more aggressive variant of follicular cancer	85% at 10 years

continued

Table 6.17 (*Continued*) Features of thyroid malignancy

Type	Age group	% of tumours	Characteristics	Prognosis
Medullary	30–50 years	Up to 10%	Associated with MEN II Does not take up iodine (alternatives = FDG positron emission tomography, octreotide, etc.).	60% at 10 years
Anaplastic	Elderly patient	Rare	Invasive tumour with haemorrhage, calcification and necrosis Commonly nodal disease at presentation Does not take up iodine	6 months
Lymphoma	3× risk in females, 60–80 years	Rare	80% in patients with Hashimoto thyroiditis, most is diffuse large B-cell lymphoma Rapidly enlarging neck mass	95% at 5 years (without metastases)

Box 6.51 STAGING THYROID CANCER

T1 <2 cm
T2 2–4 cm
T3 Minimal local invasion
T4 Extensive local invasion or anaplastic type
N1a Level VI nodes only
N1b Any other level

THYROID NODULES

Up to 80% of people have nodules on US, but <10% are malignant. FNA is diagnostic in about 90%, but reserved for nodules >1–1.5 cm.

Box 6.52 ULTRASOUND OF THYROID NODULES

Kwak, J.Y. et al. 2011. Thyroid imaging reporting and data system for US features of nodules: A step in establishing better stratification of cancer risk. *Radiology* 260:892–899.

US

- Features of malignancy: frank invasion, solid hypoechoic mass, ill-defined margin, micro-lobulated margin, microcalcifications, taller than wide.
- In benign nodules, look for a complete hypoechoic halo (incomplete halo could be malignant), peripheral vascularity.
- Cystic nodules are usually benign (Note: 20% of papillary cancers are cystic).
- Comet-tail artefact is seen in colloidal cysts (benign).

Box 6.53 THYROID IMAGING REPORTING AND DATA SYSTEM (TIRADS)

TIRADS aims to provide a practical system for categorising thyroid nodules and stratifying the malignant risk. Comparable to breast imaging reporting and data system (BIRADS) in breast imaging (U = ultrasound).

U1—normal appearances (i.e. no nodule).
U2—benign nodule.
U3—probably benign (follow-up).
U4—probably malignant (biopsy). U4 is subdivided into: 4a, one malignant feature; 4b, two malignant features; 4c, three to four malignant features.
U5—five malignant features
U6—known malignancy

ORBITS

Table 6.18 A differential diagnosis for the orbital spaces

Space	Contents	Differential
Extra-conal	Fat	Infection
	Lacrimal gland	Neurofibroma
	Bony orbit	Adenocarcinoma
		Mucoepidermoid
		Adenoid cystic carcinoma
		Bone cancer
		Lymphoma
		Pseudotumour
		Wegener granulomatosis
		Sarcoidosis
		Meningioma
Conal	Extraocular muscle itself	Rhabdomyosarcoma
		Pseudotumour
		Metastases
		Lymphoma
		Leukaemia
		Thyroid eye disease
		Acromegaly
		Orbital myositis
		Sarcoidosis
		Sjögren syndrome
		Wegener granulomatosis
		Grave disease
Intra-conal	Fat	Venolymphatic malformation
	Nodes	Haemangioma
	Vessels	Arteriovenous malformation
	Nerve	Meningioma
	Nerve sheath	Glioma
		Lymphoma

CAVERNOUS HAEMANGIOMA OF THE EYE

This is a vascular malformation of the eye—it is encapsulated (unlike an infantile capillary haemangioma), rounded and well defined. It is the most common benign intra-orbital tumour in adults. Slowly progressive, painless proptosis is the typical presentation.

CT

- Typically, a lateral intra-conal lesion with patchy enhancement that fills in on delayed images.
- Orbital walls mould around the mass with no bony destruction.

CAPILLARY HAEMANGIOMA OF THE EYE (INFANTILE)

These typically regress after 2 years. They increase in size with Valsalva and large lesions consume platelets.

CT

- Lobular lesion that enhances intensely

MRI

- Prominent curvilinear flow voids

GLOBE CALCIFICATION

Either bilateral (drusen—incidental and asymptomatic) or unilateral (choroidal osteoma—distal to the optic disc and associated with tuberous sclerosis). The extra-ocular muscles commonly calcify in the elderly.

CT

- Drusen appear as flat discs of calcification overlying the optic nerves.

ORBITAL CELLULITIS/ABSCESS

Commonly, it arises due to adjacent sinusitis (also trauma, foreign body, etc.).

CT

- Inflammation of the peri-orbital fat.
- With or without focal fluid collection showing rim enhancement.
- Pre-septal infection is confined to the tissues anterior to the septum (the point of attachment of the eyelid).

- Post-septal infection is usually extra-conal and may be complicated by subperiosteal phlegmon/abscess, ophthalmic vein/cavernous sinus thrombosis, epidural or subdural empyema, cerebritis or meningitis.

Box 6.56 CAUSES OF BILATERAL ENLARGEMENT OF THE LACRIMAL GLANDS

- Lymphoma
- Leukaemia
- Sarcoidosis
- Sjögren syndrome

OPTIC NERVE GLIOMA

This is the most common cause of optic nerve enlargement and is mostly found in children <10 years of age (80% <20 years of age). It is more common in patients with NF1 and may be bilateral.

MRI

- Mild high signal on T2 with variable (poor patchy) enhancement.
- The nerve is kinked/buckled, sausage-shaped or fusiform.
- Widens optic canal if there is intracranial extension.

OPTIC NERVE SHEATH MENINGIOMA

Benign and slow growing, these arise from the arachnoid layer. They encircle and grow along the nerve sheath. See Table 6.19.

Table 6.19 Optic nerve glioma versus meningioma

Optic nerve glioma	Optic nerve sheath meningioma
80% <20 years of age	Middle-aged women
Variable enhancement	'Tram track' enhancement
Calcification rare	Calcification in up to 50%
Buckling of the nerve (fusiform thickening)	Straight nerve (tubular thickening)
Often asymptomatic	Visual impairment early

MRI

- Mass surrounding the intra-orbital optic nerve that enhances more than the nerve itself, 'tram track' enhancement.
- Calcification in up to 50%.
- Look for erosion or hyperostosis of the optic canal.

OPTIC NEURITIS

In total, 60% of those with optic neuritis go on to have a diagnosis of MS. In this group, 50% will have a lesion on MRI. A total of 70% are unilateral in adults, and 60% are bilateral in children.

MRI

- Enlarged and enhancing optic nerve
- Typically hyperintense on T2
- White matter lesions for MS

ORBITAL LYMPHATIC MALFORMATION

Also known as lymphangioma or cystic hygroma, they are the most common vascular orbital tumour. They usually affect children aged 3–15 years and tend to bleed. Bleeds cause sudden proptosis. They are associated with chromosomal abnormalities including Turner syndrome, trisomies and Noonan syndrome.

CT

- Multi-cystic lesion with fluid–fluid levels (from recurrent haemorrhage)
- More commonly extra-conal
- Phleboliths with venous malformations

MRI

- High T1 and T2
- Typically no enhancement

ORBITAL PSEUDOTUMOUR

This affects adults and is due to lymphocytic infiltration. It causes a painful, proptosed and paralysed eye. The lacrimal gland is the most frequently affected. It is associated with retroperitoneal fibrosis, Wegener granulomatosis, sarcoidosis and fibrosing mediastinitis. It may affect other parts of the skull base, meninges, nasopharynx, etc. The main differential is lymphoma. A response to steroids suggests pseudotumour. Tolosa–Hunt syndrome is a variant of pseudotumour extending through the superior orbital fissure to the cavernous sinus, producing painful ophthalmoplegia (palsy of III, IV, V and VI). See Figure 6.30.

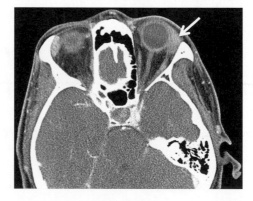

Figure 6.30 Post-contrast CT scan of the orbits showing asymmetrical enlargement of the left lacrimal gland (white arrow) in a patient with known sarcoidosis. A basic knowledge of orbital anatomy will help narrow the differential, see Table 6.18.

MRI

- Low signal mass on T2 (due to fibrosis, tumours are usually high signal on T2)
- Diffuse enhancement

- Sparing of the tendinous insertions of the extraocular muscles
- 85% unilateral (Table 6.20)

Table 6.20 Orbital pseudotumour versus Grave disease

	Pseudotumour	Thyroid ophthalmopathy
Symptoms	Unilateral, painful ophthalmoplegia	Bilateral, painless ophthalmoplegia
Demographic Features	Young adult females	Old adults
	Isolated involvement of lateral rectus	Inferior rectus in Graves
	Enhancement of the fat with contrast, fat stranding	Increased retro-orbital fat
	Involvement of the lacrimal gland	

RETINAL DETACHMENT

CT

- Characteristic V shape on cross-sectional imaging, the apex of the V is at the optic disc.

THYROGLOSSAL DUCT CYST

This is the most common congenital midline neck mass. It accounts for 90% of congenital neck lesions. The foramen caecum (at the tongue base) connects to the thyrohyoid membrane, ending at the thyroidal isthmus. If this does not involute during development, it forms a tract/sinus along which thyroid tissue can arrest. Commonly infrahyoid (65%) and 15% are suprahyoid. There is rarely malignant transformation to SCC.

MRI

- Best on sagittal imaging.
- Homogeneous high signal on T2, low on T1.
- Wall may enhance if the cyst is infected.
- Calcification or nodular tissue suggest malignancy.

UVEAL MELANOMA

This is the most common ocular tumour in adults. It arises from the choroid. For tumours >12 mm, the mortality is 70%.

US

- 'Cottage loaf' appearance

CT

- Hyperdense mass
- Nearly always unilateral
- Check for liver metastases

MRI
- High signal on T1 (due to melanin), low on T2

MANDIBLE AND MAXILLA

Table 6.21 Cystic lesions of the maxilla and mandible—ask yourself three questions: what is the relation to the tooth? Is it a unilocular or multilocular cyst? How old is the patient?

Cyst characteristic	Differential
Unilocular, related to the dentition	Periapical/radicular cyst (painful)
	Dentigerous cyst (at the crown of an unerupted tooth)
Unilocular, not related to dentition	<30 years of age: odontogenic keratocyst, simple bone cyst
	>40 years of age: ameloblastoma, metastases, myeloma
Multilocular cyst	<30 years of age: aneurysmal bone cyst or odontogenic keratocyst
	Multiple cysts: odontogenic keratocyst, Gorlin syndrome
	>30 years of age: ameloblastoma

AMELOBLASTOMA

This is the most common odontogenic tumour. It is benign but locally aggressive. It cannot be differentiated from a dentigerous cyst or odontogenic keratocyst with imaging.

PLAIN FILM
- Large, multilocular, expansile lucent lesion in the posterior mandible.
- 'Honeycomb/soap bubble' appearance.
- Typically involves the lower premolars and molars.

MRI
- Contains a soft tissue element that enhances
- Cyst wall also enhances

BROWN TUMOUR

Lesions associated with hyperparathyroidism. The mandible is the most common location to find a Brown tumour.

PLAIN FILM
- Expansile lytic lesion
- Narrow zone of transition

CEMENTOMA

Benign, mineralised lesion with a lucent halo. It is self-limiting and usually incidental unless infected.

PLAIN FILM

- Multiple expansile sclerotic lesions with adjacent lucency centred on the tooth apices.
- It is the only lytic and sclerotic lesion in this location.
- Bilateral and symmetrical.

DENTIGEROUS CYST

Due to excessive fluid accumulation associated with the cap of unerupted molars (key to diagnosis). In total, 80% are mandibular and they rarely become malignant. The key features of cystic lesions in the maxilla and mandible are summarised in Table 6.21.

PLAIN FILM

- Well-corticated, unilocular cyst associated with an unerupted molar.
- Look for a fracture or evidence of infection.
- Can be very large, taking over the whole mandibular ramus and displacing teeth.

GIANT CELL GRANULOMA

Reactive inflammatory process due to infection or trauma. It affects the mandible more than the maxilla. It is associated with gingivitis, fibrous dysplasia and Paget disease.

PLAIN FILM

- Multilocular, well-defined cyst with a thin sclerotic margin

CT

- Heterogeneous contrast-enhancing mass

ODONTOGENIC KERATOCYST

Aggressive behaving cystic mandibular/maxillary lesion, linked to Gorlin–Goltz syndrome (multiple keratocysts, kyphoscoliosis, bifid ribs and meningiomas).

PLAIN FILM

- Expansile unilocular cystic mass with a sclerotic rim
- May displace or extrude teeth

PERIAPICAL/RADICULAR CYST

This is the most frequently encountered mandibular cyst. It occurs due to caries or infection and is painful.

PLAIN FILM

- Found at root of the affected tooth
- Unilocular, <1 cm and with a sclerotic margin
- May form an abscess

SPINE

> **Box 6.57 TERMINOLOGY FOR DESCRIBING DEGENERATIVE DISC PATHOLOGY**
>
> **Focal protrusion**
> Disc material protrudes so that the displaced material is <25%/90° of the body circumference on axial slices.
>
> **Broad-based protrusion**
> Disc material protrudes so that the displaced material is >25%/90° of the body circumference on axial slices.
>
> **Bulge**
> Annulus extends >3 mm beyond the vertebral body margin >50%/180° of the body circumference.
>
> **Extrusion**
> Disc material is expelled from its containment through an aperture (i.e. it has a neck).
>
> **Sequestrated disc or free fragment**
> A fragment of disc that has separated from its parent entirely and is therefore found away from the level of the pathological disc.
>
> **Annular fissure**
> Separation of annular fibres, may occur in the radial, transverse or concentric plane. High signal on T2 magnetic resonance imaging sequences and may enhance post-contrast.

> **Box 6.58 TERMINOLOGY FOR DESCRIBING THE LOCATION OF DEGENERATIVE DISC PATHOLOGY**
>
> **Central**
> Overlying the posterior longitudinal ligament. Protrusion tends to be either side of this. Central protrusions are more common in the cervical spine, especially at C6–7 and C5–6.
>
> **Paracentral/lateral recess**
> This is the most common site for disc protrusion.
>
> **Foraminal**
> Disc material is present in the intervertebral foramen with inevitable compromise of the exiting nerve root/dorsal root ganglion. Up to 10% of herniations affect the foraminal zone.
>
> **Extra-foraminal**
> External to the neural exit foramen. This is an unusual site for protrusion.

DISC DEGENERATION AND PROTRUSION

Herniated material may be contained by the posterior longitudinal ligament (PLL) or be accompanied by a PLL tear. In total, 90% of discs improve clinically with 8–10 weeks of symptomatic treatment, 50% improve on MRI and 10% get worse.

MRI

- Axial and sagittal T2 and T1 slices are key to diagnosis.
- Look for disc material herniating into the canal, lateral recess or exit foramina.
- Lateral disc protrusion passes into the exit foramen and compresses the exiting root (symptoms are the same as a central protrusion at the level above).
- Check for signal change within the cord on T2 (i.e. cord compression).
- Check for associated facet joint degeneration and thickening of the ligamentum flavum.
- Sequestrated fragments may migrate caudally/cranially/become intradural.
- Sequestered fragments may become surrounded by granulation tissue and enhance with contrast.
- Post-operatively, look for non-enhancing disc material (recurrence); enhancement of disc material suggests fibrosis and scarring.

Box 6.59 FURTHER READING

Hayashi, D. et al. 2012. Imaging features of postoperative complications after spinal surgery and instrumentation. *Musculoskeletal Imaging* 199:W123–W129.

END-PLATE DEGENERATION

Connected to back pain, though the precise link is controversial.

MRI

- Disc degeneration with signal change paralleling the end plates.
- Signal characteristics are commonly classified according to the Modic system (Table 6.22).

Table 6.22 The Modic classification system for degenerative end-plate changes

	T1	T2	Pathology
1	↓	↑	Inflammation
2	↑	↔ or ↑	Fatty replacement
3	↓	↓	Sclerosis

ENDPLATE INFRACTION

Also known as a Schmorl node. There is herniation of the nucleus pulposus through the end plate. May follow an end-plate fracture.

CT

- Most seen between T7 and L2
- Can be large, cyst-like and may develop at any age

Box 6.60 FACETAL CYSTS

Facet joints degenerate like any other synovial joint. Facetal cysts may form containing fluid, blood or air and thus demonstrate a variable signal on magnetic resonance imaging.

OSSIFIED POSTERIOR LONGITUDINAL LIGAMENT

Represents heterotopic bone from repeated trauma to the PLL. It tends to occur in the cervical spine, causing canal stenosis and myelopathy.

CT

- CT preferred for pre-operative planning
- Multilevel ossification of the PLL with narrowing of the spinal canal
- Typically minimal disc disease

SPINAL STENOSIS

This often coexists with disc disease. Central stenosis is mostly the result of bilateral facet joint degeneration causing a slip. Other than degeneration, possible causes include Paget disease, spondylolisthesis and trauma. Superior facet hypertrophy may cause a lateral recess stenosis.

MRI

- Facet joint degeneration (loss of disc space) and hypertrophy
- Spondylolisthesis
- Thickening/buckling of the ligamentum flavum

SPONDYLOLISTHESIS

Mostly due to either degenerative disease (facet joint hypertrophy and slip) or, in 10%, pars defects (i.e. spondylolysis). It is commonly asymptomatic. Pars defects are thought to arise from microtrauma in childhood (e.g. gymnastics, etc.). The defect in the pars contains fibrous material.

PLAIN FILM

- Scotty dog sign on oblique lateral, Napolean's hat sign on AP

CT

- Displacement of the posterior margin of the vertebral body.
- Graded with the Meyerding scale (I–IV) for each 25% of slippage.
- Complete slippage so the body above lies below the superior end plate of the lower body is 'spondyloptosis'.

BOX 6.61 FIVE THINGS TO LOOK FOR IN THE CERVICAL SPINE WITH RHEUMATOID ARTHRITIS (RA)

1. **Atlantoaxial instability** (C1 transverse ligament destruction by pannus). Frank instability in 5% with RA. Shown by pre-dentate space >2.5 mm in adult.
2. **Atlantoaxial impaction**: severe atlantoaxial subluxation with collapse of the C1–2 facets and basilar invagination. Look for anterior slip of C1 so the anterior border of C1 lies anterior to the inferior border of C2.
3. **Basilar invagination** (tip of dens >5 mm above McGrigor's line, drawn between superior border of the hard palate to the inferior border of the occiput).

4. **Cord compression**, especially in flexion. In the long term, the effect is myelomalacia. Associated with an increased risk of sudden death.
5. **Loss of disc height**.

CORD

Box 6.62 A MODEL FOR THE DIFFERENTIAL DIAGNOSIS OF CORD LESIONS

- Intramedullary (i.e. confined to the cord)
- Intradural (i.e. within the dura but outside the cord itself)
- Extradural (i.e. outside the dura)

Box 6.63 A BASIC DIFFERENTIAL FOR PRIMARY CORD MALIGNANCY

- In adults mostly ependymoma
- In children, NF1 astrocytoma
- In Von Hippel–Lindau disease then haemangioblastoma

ARACHNOIDITIS

Changes following inflammation. Mostly iatrogenic after spinal surgery, but also associated with TB.

MRI

- Nerve roots gathered either centrally or peripherally ('empty thecal sac')
- With or without thickening of the thecal sac and enhancement

ARACHNOID CYST

Usually incidental and asymptomatic.

MRI

- Cyst contents match CSF signal on all sequences
- No restriction on DWI

ARTERIOVENOUS FISTULA (AVF)

Disrupted venous drainage causes cord oedema. Associated with hereditary haemorrhagic telangiectasia (Osler–Weber–Rendu disease). They may be amenable to embolisation.

MRI

- Cord oedema (hyper-intense on T2) with flow voids
- No nidus (distinguishes from an AVM)

ARTERIOVENOUS MALFORMATION (AVM)

This is the most common vascular malformation of the cord. There is an abnormal direct communication between the arteries and veins of the cord with a central nidus. In total, 5% are associated with hereditary haemorrhagic telangiectasia.

MRI

- The hallmark is a prominent draining vein (seen in 50%).
- Tangle of low-signal flow voids best seen on T2.
- GE most sensitive in order to demonstrate blood products.

INTERVENTION

- May be amenable to embolisation

BOX 6.64 CENTRAL NERVOUS SYSTEM TUMOURS THAT SEED TO THE SUBARACHNOID SPACE

- Medulloblastoma
- Ependymoma
- Germinoa
- Glioblastoma multiforme
- Choroid plexus pappiloma/carcinoma
- Pinoblastoma/pineocytoma
- Angioblastic meningioma

ASTROCYTOMA

This represents 30% of intramedullary tumours. It is more common in children.

MRI

- Eccentrically placed low T1, high T2 lesion
- Most often in the thoracic cord, then cervical
- Cord expansion
- Multisegmental involvement is common
- Patchy tumoural enhancement
- Associated with syrinx and cysts
- Associated with scoliosis in children

CAVERNOUS MALFORMATION

Cavernomas are unusual in the spine. Made up of dilated vascular sinusoids and are devoid of smooth muscle and elastic fibres. Not seen on conventional angiography.

MRI

- Bright on T1 and T2
- Central, speckled, 'popcorn'/bubbly, high-signal appearance, with low-signal (haemosiderin) rim from previous bleeds
- More common in the cervical/thoracic regions
- Cord oedema if recent haemorrhage

> **Box 6.65 CAUDAL AGENESIS/REGRESSION SYNDROME**
>
> This spectrum of abnormalities is associated with diastematomyelia, intraspinal lipomas, dermoids and dermal sinuses. Extraspinal-associated anomalies include absent lower vertebrae, anal atresia, genital malformation, renal anomalies and fusion of the lower limbs. In total, 16% of cases are the offspring of diabetic mothers.

DERMOID

Spinal dermoids are normally symptomatic by adolescence. Dermoids contain all layers of the ectoderm and a third are associated with a dermal sinus tract. Rupture may cause a chemical meningitis.

CT

- Lesion may contain fat/calcification
- Minimal peripheral enhancement—dense enhancement suggests infection
- Dermal sinus tract

MRI

- T1/T2 hyperintensity if fat containing
- Enhancement as for CT
- With or without restriction on DWI

DIASTEMATOMYELIA

The cord is split in the sagittal plane. Expect to find vertebral segmentation anomalies and overlying skin lesions. There is a 30% prevalence with myelomeningocele and 5% with congenital scoliosis. Diplomyelia is a duplicated spinal cord, held in a single dural sac. It is very rare and may be considered a severe form of diastematomyelia.

PLAIN FILM

- Vertebral segmentation abnormalities
- Look for a bony spur at the site of diastematomyelia

US

- May be seen on pre-/post-natal US

MRI (FIGURE 6.31)

- Two cords (may be asymmetrical in size)—usually a single cord above/below the lesion, separated by a fibrous or bony spur
- May have a single or dual dural sac
- Syringohydromyelia in 50%

EPENDYMOMA

This is the most common primary tumour of the spinal cord (up to 60%). Myxopapillary ependymoma is a subtype found in the filum terminale (the most common primary tumour at the conus).

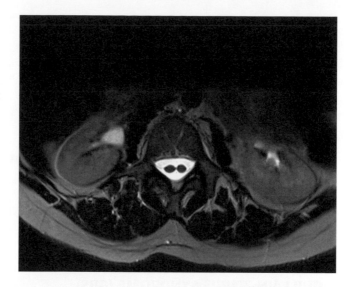

Figure 6.31 Axial T2-weighted MRI of the lumbar spine showing two roughly equally sized hemicords separated by a fibrous band, in keeping with diastematomyelia.

MRI

- Low/intermediate T1, foci of high signal T2.
- Most common in the cervical cord.
- Extends over a large area (four vertebrae length is the average).
- Low-signal rim due to repeated haemorrhage—a rim of extreme hypointensity (haemosiderin) at the poles of the tumour may be seen on T2, the 'cap' sign.
- Lesions enhance and are associated with bone remodelling, therefore causing posterior scalloping.
- Expansion is seen more commonly than with demyelination.

EPIDERMOID

Contains skin appendages only (unlike dermoid). Congenital or acquired—if the latter, it is nearly always found at the cauda equina (e.g. post-lumbar puncture). Asymptomatic or gradual progressive radiculopathy.

CT

- Internal density similar to CSF
- Rarely calcification or enhancement
- Enhancement suggests infection

MRI

- Iso-intense to CSF/mildly hyper-intense on T2
- Commonly restrict on DWI

EPIDURAL ABSCESS

These mostly arise from adjacent osteomyelitis (80%), usually from *Staphylococcus aureus*. They spread craniocaudally via the extradural route and may cause cord compression.

MRI

- T2 hyperintense mass in the epidural space
- Peripheral enhancement post-contrast
- Adjacent cord signal may be abnormal from infection spread, compression or ischaemia

EPIDURAL HAEMATOMA

Due to e.g. trauma, disc herniation, vascular anomaly, iatrogenic, etc.

MRI

- Lentiform/fusiform collection in the spinal canal hyperintense on T1 and T2 (depending on age)
- May show mild peripheral enhancement

GUILLAIN–BARRÉ SYNDROME (GBS)

Autoimmune demyelination stimulated by viral infection or vaccination. It affects the peripheral nerves, nerve roots and cranial nerves. It presents with sensory loss and an ascending paralysis. Symptoms tend to peak after about 30 days and then improve, with two-thirds recovering completely.

MRI

- Marked enhancement of the cauda equina with or without smooth, mild root thickening
- May also affect the grey matter horns of the cord and rarely brainstem

Box 6.66 CAUSES OF DIFFUSE LEPTOMENINGEAL ENHANCEMENT
• Guillain–Barré syndrome
• Metastases
• Leukaemia
• Chemotherapy
• Infection

HAEMANGIOBLASTOMA

This is a low-grade, vascular tumour that is most commonly sporadic. About a third are associated with VHL.

MRI

- Intramedullary cystic lesion with an enhancing tumour nodule.
- The appearance is similar to an AVM, but in this case there is cord expansion and a cystic component.
- Look for flow voids with large lesions.
- Typically causes a large associated secondary syrinx.

INFARCTION

Mostly iatrogenic (e.g. post-abdominal aortic aneurysm repair or inadvertent intra-arterial injection of steroid; beware root injections).

MRI

- Lesion much like a cerebral infarct—focal high signal on T2 and DWI
- Cord oedema
- Myelomalacia in the long term

LIPOMA

Most lipoma are found at the filum terminale and are usually symptomatic by 5 years. Intradural lipomas are rare.

MRI

- Linear streak of T1 and T2 hyperintensity in the filum
- Signal loss with fat suppression

LIPOMYELOMENINGOCELE/LIPOMYELOCELE

This is a midline spinal bone defect with a skin covering (i.e. closed defect) in the lumbosacral region. There may be a dermal sinus, hairy patch or haemangioma above the intergluteal fold. May be incidental.

- Lipomyelocele—the lipoma/placode interface is inside the spinal canal.
- Lipomyelomeningocele—lipoma/placode interface is outside the spinal canal.

PLAIN FILM

- Multi-level spinal dysraphism (wide laminae)
- Associated anomalies—segmentation anomalies, sacral dysgenesis

MRI

- T1/T2 hyperintense (i.e. fat) lesion herniation from spinal canal with neural placode immediately below last normal-appearing lamina.
- Additional findings may include intramedullary/intradural/extradural lipoma or tethered cord.

MYELOMENINGOCELE/MYELOCELE

Due to failure of neural tube closure (i.e. 'spina bifida'). The end result is an open midline defect where the meninges, CSF and unfolded cord ('neural placode') are exposed and uncovered by skin. Most (>40%) are lumbosacral.

- Myelomeningocele—placode bulges above the skin surface (enlarged subarachnoid space behind pushes neural tissue out). These are most common and usually associated with Chiari II malformations.
- Myelocele—placode is flush with the skin.

PLAIN FILM
- Wide laminae (spinal dysraphism) seen on AP spine
- Kyphoscoliosis, segmentation anomalies

US
- Prenatal diagnosis—wide laminae, myelomeningocele sac
- Brain abnormalities associated with Chiari II

MRI
- Look for additional findings—diastematomyelia, syrinx, evidence of Chiari II malformation.

LUPUS

This is a necrotising arteritis that may cause cord ischaemia/transverse myelitis. Symptoms are relieved by steroids.

MRI
- Mild cord expansion, high signal on T2, with a longer segment of cord involvement than MS, typically spanning four to five vertebral bodies
- No significant enhancement post-contrast

MENINGIOMA

In total, 80% are found in women and can be malignant. They are generally solitary, but if multiple, then consider NF2.

MRI
- Mostly thoracic cord upwards (rarely lumbar).
- Most common tumour at the foramen magnum.
- Iso-intense/hypo-intense T1 and slightly hyper-intense T2.
- Most contain calcification (they are the only cord tumour to calcify).
- Broad-based tumour with a dural tail.
- Avid contrast enhancement.
- A solitary posterior cord tumour is more likely meningioma than schwannoma.

Box 6.67 INTRADURAL EXTRAMEDULLARY MASSES ('MNM')
Meningioma **N**erve sheath tumour **M**etastasis

METASTASES—INTRADURAL, EXTRAMEDULLARY

These are rare—most are from the subarachnoid seeding of a CNS primary. They may also arise from e.g. breast, lung, melanoma or lymphoma, and may present as carcinomatous meningitis.

MRI

- Post-contrast, whole spine
- Diffuse dural thickening, small nodules or a mass in the inferior thecal sac

METASTASES—VERTEBRAL

Mostly from breast, lung and prostate cancer. They mostly occur in the thoracic spine and are multiple in 90%. The main differentials are the primary vertebral tumours: chordoma, giant cell tumour, haemangioma and sarcoma.

MRI

- Marrow replacement with sparing of the disc (i.e. dark marrow on T1 [loss of usual fat] and bright on T2).
- Lesions restrict on DWI and light up on STIR.
- If the disc is not spared, it is most likely infection.

Box 6.68 DIFFUSE LOW T1 SIGNAL IN A VERTEBRAL BODY

- Diffuse metastatic disease
- Haemopoietic malignancy (lymphoma, leukaemia)
- Severe anaemia
- Myelofibrosis

Box 6.69 VERTEBRAL METASTASES VERSUS OSTEOPOROTIC WEDGE FRACTURES

- Expect a wedge-shaped fracture if benign.
- No involvement of the posterior elements (pedicles) if benign.
- Old benign fractures have a normal marrow signal.

MULTIPLE SCLEROSIS

MS is the most common cause of intramedullary inflammation. Up to 12% of patients have cord involvement only, and the cervical cord is most commonly affected. If cord MS is the main feature, it suggests progressive disease. Involvement of the spinal cord and/or optic pathways without brain involvement is known as Devic disease.

MRI

- Sagittal FLAIR and T2 most useful.
- High signal within the cord (two-thirds in the cervical cord).
- Contrast enhancement suggests disease activity with or without cord expansion when acute.
- Expect atrophy once the lesion burns out.

NERVE ROOT AVULSION

Typically occurs at the site of connection to the cord, most commonly in cervical cord (i.e. brachial plexus). Thoracic and lumbar roots are rarely avulsed. Erb palsy is avulsion of the C5–7 roots (e.g. from birth trauma). Diagnosis made with MRI or CT myelography.

MRI

- Pseudomeningocele is the most reliable indicator of a preganglionic avulsion.
- Brachial plexus thickening (i.e. oedema) is most useful for identifying a post-ganglionic injury.

NEUROFIBROMA

Linked to NF1. In NF1, they emerge from multiple consecutive neural foramina, in which case they are said to be 'plexiform'—pathognomic for NF1. Unlike schwannomas, they encase the nerve roots.

PLAIN FILM

- Neurofibromas cause ribbon ribs.
- Scalloped vertebral bodies are from dural ectasia.

MRI

- Diffuse elongation or fusiform enlargement of multiple nerves, which enhance intensely
- Target sign—central hypointensity on T2 with peripheral hyperintensity

---

Box 6.70 CAUSES OF DURAL ECTASIA (I.E. WIDENING OF THE DURAL SAC)

- Marfan syndrome
- Ehlers–Danlos syndrome
- Neurofibromatosis type 1
- Ankylosing spondylitis
- Osteogenesis imperfecta
- Trauma
- Post-surgery
- Tumours
- Scoliosis

RADIATION MYELITIS

Results from damage to the cord following radiation treatment. The incidence peaks 6–12 months after radiotherapy with progression of symptoms. It occurs within the radiation field—look for fatty bone marrow changes to indicate the extent of the radiation field.

MRI

- Fusiform cord expansion and intramedullary T2 hyper-intensity
- Cord atrophy in chronic phase
- Variable enhancement post-contrast

SCHWANNOMA

This is the most common primary spinal tumour, typically in the cervical region. It usually arises from the dorsal sensory nerve root, is extrinsic to the nerve and is solitary and benign. Symptoms arise from compression of adjacent structures.

MRI

- Dumbbell-shaped lesion that has both intra- and extra-dural components.
- May appear as a posterior mediastinal mass causing rib splaying.

SYRINX

This is a non-specific term, commonly taken to mean dilatation of the central canal of the cord. Severe central cord oedema (without central canal dilatation) is known as a pre-syrinx.

MRI (FIGURE 6.32)

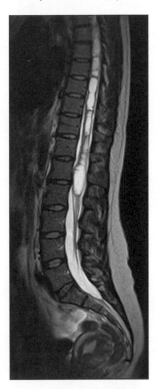

Figure 6.32 Sagittal T2 magnetic resonance image of the thoracolumbar spine showing marked dilatation of the central canal of the cord, which is filled with fluid of equal intensity to surrounding CSF, in keeping with a syrinx. The cause of the syrinx is not shown.

- Dilated central canal, the signal of the syrinx contents should match CSF.
- Signal may be patchy due to flow artefact.
- If there is no cause for the syrinx demonstrated, a tumour should be excluded and contrast administered.

TRANSVERSE MYELITIS

This is non-specific, acute cord inflammation. There are numerous causes, including lupus. Myelopathy describes the symptoms; these may involve motor, sensory and autonomic pathways and progress rapidly. By definition, there is no extra-axial lesion causing cord compression.

MRI

- May be normal.
- Iso-/hypo-intense T1, poorly defined hyper-intense T2, variable enhancement post-contrast.
- Typically occupy greater than two-thirds of the area of the cord and commonly extends over three to four segments.

Box 6.71 LONG, DIFFUSE, HIGH T2 INTRAMEDULLARY SIGNAL ('T VOID')
Transverse myelitis **V**asculitis (including lupus) **O**edema **I**nfarction (look for H-shaped hyperintensity) **D**emyelination (mostly posterior/posterolateral within the cord)

TRAUMA

Contusion from e.g. a bone fragment or compression at the site of a fracture. The junction of the cervical and thoracic cord is a relatively weak spot of cord avulsion.

MRI

- Cord oedema or haemorrhage is a poor prognostic indicator.
- May occur with flexion/extension-type injuries.

Index